Healthy Sleep Habits,
Happy Child

ALSO BY THE AUTHOR

Crybabies

Sweet Baby: How to Soothe Your Newborn

Your Fussy Baby

Healthy Sleep Habits, Happy Child

A STEP-BY-STEP PROGRAMME FOR A GOOD NIGHT'S SLEEP

DR MARC WEISSBLUTH

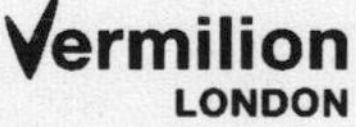

This book is dedicated to
Linda Weissbluth

10

First published in 2005 by Vermilion,
an imprint of Ebury Publishing

This edition first published in the United States in 2003 by Ballantine

Ebury Publishing is a Random House Group Company

The Random House Group Limited Reg. No. 954009

Addresses for companies within the Random House Group can be found at: www.randomhouse.co.uk

A CIP catalogue record for this book is available from the British Library

The Random House Group Limited supports The Forest Stewardship Council (FSC®), the leading international forest certification organisation. Our books carrying the FSC label are printed on FSC® certified paper. FSC is the only forest certification scheme endorsed by the leading environmental organisations, including Greenpeace. Our paper procurement policy can be found at www.randomhouse.co.uk/environment

Printed and bound by CPI Group (UK) Ltd, Croydon, CR0 4YY

ISBN 9780091902551

Grateful acknowledgement is made to the following for permission to reprint the following material:

The American Psychological Association: an article by Carl D. Williams entitled 'Case Report: The Elimination of Tantrum Behaviour by Extinction Procedures' which appeared in Journal of Abnormal and Social Psychology, 1959. Copyright © 1959 by the American Psychological Association. Reprinted by permission of the publisher and author.

Karen Pierce, MD: Chapter 12, entitled 'Competent Parents, Competent Child' by Karen Pierce, MD. Copyright © 1999 by Karen Pierce, MD. Reprinted by permission of the author. All rights reserved.

Contents

FOREWORD xi
HOW TO USE THIS BOOK xiii
INTRODUCTION xv

Part I. How Children Sleep

Chapter 1. Why Healthy Sleep Is So Important 5

Chapter 2. Healthy Sleep and Sleep Strategies 14

Healthy Sleep 14
Sleep Duration: Night and Day 16
Naps 26
Sleep Consolidation 39
Sleep Schedule, Timing of Sleep 45
Sleep Regularity 49
Sleep Positions, SIDS 57
The Benefits of Healthy Sleep: Sleep Patterns, Intelligence, Learning and School Performance 59
Sleep Strategies 63
Drowsy Signs 63
Soothing to Sleep 63
Resources for Soothing 73
Bedtime Routines 75
Breast-feeding versus Bottle-feeding and Family Bed versus Cot 76
Breast-feeding the Fussy Baby (by Nancy Nelson, RN, IBCLC) 87
Solid Foods and Feeding Habits 99
Solutions to Help Your Child Sleep Better: 'No Cry', 'Maybe Cry,' or 'Let Cry' 103

Prevention versus Treatment of Sleep Problems 104
Action Plan for Exhausted Parents 106

Chapter 3. Sleep Problems and Solutions 111
Disturbed Sleep 111
Sleep Log 118
Morning Wake-up Time Is Too Early 119
Morning Nap Is Absent, Too Short, Too Long or at the Wrong Time 121
Afternoon Nap Is Absent, Too Short, Too Long or at the Wrong Time 123
Third Nap Is Absent, Too Short, Too Long or at the Wrong Time 124
Needs Two but Can Get Only One 125
Needs a Nap but Refuses to Nap 126
Bedtime Is Too Late: Sometimes or Always a Battle 130
Night Waking, Difficulty Staying Asleep 130
More Than One Child Creates Bedtime Problems 131
Unable to Fall Asleep 131
Afraid of the Dark or Being Alone 131
Will Not Stay in His Cot or Bed 132
Will Not Sleep Anywhere Else 133
Only One Bedroom 133
Transition from Family Bed to Cot 134
Action Plan for Exhausted Parents 134

Chapter 4. Sleep, Extreme Fussiness/Colic, and Temperament 137
How to Use This Chapter 137
Introduction 138
Sleep and Extreme Fussiness/Colic 138
Temperament at Four Months 160
Connecting Sleep, Extreme Fussiness/Colic, and Temperament 166
Post-colic: Preventing Sleep Problems After Four Months of Age 176

Summary and Action Plan for Exhausted Parents 184

Part II. *How Parents Can Help Their Children Establish Healthy Sleep Habits: You Can Prevent Sleep Disturbances from Infancy to Adolescence*

Chapter 5. Months One to Four 195
Newborn: The First Week 197
Weeks Two to Four: More Fussiness 201
Weeks Five to Six: Fussiness/Crying Peaks 204
Weeks Seven to Eight: Earlier Bedtimes and Longer Night Sleep Periods Develop 218
Months Three to Four: Extreme Fussiness/Colic Ends. Morning Nap Develops at 9:00 to 10:00 A.M. 224
Preventing and Solving Sleep Problems 230
Action Plan for Exhausted Parents 240

Chapter 6. Months Five to Twelve 244
Months Five to Eight: Early Afternoon Nap Develops at 12:00 to 2:00 P.M. Variable Late Afternoon Nap at 3:00 to 5:00 P.M. 244
Month Nine: Late Afternoon Nap Disappears. No More Bottle-feeding at Night 266
Months Ten to Twelve: Morning Nap Starts to Disappear but Mostly Two Naps 267
Preventing and Solving Sleep Problems: Months Five to Twelve 271
Action Plan for Exhausted Parents 306

Chapter 7. Months Thirteen to Thirty-six 308
Months Thirteen to Fifteen: One or Two Naps 308
Months Sixteen to Twenty-one: Morning Nap Disappears 311
Months Twenty-two to Thirty-six: Only a Single Afternoon Nap 313
Preventing and Solving Sleep Problems 317
Action Plan for Exhausted Parents 337

Chapter 8. Preschool Children 338

Years Three to Six: Naps Disappear 338

Preventing and Solving Sleep Problems 344

Action Plan for Exhausted Parents 357

Chapter 9. Schoolchildren and Adolescence 358

Years Seven to Twelve: Bedtime Becomes Later 358

Adolescence: Not Enough Time to Sleep, Especially in the Morning 360

Preventing and Solving Sleep Problems 368

Part III. Other Sleep Disturbances and Concerns

Chapter 10. Special Sleep Problems 377

Sleepwalking 377

Sleep Talking 378

Night Terrors 378

Nightmares 379

Head Banging and Body Rocking 381

Bruxism 381

Narcolepsy 382

Poor-Quality Breathing (Allergies and Snoring) 382

Hyperactive Behaviour 393

Seasonal Affective Disorder 397

Bed-wetting 398

Chapter 11. Special Events and Concerns 399

Changes with Daylight Saving Time 399

New Sibling 399

Twins, Triplets and More 400

Moving 412

Holidays and Crossing Time Zones 414

Frequent Illnesses 417

Mother's Return to Work 419

Home Office 421

Dual-Career Families 425

Adoption 428

Injuries 430

Overweight, Exercise and Diet 432

Child Abuse 434
Atopic Dermatitis and Eczema 435
Chapter 12. Competent Parents, Competent Child, by Karen Pierce, M.D. 436
Self-esteem 438
Good-Enough Parenting 440
Development of Internal Controls 442
Saying No Helps Your Child 443
My Child Has Sleep Problems. What Do We Do Now? 445
When Other Issues Get in the Way 447
Summary 453
Chapter 13. The Pros and Cons of Other Approaches to Sleep Problems 454
Proper Association with Falling Asleep (Richard Ferber's Theory) 454
Unrestricted Breast-feeding and the Family Bed (William Sears's Theory) 455
Summary 456
REFERENCES 458
INDEX 493

Foreword

A friend recommended this book to me when my first child, Presley, was seven months old. I was still nursing, but getting ready to stop, and definitely ready to stop the 4:00 A.M. feeding. Also, we had let Presley get into the bad habit of only wanting to nap *on* someone. This was great when I needed an excuse for a nap, but not so convenient on busy days.

I devoured the book in a matter of hours and put the principles into practice immediately – with instant results. I especially liked how Dr Weissbluth taught me to watch out for my child's sleepy signs and then encouraged me to get him to bed before he was overtired. I was also very comforted by Dr Weissbluth's explanation of sleep as one of your child's basic needs. You offer healthy food to your child when she's hungry. You must also offer healthy sleep when your child is tired – even if she doesn't know it or thinks she doesn't want it (just like my kids won't usually choose vegetables!)

As a correspondent for *Good Morning America,* I was able to contact and interview Dr Weissbluth as part of my series Baby's First Year. I feel tremendously lucky to have Dr Weissbluth as a resource in my life (yes, there are some perks!) Dr Weissbluth has become a trusted adviser not only on the topic of sleep, but also on potty training and discipline.

Dr Weissbluth, thank you for being a mentor and friend. I wish I could say my kids never wake up at night or always go to sleep without a power struggle. We have our ups and downs – but that's parenthood. What I do have is a structure for sleep, which we're always trying to get back to after travelling or any other disruption in our routine. It really helps to have that and to know it works – especially when *you* are bleary-eyed at 2:00 A.M. I love Dr Weissbluth's philosophy that the most important thing to have is a well-rested *family*. And fortunately, thanks to *Healthy Sleep Habits, Happy Child*, most days (and nights) we do!

– Cindy Crawford

How to Use This Book

If you are still pregnant, it is important for both parents, not just the mother-to-be, to read the Introduction and Chapters 1, 2, 4 and 5. Try to read all of this before your baby is born because no matter how tired you may feel now, you will be even more tired once your baby has arrived. Trying to read anything then is difficult, to say the least. In these chapters you will gain an understanding as to why healthy sleep is valuable, how to satisfy your baby's need to sleep, how to cope with fussiness or crying in the evening and how to prevent sleep problems.

If you have already delivered your baby, it is likely that you are exhausted, feeling a little lost, or both. Shortly after the birth, you may have 'baby brain' and be unable to concentrate, focus, or develop a plan of action because you are so sleep-deprived. And if you are breast-feeding, it is possible that you feel physically drained. It is absolutely necessary for husbands, who never have 'baby brain', to read portions of this book and to act as a coach for their wives. First, even if your baby was not very fussy or crying much in the evenings, please read Chapter 4, because all babies have some fussiness. Then go to the sleep problems discussed in Chapter 3; first read about the problem and then consult the Action Plan for Exhausted Parents. Finally, read the Action Plan for Exhausted Parents in the chapters before and after the chapter for your child's age, because chronological age is only a rough guide both for sleep problems and their solutions. If your child has snoring or mouth breathing during sleep or has very dry and itchy skin, read the appropriate sections in Chapter 10 or 11.

Introduction

Why won't my child sleep better? Where does he get all his energy? He really never seems tired; he just goes and goes and goes until he crashes. I'm burned out and I know he must be exhausted. Of course, he never slept well, even when he was a baby. He was up at all hours during the night, every night. Naps? Forget them. Yes, he took catnaps, but only in my arms or in the car. I just thought it was normal because no baby wants to sleep with so many interesting things going on around him. Anyway, I didn't want to hear all that crying when he didn't want to sleep. But now he's two, and I'm getting tired of those constant bedtime battles. There are times when I wish he would simply just settle down and be less wild.

Sound familiar?

All kids occasionally are firecrackers when things are not going their way. But why do some kids have much shorter fuses than others?

Healthy Sleep Habits, Happy Child will explain how fatigue caused by poor-quality sleep makes some children drop off more often or explode with more force than others. It will also explain how chronic fatigue can reduce your child's ability to succeed in school. This book will show how you can nurture, enhance and maintain calm and alert behaviour in your child by instilling good sleep habits.

I will lead you on a tour through the shadows of your child's night and shine my torch on the most frustrating nocturnal problems that can disrupt sleep. The first leg of our journey covers terrain that may not be familiar even to experienced parents. Part I, How Children Sleep, describes healthy sleep, disturbed sleep, sleep problems and common myths about sleeping. It also covers some sad territory that has not been explored previously: the harmful effects of disturbed sleep when everyone in the family suffers from fatigue. The second part of our journey, How Parents Can Help Their Children Establish Healthy Sleep Habits, is an age-specific guide to understanding sleep patterns and solving common sleep problems in your child. Finally, in Part III, we explore Other Sleep Disturbances and Concerns. When we finish our tour, you will be able to direct your own child toward healthy sleep habits.

SLEEP DEPRIVATION HARMS CHILDREN

Sleep deprivation can be prevented and treated.

What do I mean by healthy sleep?

Do you know how to get a good night's sleep and feel rested? I think I do. But sometimes I go to bed too early, sometimes too late – and I'm supposed to know a lot about sleeping! The truth is that no one really knows exactly how to programme good sleep so that we always feel rested. In fact, we're really in the dark ages when it comes to understanding how sleep works. Interestingly enough, adult volunteers in early sleep studies were kept in deep, dark caves. This was done to eliminate day- and night-time cues so that researchers could study how sleep affects our body and our feelings. Of course, sleep researchers now use specifically designed laboratories and trick clocks that run faster or slower than 'real' time to observe how our biological rhythms, or 'internal clocks', work when external time cues are removed. Studies also have been performed on shift workers and Air Force pilots who often cross time zones and suffer from jet-lag syndrome to observe how time differences affect sleep patterns.

But children's sleep habits have not been studied in such detail. Obviously, it's a bigger problem if a bomber crew carrying nuclear weapons is inattentive because of a lack of sleep or jet-lag syndrome than if a child has fatigue-driven temper tantrums. But if it's your child, you might not agree!

I have studied both healthy and disturbed sleep in thousands of children as founder of the original Sleep Disorders Center at Children's Memorial Hospital in Chicago. I have helped hundreds of families understand how their children's sleep habits are directly connected to how they behave and how they will do in school. Based on this research, my general paediatric practice spanning more than thirty years and life with my own four sons and two grandchildren, I have discovered that there is hope for bleary-eyed parents. In fact, both you and your child can benefit from this knowledge. I personally benefited from my sleep research: I used to think naps were a waste of time. I wanted to spend time with my boys, and I had all those chores to do. The result? I was combative and irritable from accumulated sleeplessness. Now I think my whole family benefits when I take the naps I need.

Prevention and treatment of unhealthy sleep habits in infants and young children are important because if they are uncorrected, they will persist. There is no automatic correction. Children do not simply outgrow these problems. The good news is that the harmful effects of unhealthy sleep are reversible when parents provide treatment. The younger the child, the more successful you will be in reversing the ill effects of unhealthy sleep.

Preventing the development of unhealthy sleep patterns is something all parents can do. But it requires that they start early, paying attention to their baby's evolving natural sleep rhythms and to synchronise their soothing-to-sleep behaviour with the time when the sleep process first begins. Perfect timing produces no crying. This book is designed to educate parents as to how they can accomplish perfect timing and prevent sleep problems in their child. But to achieve perfect timing requires practice, so it is possible, especially if this is your first child, that there may be a little crying when your baby becomes overtired.

Treatment of sleep problems is more difficult than prevention for the simple reason that both the child and the parents are stressed from being overtired. Overtired children are fatigued, and the body's natural response is to fight the fatigue by producing a stimulating chemical. This response was important for survival, as primitive man had to flee, fight or continue hunting even when overtired. This 'second wind' of stimulating energy causes a hyperalert or hypervigilant state, which prevents easy entry into sleep or sleeping for long periods. That's why overtired children appear 'wired', unable to fall asleep easily or stay asleep. But why the crying?

First, severe fatigue itself can be painful. Second, changing established habits is very disturbing. After the first few months of life children can protest against changes in routine by crying; they would rather play with their parents than sleep.

No parent wants her child to cry. The truth is that encouraging healthy sleep habits will prevent a lot of crying in the long run. It is possible that the treatment of unhealthy sleep habits may *initially* increase crying around sleep times, but subsequently it will eliminate crying altogether. Some treatments will involve no crying.

How is a parent able to trust what they read in books, magazines or on the Internet? When you compare advice on sleeping and crying from different writers, ask yourself on what are they basing their advice. Besides practising general paediatrics since 1973, conducting and publishing original research, and lecturing on crying and sleeping problems in children since 1981, I have helped my wife raise our four sons.

These experiences have led me to the conclusion that sleeping patterns, temperament and infant fussing or crying are all connected. And in young babies, these features are mostly biologically determined. Other studies have confirmed these observations, so I am reasonably confident that children are born with a package of interrelated initial predispositions or tendencies.

In the same way that we know how much calcium your

baby needs for his bones to grow stronger, we know how important healthy sleep is for the growing brain. Calcium deficiency in childhood harms bone development, but the problems of osteoporosis may not show up until much later in adult life. So if your child eats a calcium-deficient diet, the problem is 'hidden' because there are no immediately apparent ill effects. Likewise, sleep deficiency in childhood may harm neurological development; the problems remain 'hidden', not showing up until later. I think it is possible that unhealthy sleep habits contribute to school-related problems such as attention deficit hyperactivity disorder (ADHD) and learning disabilities. I also suspect chronically tired children become chronically tired adults who suffer in ways we can't measure: less resiliency, less ability to cope with life's stress, less curiosity, less empathy, less playfulness. The message here is simple: sleep is a powerful modifier of mood, behaviour, performance and personality.

WARNING

If your child does not learn to sleep well, he may become an incurable adult insomniac, chronically disabled from sleepiness and dependent on sleeping pills.

One of the world's foremost researchers in sleep, William C. Dement, taught me at Stanford University Medical School, USA in 1967 that we exist in three distinctly different biological domains: awake, REM sleep and non-REM sleep. Although all three domains interact with one another, there are specific problems that can occur within each domain.

According to Dr Dement, traditional medical science focused on only the first domain, wakefulness. His major point was that we are fundamentally different when we are asleep than when we are awake. The body's clock knows when we should be asleep and adjusts our brain, our temperature and our hormone levels to the sleep mode. In sleep mode, we do not respond, think or feel as we do when awake. If you do not believe this, ask any mother of a six-week-old infant how she is when she is up at night soothing her baby!

There has been much misunderstanding about 'insecurity' and 'crying to sleep' because of a failure to make the distinction between (1) *the importance of sleeping well when we are in a biological sleep mode* and (2) *the importance of security of attachment when we are in a biological awake mode*. This failure is understandable, because most child psychologists and child psychiatrists have not had the opportunity to do research or to receive training regarding the benefits of healthy sleep. They do not understand that the sleeping brain is different from the awake brain. Even today, very little teaching regarding sleep takes place; only about five hours during the three-year training programme for paediatricians in the United States. Sadly, 'expert' advice in popular magazines or books often reflects this lack of knowledge.

Because there is a basic difference between the sleeping brain and the awake brain, different types of problems can develop. When the brain enters the biological domain of sleep, problems such as night terrors might appear. Night terrors and other sleep problems simply do not occur when the brain shifts to the awake domain.

Similarly, we are fundamentally different when we are awake.

When our children are awake, we worry about problems such as temper tantrums, fighting, not sharing or not eating well. Also, we sometimes wonder if we are making the appropriate emotional connection. Are our children getting enough love? Are they happy? Are they securely attached, or do they feel insecure? How we interact with our children while we feed them, bathe them, dress them and play with them is very important. Insecurity of attachment as a concept makes no sense when the brain shifts to the sleep domain.

BE PATIENT

It takes time for your child to develop strength, coordination, balance and confidence to 'learn' to walk.

It takes time for your baby to develop night sleep consolidation, regular and long naps, and self-soothing skills to 'learn' to sleep well.

We know that the process of falling asleep and staying asleep is learned behaviour, and that the learning will occur naturally, just like learning how to walk, if parents do not interfere. Difficulties in learning how to walk used to occur when walkers were popular, because they interfered with the natural evolution of a normal gait. Difficulties in learning how to sleep occur when parents do not respect and protect the child's natural, periodic need to sleep. With practice, all parents will clearly see that perfect timing produces no crying!

New parents need to practise before they achieve perfection, and they need to be patient. Because of new parents' inexperience and the baby's shifting sleep rhythms, there will be incidents when the timing will be off and the baby will become painfully overtired. Then there may be some crying. This book will provide a guide to help coach you to catch the rising wave of sleepiness before the child crashes into an overtired state. *Making children cry is* not *the way to help them learn to sleep.*

Helping babies and children sleep well is not just mothers' work; fathers also play an important role in helping to establish healthy sleeping. Traditionally, mothers have suffered the burden of sleep deprivation because they were doing night duty alone. They were on call day and night much more than the fathers were, and when there were problems occurring on the night shift, guess who was expected to handle it? When babies do not sleep well, guess who gets the blame? I have tried to correct this situation by discussing how important it is – for the sake of the child, the marriage and the family – to get the father actively involved.

In *Healthy Sleep Habits, Happy Child*, you will learn in detail how to prevent and treat sleeping problems. The discussion of prevention includes a detailed map to help you decide whether the path of breast-feeding or the family bed will be important on your journey to prevent sleep problems. The discussion of treatment has been expanded to include a comparison of different treatment strategies: extinction (ignoring), graduated extinction (controlled crying, check and console), scheduled awakenings, bedtime routines, day correction of bedtime problems, relaxation and white noise. To make this book easier to use, Action Plans for Exhausted Parents have been included at the end of every chapter for handy reference and guidance. Throughout the book I mention husbands, wives, marriage or marital problems merely for convenience, but I wish to embrace all partner and parent-child relationships.

Healthy Sleep Habits, Happy Child

PART I

How Children Sleep

CHAPTER 1

Why Healthy Sleep Is So Important

Infants and children who are still of tender age [may be] attacked by . . . wakefulness at night.
– Aulus Cornelius Celsus, A.D. 130

Sleeplessness in children and worrying about sleeplessness have been around for a long time.

Healthy sleep appears to come so easily and naturally to newborn babies. Effortlessly, they fall asleep and stay asleep. Their sleep patterns, however, shift and evolve as the brain matures during the first few weeks and months. Such changes may result in 'day/night confusion' – long sleep periods during the day and long wakeful periods at night. This is bothersome, but it is only a problem of timing. The young infant still does not have any difficulty falling asleep or staying asleep. After several weeks of age, though, parents can shape natural sleep rhythms and patterns into sleep habits.

It comes as a surprise to many parents that healthy sleep habits do *not* develop automatically. In fact, parents can and do help or hinder the development of healthy sleep habits. Of course, children will spontaneously fall asleep when totally exhausted – 'crashing' is a biological necessity! But this is unhealthy, because extreme fatigue (often identified by 'wired' behaviour immediately preceding the crash) interferes with normal social interactions and even learning. You should not assume that it is 'natural' for all children to get peevish, or irritable at the end of the day. Well-rested children do not behave this way.

Before electricity, radio, television, computers or commuting long distances to work, children went to sleep earlier than children do today. Our current popular late bedtimes may be no more 'natural' than the outdated 'natural' belief that fatter babies are healthier babies. Commonly held or popular beliefs about what is natural, normal or healthy are not always true. In addition, when you think of child rearing, it may appear 'natural' for you to consider parenting practices performed in traditional cultures. That is, breast-feed frequently day and night and sleep with your baby, wear your baby in a sling or soft carrier, always be close to your baby and always respond to your baby. This is not always practical for some families, and even for those families who choose this 'natural' style, their baby's extreme fussiness/crying/not sleeping or 'unnatural' factors can interfere.

'NATURAL' VERSUS 'UNNATURAL'

'Natural'

All babies have spells of fussing and crying.

These spells distress all parents.

All parents want to soothe their baby.

The more the baby fusses or cries, the less she sleeps.

The less the baby sleeps, the less the parents sleep.

The less the parents sleep, the harder it is for them to soothe their baby.

Relatives and friends want to help soothe the baby and are expected to assist parents.

Breast-feeding and sleeping with your baby are powerful ways to soothe your baby.

'Unnatural'

Urban stimulation (noises, voices, delivery trucks, shopping trips, errands) may interfere with baby's sleeping.

Day care (not being able to put your child to sleep when just starting to become tired, or too much stimulation) may interfere with baby's sleeping.

<u>Social isolation</u> forcing only the mother to be wholly responsible to take care of soothing and sleeping may cause intense stress for the mother.

<u>Busy modern lifestyles</u> means that parents have many things to do and little time to do them; sometimes they have to take their baby with them even at sleep times.

<u>Mothers have to work outside the house</u>, miss playing with their baby and keep their baby up too late at night.

<u>Fathers or mothers have a long commute</u> and return home from work late, want to play with their baby and keep their baby up too late at night.

<u>Grandparents</u> interfere with sleep routines.

Dr Christian Guilleminault, who along with Dr William C. Dement was the founding editor of the world's leading journal of sleep research, taught me to consider five fundamental principles of understanding sleep:

1. **The sleeping brain is not a resting brain.**
2. **The sleeping brain functions in a different manner from the waking brain.**
3. **The activity and work of the sleeping brain are purposeful.**
4. **The process of falling asleep is learned.**
5. **Providing the growing brain with sufficient sleep is necessary for developing the ability to concentrate and an easier temperament.**

Sleep is the power source that keeps your mind alert and calm. Every night and at every nap, sleep recharges the brain's battery. Sleeping well increases brainpower just as lifting weights builds stronger muscles, because sleeping well increases your attention span and allows you to be physically relaxed and mentally alert at the same time. Then you are at your personal best.

As you will discover as you read this book, when children learn to sleep well, they also learn to maintain *optimal wakefulness*. The notion of optimal wakefulness, also called optimal alertness, is important, because we tend to think simplistically of being either awake or asleep. Just as our twenty-four-hour cycle consists of more than just the two states called daytime and night-time, there are gradations – which we call dawn and dusk – in sleep and wakefulness.

In sleep, the levels vary from deep sleep to partial arousals; in wakefulness, the levels vary from being wide awake to being groggy.

The importance of optimal wakefulness cannot be overemphasised. If your child does not get all the sleep he needs, he may seem either drowsy or hyperalert. If either state lasts for a long time, the results are the same: a child with a difficult mood and hard-to-control behaviour, certainly not one who is ready and able to enjoy himself or get the most out of the myriad learning experiences placed before him.

With our busy lifestyles, how can we keep track of nap schedules and regular bedtime hours? Is it really true that I can harm my baby by giving him love at night when he cries out for me? How can I be sure that sleep is really that important? Am I a bad parent if my child cries? If he cries at night, isn't he feeling insecure? These are questions many parents ask me. Parents will often mention that articles or books they have read seem to support different ideas, and so they conclude by saying that since this whole issue is 'so controversial,' they would rather let matters stay as they are. If you think your child is not sleeping well and if you disagree with the suggestions in this book, then ask yourself how long you should wait for improvement to occur. Three months? Three years? If you are following the opinion of a professional who says you must spend more time with your child at night to make him feel more 'secure,' ask that professional, 'When will I know we are on the right track?' Don't wait for ever. Consider what Dr Charles E. Sundell, the physician in charge of the Children's Department in the Prince of Wales General Hospital in England, wrote in 1922: 'Success in the treatment of sleeplessness in infants is a good standard by which to estimate the patience and skill of the practitioner.' He also wrote: 'A sleepless baby is a reproach to his guardian, and convicts them of some failure in their guardianship.' So don't think that worrying about sleeplessness is just a contemporary issue.

The truth is, modern research regarding sleep/wake states only confirms what careful practitioners such as Dr Sundell observed over eighty years ago. He wrote:

> The temptation to postpone the time for a baby's sleep, so that he may be admired by some relative or friend who is late in arriving, or so that his nurse may finish some work on which she may be engaged, must be strongly resisted. A sleepy child who is kept awake exhausts his nervous energy very quickly in *peevish restlessness*, and when preparations are at last made for his sleep *he may be too weary to settle down* . . .
>
> *Regularity of habits* is one of the sheet-anchors by which the baroque of an infant's health is secured. The re-establishment of a regular routine, after even a short break, frequently calls for *patient perseverance* on the part of the nurse, but though the child may protest vigorously for several nights, *absolute firmness seldom fails to procure the desired result.*

Each baby is unique. They're like little snowflakes. Babies are born with individual traits that affect the amount of physical activity, the duration of sleep and the length of periods of crying they will sustain. But babies also differ in more subtle ways. Some are easier to 'read'; they seem to have predictable schedules for feeding and sleeping. These babies also tend to cry less and sleep more. Regular babies, that is, those whose behaviours seem to follow a pattern that occurs without much variation, are more self-soothing; they fall asleep more easily, and when they awaken at night they are more able to return to sleep unassisted. But don't blame yourself if you have an irregular baby who cries a lot and is less self-soothing. It's only luck, although social customs may affect how you feel about it.

In those societies where the mother holds the baby close all the time, and her breasts are always available for nursing and soothing, there are still great differences among babies in terms of fussiness and crying. The mother compensates by increasing the amount of rhythmic, rocking motions or nursing. She may not even expect the baby to sleep alone, away from her body. As she grows up, a child might share the bed with her parents for a long time. This is not necessarily good or bad; it's just *different* from the expectations of most middle-class Western families.

So not only do babies sleep differently, but every society's expectations condition parents' feelings in different ways. Remember, there are no universally 'right' or 'wrong' ways, or 'natural' versus 'unnatural' styles, of raising children. Less-developed societies are not necessarily more 'natural' and thus 'healthier' in their child-rearing practices. After all, strychnine and cow's milk are equally 'natural', but they have altogether different effects when ingested.

How much we are bothered by infant crying or poor sleep habits might partially reflect our own expectations about how to be 'good' parents. Do we want to carry the baby all the time, twenty-four hours a day, or do we want to put the baby down sometimes to sleep?

Here's a true story. A Saudi Arabian princess came to my office for a consultation, accompanied by her English-trained Saudi paediatrician, her English-trained Saudi nanny and two other women, to discuss sleeping habits for the royal family's children. The paediatrician described child care arrangements that had been popular among British aristocrats in the nineteenth century. Like trained baby nurses in nineteenth-century England, the Saudi Arabian nanny was always able to hold the princess's baby while the child was sleeping for the simple reason that the Saudi nurse had her own servants! These subordinate nannies were not as well trained and were assigned the menial domestic chores associated with child rearing.

The majority of parents do not have child care staffs. They have to rely on their own skills. So if we are greatly bothered by our baby's crying or our guilt about not being 'good' parents, this may interfere with our developing a sense of competence. We may feel that we cannot influence sleep patterns in our child. Unfortunately, this way of thinking can set the stage for future sleep disorders.

Sleep problems not only disrupt a child's nights, they disrupt his *days*, too, by making him less mentally alert, more inattentive, unable to concentrate, and easily distracted. They also make him more physically impulsive, hyperactive or lazy. But when children sleep well, they are optimally awake and alert, able to learn and grow up with charm and humour. When parents are too irregular, inconsistent or oversolicitous, or when there are unresolved problems between the parents, the resulting sleep problems converge, producing excessive night-time wakefulness and crying.

Please do not simply assume that children must pass through different 'stages' at different ages, and that these stages inevitably create sleep problems. The truth is that after three or four months of age, all children can begin to learn to sleep well. The learning process will occur as naturally as learning how to walk.

The bad news is that some *parents* create sleep problems. The good news is that parents can prevent sleep problems as well as correct any that develop.

Parents who favour a more gradual approach (controlled crying or graduated extinction) over an abrupt approach (ignoring or extinction) often complain of frequent 'relapses'. The general reason why a gradual approach tends to be less successful in the long run is that it takes longer and there are always natural disruptions of sleep, such as illnesses or holidays. The subsequent reestablishment of healthy sleep routines using a gradual approach becomes very stressful to the parents. Several days or weeks of a gradual approach often wear down parents, so they give up and revert to their old inconsistencies. Parents who have successfully used extinction know that they might have one, and only one, night of crying after they return home from several days on holiday or from a visit to a relative's house.

The truth is that some parents swing back and forth between firmness and permissiveness so often, they cannot make any cure stick. They often confuse their wishful thinking with the child's actual behaviour. This is why a sleep log, which I will describe later, can be an important tool to help you document what you are really doing and how your child is really responding. After all, short-term 'successes' might only reflect brief periods when your child crashes at night from chronic exhaustion. Or the actual improvement in sleep habits may be so marginal that the normal disruptions of holidays, trips, illnesses or other irregularities constantly buffet the still-tired child and cause repeated 'relapses' in which he wakes often during the night or fights going to sleep.

In contrast, parents who successfully carry out an abrupt retraining programme – the cold-turkey approach – to improve sleep habits see immediate and dramatic improvement without any lasting ill effects. These children have fewer relapses and recover faster and more completely from natural disruptions of sleep routines. Seeing a cure really 'stick' for a while gives you the courage to keep tighter control over sleep patterns and to repeat the process again if needed.

I cannot emphasise enough how important it is for parents to start early to help their child learn to sleep well.

PRACTICAL POINT

If you start *early* with sleep training, you will be well along the path to *preventing* sleep problems.

When you start early, there are no long bouts of crying and no problems with sleeping. The process of falling asleep unassisted is a skill, and as with any other skill, it is easier to teach good habits first than it is to correct bad habits later. Also, as with any other skill, success comes only after a period of practice.

The many personal accounts in this book, contributed by a variety of caring, thoughtful parents, should add extra incentive to teach healthy sleep habits early or to make a change to correct your child's sleep problems right now, so that you can all get on with the best part of having children – *enjoying* them!

Some parents may need professional help to establish reasonable, orderly home routines, to iron out conflicts between parents or to help an older child with a well-established sleep problem. To maintain healthy sleep for your young child, you need the courage to be firm without feeling guilt or fear that she will resent you or love you less. In fact, the best prescription I can offer is to create a loving home with a well-rested child and well-rested parents.

> *There never was a*
> *Child so lovely but his*
> *Mother was glad to see him asleep.*
>
> – Ralph Waldo Emerson

What a difference healthy sleep can make in our children!

CHAPTER 2

Healthy Sleep and Sleep Strategies

HEALTHY SLEEP

Are your child's sleep patterns healthy? There are five elements of healthy sleep for children:

1. **Sleep duration: night and day**
2. **Naps**
3. **Sleep consolidation**
4. **Sleep schedule, timing of sleep**
5. **Sleep regularity**

When these five items are in proper balance, children get the rest they need. Let's first take a look at each one separately. Later, we will see how each element is not really independent from the others but simply part of a package called 'healthy sleep'.

As we consider the biological development of these five factors, please remember that parenting practices such as feeding do not influence how the brain develops. There are five turning points in the sleep maturation process: six weeks (night sleep lengthens), twelve to sixteen weeks (daytime sleep regularises), nine months (disappearance of night waking for feeding and a third nap), twelve to twenty-one months (disappearance of the morning nap) and three to four years (afternoon nap becomes less common).

As your baby's brain matures, the patterns and rhythm of sleep change. If you always adapt your parenting practices to these changes, your child will sleep well. Those parents who do not see these changes or make these adjustments have babies who become overtired. The biological development causing all these changes is under the control of two regulatory mechanisms. Understanding these controlling mechanisms will help you organise your thoughts and plan your actions to ensure healthy sleep for your child.

The first regulatory system controls the body's need for sleep and has been called the 'homeostatic control mechanism'. In a nutshell, this means that the longer you go without sleep, the longer you will subsequently sleep. If you lose sleep, the body tries to restore it. The body tries to make sure you are getting enough sleep. This automatic process reflects an internal biological mechanism that we do not control. It is similar to the body wanting to control its temperature; when we get hot, we automatically sweat. If we do not drink enough fluid, then we cannot sweat, and we suffer the ill effects of dehydration. However, if we drink too much caffeine and deprive the body of sleep, we also cause harm. Unfortunately, our baby's biological need for sleep is always changing, so we have to be on our toes in order not to miss shifts in sleeping requirements.

The secondary regulatory system has been called the 'circadian timing system'. It is also called the 'internal timing system' and can be thought of as a dedicated regulatory programme that switches specific genes on and off in response to the light-dark cycle. This regulatory apparatus built to turn on and off is a molecular clock that is genetically specified and it is set to the proper time by sunlight. This mechanism automatically tries to ensure that the body is sleeping at the right time, and that when you are asleep, the timing and amounts of different stages and types of sleep are correct. Signals come from a specific area within the brain to make us feel sleepy or wakeful. The pattern of these signals changes over weeks, months and years as the baby grows into an adult. The pace of these changes is especially quick during the first several months, so it is easy for a parent to get a little off tempo. Just when you think you have worked out when your baby needs to nap or be put to bed at night, the times change!

IMPORTANT POINT

The Internal Timing System is under genetic control so there is individual variation. It takes time for the Internal Timing System to express itself.

Sleep Duration: Night and Day

If you don't sleep long enough, you feel tired. This sounds very simple and obvious, but how much sleep is enough? And how can you tell if *your* child is getting enough sleep?

Under three or four months of age, infants' sleep patterns seem mostly to reflect the development of the child's brain. During these first few weeks, in fact, sleep durations equal sleep needs, since infant behaviour and sleep durations are mostly influenced by biological factors. But after about three or four months, and perhaps even at about six weeks (or six weeks after the due date, for babies born early), parenting practices can influence sleep duration and, consequently, behaviour. As I will discuss later in more detail, I believe parents can promote more pleasant, calm, alert behaviours by becoming more sensitive to their growing child's need to sleep and by helping to maintain healthy sleep habits. The goal is to recognise and respect your child's need to sleep and not do things that interfere with the natural sleep process.

Newborns and Young Infants

During their first few days, newborns sleep about sixteen to seventeen hours total each day, although their longest single sleep period is only four to five hours. It makes no difference whether your baby is breast-fed or bottle-fed, or whether it's a boy or a girl.

> **PRACTICAL POINT**
>
> **Nursing mothers often worry unnecessarily that long sleep periods deprive their baby of adequate breast milk. Weight checks with the doctor will reassure you that all is well.**

Between one week and four months, the total daily sleep duration drifts down from sixteen and a half to fifteen hours, while the longest single sleep period – usually the night – increases from four to nine hours. We know from several studies that this development reflects neurological maturation and is *not* related to the start of feeding solid foods.

Some newborns and infants under the age of four months sleep much more and others much less. During the first few months, you can usually assume that your baby is getting sufficient sleep. But if your baby cries too much or has extreme fussiness/colic, you might assist Mother Nature by trying the helpful hints for 'crybabies' described in Chapter 4.

> **PRACTICAL POINT**
>
> **When they are one or two weeks old, many infants begin to have several hour periods of increasingly alert, wakeful and fussy behaviour. This continues until about six weeks of age, after which they start to calm down. This increasingly irritable and wakeful state is often misinterpreted as resulting from maternal anxiety or insufficient or 'bad' breast milk. Nonsense! The culprit is a temporarily uninhibited nervous system that causes excessive arousal. Relax; this developmental phase will pass as the baby's brain matures. It's not your fault.**

Young infants are very portable. You can take them anywhere you want, and when they need to sleep, they will. I remember when, as a medical student at Stanford University, I was playing tennis with my wife one day and my first child was sleeping in an infant seat near the fence. A huge dump truck came crashing down the narrow street, making an awful racket. We ran over to our son, only to be surprised that he remained sweetly asleep. After six weeks of age, he became more socially aware of people around him; after about four months of age, he, like all children, became interested in barking dogs, wind in the trees, clouds and many other curious things, all of which could and did disturb his sleep.

For some infants, the time when the baby first makes a socially responsive smile (usually at six weeks of age, or six weeks after the due date, for babies born early) is when social curiosity or social learning begins. However, under about three or four months of age, most infants, like my son, are not much disturbed by their environment when it comes to sleeping. When their body says it's time to sleep, they sleep. When their body tells them to wake up, they wake up – even when it is not convenient for their parents! This is true whether they are fed on demand or according to a regular schedule. It is also true even when they are continuously fed intravenously because of birth defects of the stomach or intestines. Hunger, in fact, seems to have little to do with how babies sleep. A much more likely candidate for influencing a baby's sleeping patterns is the hormone melatonin, which is produced by the baby's brain beginning at about three to four months of age. This hormone surges at night and has the capability to both induce drowsiness and relax the smooth muscles encircling the gut. So around three or four months of age, so-called day/night confusion and apparent abdominal cramps (colic) begin to disappear.

Furthermore, infants raised in an environment where the lights are constantly on evolve normal sleep patterns, just like babies brought up in homes where the lights are turned on and off routinely. Another bit of evidence to suggest that environment has little effect on sleep patterns in children under three or four months of age comes from infants born prematurely. A child born four weeks before his due date, for example, reaches the same level of sleep development as a full-term baby four weeks *later* than the child born on time. Biological sleep/wake development does not speed up in premature babies who are exposed to more social stimulation.

What we can conclude, therefore, is that, for infants under three or four months of age, you should try to flow with the child's need for sleep. Don't expect predictable sleep schedules, and don't try to enforce them rigidly. Still, some babies do develop regular sleep/wake rhythms quite early, say at about six to eight weeks. These babies tend to be very mild, cry very little and sleep for long periods of time. Consider yourself blessed if you are one of these lucky parents.

Older Infants and Children

As children age, the amount of time they sleep tends to decrease. Figures 1 to 3 (pages 21–3) describe how much daytime sleep, night sleep and total sleep occur at different ages for older children. The bottom curve in each graph means that 10 per cent of children sleep less than the amount shown, while the top curve means that 90 per cent of children sleep less than the amount shown for each age. These curves were generated by my own research using data collected from 2,019 children, mostly white, middle-class residents of northern Illinois and northern Indiana in 1980. These graphs can help you tell whether your child's sleep is above the ninetieth per centile or below the tenth per centile. (Other studies have used only the fiftieth per centile, or average values, and do not tell you whether your child's sleep duration is slightly below average or extremely below average.) Interestingly, the results of studies of similar social classes in 1911 in California and in 1927 in Minnesota, also involving thousands of children, were the same as those in my study. In addition, studies in England in 1910 and Japan in 1925 showed identical sleep curves.

So it seems that despite cultural and ethnic differences, social changes, and such modern inventions as television, DVDs and computers that shape our contemporary lifestyles, the age-specific durations of sleep are firmly and universally rooted in our children's developing biology.

An exception to this generalisation is that adolescents in the United States are now getting less sleep. During the second half of the twentieth century, a trend towards earlier start times for school developed. This forced children to get up earlier during the school week and reduced the total number of hours available for sleeping. At the same time, it became more popular for teenagers to hold part-time jobs after school, so they were going to bed later. Also, the amount of homework has increased.

After about four months, I think parents can influence sleep durations, and as you will see, sleep durations for these older infants and toddlers are especially important.

I studied sixty healthy children in my paediatric practice at five months of age and then again at thirty-six months. At five months of age, the infants who were cooing, smiling, adaptable and regular, and curiously approached unfamiliar things or people, slept longer than infants with opposite characteristics. These easy and calm infants slept about three and a half hours during the day and twelve hours at night, or a total of fifteen and a half hours. Infants who were fussy, crying, irritable, hard to handle, irregular, and more withdrawn slept almost three hours less overall, almost a 20 per cent difference (three hours during the day and nine and a half hours at night, or twelve and a half hours total).

In addition, for all the five-month-olds studied, persistence or attention span was the trait most strongly associated with daytime sleep or nap duration. In other words, *children who slept longer during the day had longer attention spans.*

FIGURE 1: HOURS OF TOTAL SLEEP BY AGE FOR GIVEN PERCENTILES

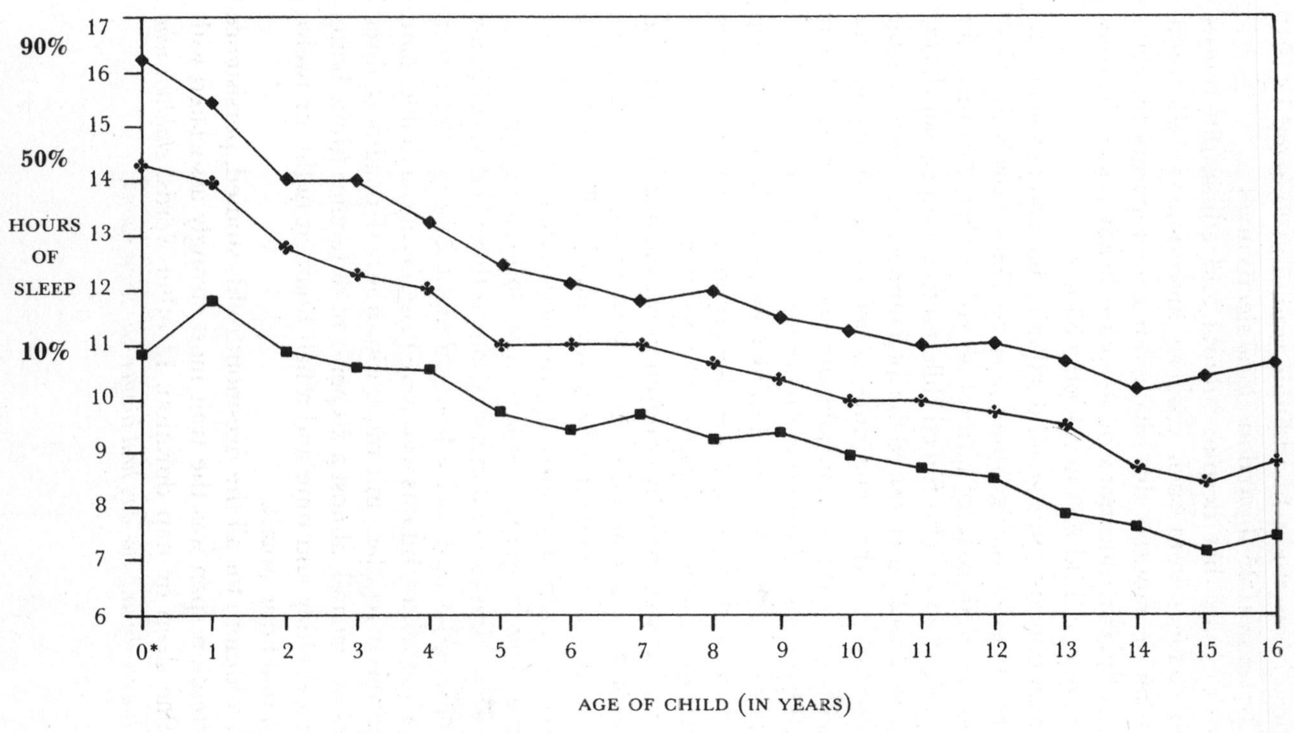

*Note: 0 represents children between 4 and 11 months of age.

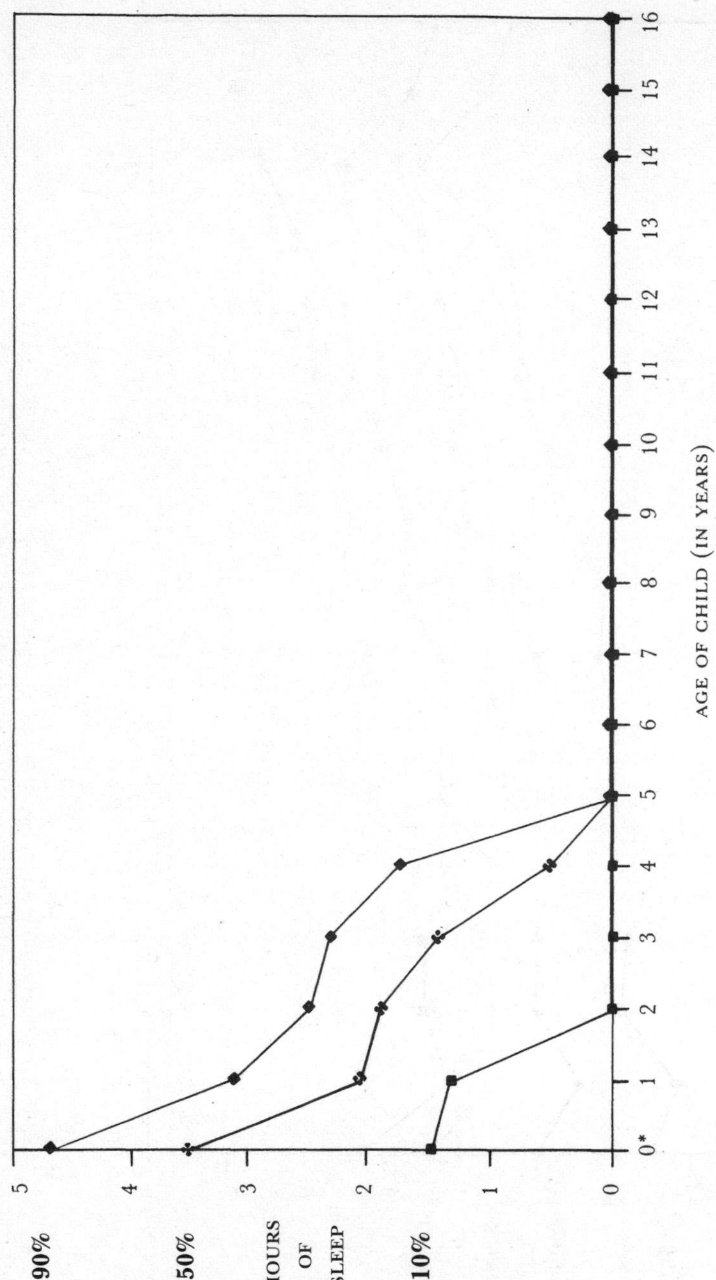

FIGURE 2: HOURS OF DAYTIME SLEEP BY AGE FOR GIVEN PERCENTILES

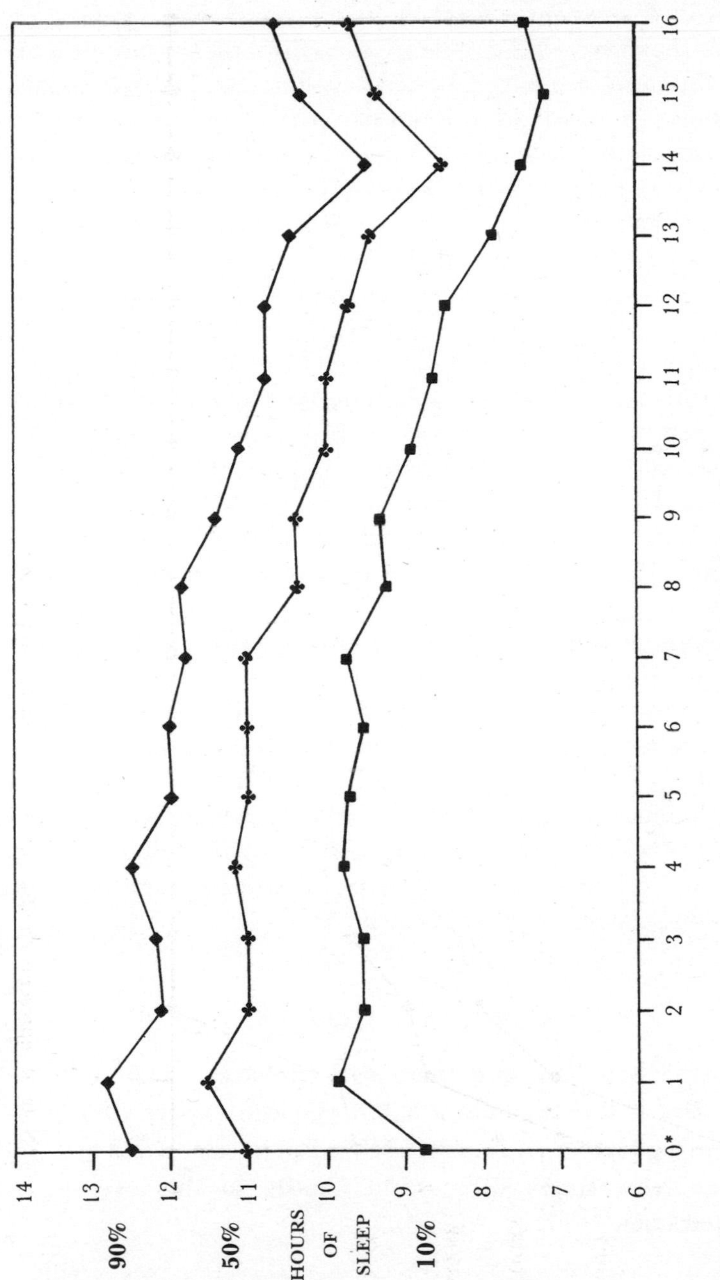

FIGURE 3: HOURS OF NIGHT SLEEP BY AGE FOR GIVEN PERCENTILES

As I will discuss in a later chapter, infants who sleep more during the day are better able to learn from their environment; this is because they have a better-developed ability to maintain focused or sustained attention. Like a dry sponge in water, they soak up information about their surroundings. They learn simply from looking at the clouds and trees, touching, feeling, smelling, hearing, and watching their mothers' and fathers' faces. Infants who sleep less in the daytime appear more fitful and socially demanding, and they are less able to entertain or amuse themselves. Toys and objects are less interesting to these more tired children.

By three years of age, the easier-to-manage children in my study who were mild, positive in mood, adaptable and approachable towards unfamiliar people slept twelve and a half hours total. The difficult-to-manage children – those who were intense, more negative, less adaptable, and withdrawing – slept about one and a half hours less, almost the equivalent of a daytime nap.

An important conclusion is that three-year-olds who nap are more adaptable than those who do not. But napping did not affect the length of sleep at night. Comparing nappers and non-nappers, night sleep duration was ten and a half hours in both groups. Those who napped, however, slept about two hours longer during the day, so their total sleep was twelve and a half hours. Therefore, it simply is not true that children who miss naps will make up for it by sleeping more at night. In fact, the sleep they miss is gone for ever.

PRACTICAL POINT

Missing a nap here and there will probably cause no harm. But if this becomes a habit, you can expect your child to lag further and further behind in his sleep and to become increasingly difficult to handle in this over-fatigued state.

SLEEP DURATION OF THREE-YEAR-OLDS

		Sleep Durations (Hours)		
		Day	*Night*	*Total*
Group A	Easy to manage	1.9	10.6	12.5
	Difficult to manage	0.9	10.4	11.3
Group B	Children who do not nap	–	10.5	10.5
	Children who nap	2.0	10.5	12.5

All in all, at age three, the children who slept more were more fun to be around, more sociable and less demanding. The children who slept less not only tended to be more socially demanding, bratty and fussy, but they also behaved somewhat like hyperactive children. Later, I will explain how these fatigued, fussy brats are also more likely to become fat kids.

One recent study examined the effects of a single night of sleep restriction in a group of children between ten and fourteen years old. The researchers noted that there were impairments in verbal creativity, abstract thinking/concept formation, and in complex problem solving. These higher cognitive abilities appear to be essential for academic performance and success. In contrast, there were no deficits on rote performance or less-complex memory and learning tasks. The ability to maintain routine performance despite being sleepy is familiar to every adult who sometimes gets very tired but nevertheless is able to perform the routine aspects of his or her job fairly well. My interpretation of this study is that chronic sleepiness in infants and young children impairs cognitive development, but this will not become apparent until the child is much older and challenged by more complex tasks. Of course, cognitive development starts in babies, not at ten to fourteen years of age, but the deficits from sleep deprivation remain hidden in young children. When younger, the challenges are at a much lower level, and these chronically sleep-deprived children may still do well with spelling, writing, reading and simple arithmetic. Later, when older, the more demanding academic challenges unmask the cognitive deficits.

Looking at our sleep curves again, we see that throughout early and middle childhood, the duration of sleep declines until adolescence, when the curve shown in Figure 1 on page 21 levels off and then slightly increases. This increase has been noted in other studies and suggests that teenagers need more sleep than pre-teens. Yet academic demands, social events and school sports combine during adolescence to pressure teenagers to stay up later and later. Also, there are biological shifts in adolescents that seem to encourage more wakefulness in the evening. This is the time when chronic and cumulative sleep losses begin to take their toll, and can make a normally rough period in life unbearably rocky.

Naps

Having grown up in a highly achievement-oriented society, most American adults are likely to view naps as a waste of time. We tend to think that the adults who nap are lazy, under-motivated, ill or elderly. In turn, we do not attach much positive benefit to daytime sleep in our infants and young children. Let me explain why naps are indeed very important for learning, or cognitive development, in children.

Naps are not little bits of night sleep randomly intruding upon children's awake hours. Actually, night sleep, daytime sleep and daytime wakefulness have rhythms that are partially independent of one another. During the first three to four months of life, these rhythms develop at different rates, so they may not be in synchrony. Only later do these sleep/wake rhythms become linked with fluctuations in body temperature and activity levels.

For example, most of us have experienced drowsiness in the afternoon. This sensation is partially related – but only partially – to how long you have been up and how long you slept the night before. Our mental state fluctuates during the day between alert and drowsy, just as fluctuations occur during the night between light and deep sleep stages. As adults, an afternoon nap is most refreshing when we take it at the time when we are biologically most drowsy. Here is how to figure out your best naptime. Take the midpoint between the time when you most easily fall asleep at night (example: 10:00 P.M.) and most comfortably awaken naturally in the morning (example: 8:00 A.M.). Then, twelve hours from the midpoint is your best naptime (example: 3:00 P.M.). If you lived in the siesta belt, you might rest or take a nap, but for the rest of us it's a coffee break.

There is an important reason, though, why some adults do not nap: sleep inertia.

Sleep Inertia

Sleep inertia is a feeling of disorientation, confusion, pain, discomfort, impaired mood, and the inability to concentrate or think well that occurs upon awakening, especially from naps. In children, sleep inertia appears to be more severe and more prolonged for those who are more overtired. It appears that sleep is intruding into wakefulness and this overlap state is painfully uncomfortable. One mother described it as a 'fugue' state, another as a 'demonic' state. The children are out of control, panicky, crying, or screaming hysterically. Parents would often call me after three-day holiday weekends, during which their children became severely overtired, and tell me that they were sure their child had a painful ear infection because their child awoke crying. They often added that they were sure their child was not overtired because the child had just completed an extra-long nap! The ears were perfect. The children had simply missed some naps or had been allowed to stay up too late during the holiday.

Understanding that the rhythms of night sleep, daytime sleep and daytime wakefulness are somewhat independent from one another leads to two important ideas.

First, in a child under three or four months of age, these rhythms are not in synchrony with each other, and the baby may be getting opposing messages from different parts of the brain. The sleep rhythm says 'deep sleep', while the wake rhythm says 'alert' instead of 'drowsy'. Wakeful but tired, the confused child cries fitfully; we might call this behaviour colic or fussiness. Opposing messages from different parts of the brain may cause ambiguous stages such as sleep inertia. In research with adults and animals, this has been called 'dissociated states of wakefulness and sleep', or 'Status Dissociatus'. For example, some birds can swim or fly when they are completely asleep! Narcolepsy is the intrusion of REM sleep into wakefulness. Sleepwalking, night terrors and crying out at night occur during the overlap state of wakefulness and non-REM sleep. Because adult wake/sleep states may overlap, be incomplete, or switch rapidly between states, it is entirely possible that during the first four months, when sleep states are developing, partial states express themselves out of phase and with other states, creating overlap problems that we refer to as fussiness, colic or sleep inertia. For example, it is known that babies can suck, smile and cry with their eyes open during REM sleep, so while they appear to be awake, they are actually asleep. We can call this 'indeterminate sleep' or 'ambiguous sleep', which reflects the immaturity of the young brain. After about four months of age, these ambiguous states are less common.

Second, if these sleep/wake rhythms are somewhat independent, they may have different functions: learning for the wake cycle, physical and emotional restoration for the sleep cycle. Daytime sleep and night-time sleep may be different in this regard. I believe that *healthy naps* lead to optimal daytime alertness for learning – that is, naps adjust the alert/drowsy control to just the right setting for optimal daytime arousal. Without naps, the child is too drowsy to learn well. Also, when chronically sleep-deprived, the fatigued child becomes fitfully fussy or hyperalert in order to fight sleep, and therefore cannot learn from his environment.

Not only are naps different from night sleep, but not every nap is created equal. There is more REM sleep in the morning nap compared to the afternoon nap. Research suggests that high amounts of REM sleep, under the influence of low melatonin levels, help direct the course of brain maturation in early life. Also, adult studies have suggested that REM sleep is especially important for restoring us emotionally or psychologically, while deep, non-REM sleep appears to be more important for physical restoration. Let's get all the REM sleep we can for our babies!

Because naps have their own function and do their job best when they occur at the right time, I suggest that if a nap has been missed, try to keep your child up until the next sleep period in order to maintain the timeliness of the sleep rhythm. This suggestion has to be balanced with the general theme of avoiding the overtired state, so the next sleep period (nap or night) might begin a little earlier.

My studies show that at four months of age, most children take either two or three naps. The third nap, if taken, tends to be brief and in the early evening. But by six months of age, the vast majority of children (84 per cent) are taking only two naps; by nine months of age virtually all children are taking just one or two naps. About 17 per cent of children have started taking only a single nap by their first birthday, and this percentage increases to 56 per cent by the age of fifteen months. By twenty-one months, most children are down to just a single nap.

The morning nap develops before the afternoon nap, but it also disappears before the afternoon nap. The single nap that is present by twenty-one months and resurfaces in adolescence or adulthood is always the afternoon nap. Infants and young children have much more REM sleep at night than older children, and the morning nap has more REM sleep than the afternoon nap; this suggests that in some infants, the morning nap may be viewed as a sort of continuation of night sleep. Later I will discuss how we can help babies sleep better by keeping the interval of wakefulness between the wake-up time and the start of the first nap very short. This strategy may work because we are really allowing night sleep to continue longer.

Another thing that I've discovered is that up until about

twenty-one months of age, some babies are born to be short nappers and some are inherently long nappers.

IMPORTANT POINT

Not all sleep periods are created equal!

Parents can interfere with a child's long naps by messing up the child's schedule, but they cannot make short nappers into long nappers. Here are some important facts about short nappers: at six months of age, 80 per cent of babies nap between two and a half and four hours total each day. Napping more than four total hours each day occurs in 15 per cent of babies. However, in 5 per cent of babies, the total daytime sleep each day is less than two and a half hours. If you look at brief naps slightly differently and include babies who sleep a total of two and a half hours or less each day, then 18 per cent of babies fall into this category. These short nappers tend to keep this pattern for the next twelve to eighteen months! This truth is especially frustrating to mothers whose first child was a long napper and they remember having long breaks during the day to do whatever they wanted. If their second child is a short napper, they may incorrectly think they are doing something wrong.

If parents can cause problems that interfere with good naps, why can't parents make their babies sleep longer? This question provides a good example of the asymmetry between sleep and wakefulness. Sleep is not the absence of wakefulness; rather, the brain automatically and actively turns on the sleep process and simultaneously turns off wakefulness. You, and your child, can force wakefulness upon sleep, but you cannot force sleep upon wakefulness. You, and your child, can motivate or force yourself and him into a more wakeful or alert state, but you cannot will anyone into a deeper sleep state. So sleep and wake states are different but not opposite. Parents have the opportunity to *permit* the maximum amount of sleep to occur; this amount reflects their child's actual need for sleep. As stated before, a baby's nap pattern is largely an individual trait that stays stable until about twenty-one months.

Evidence of the individuality of this trait comes from studies on twins and argues for a strong genetic component to the control of sleep in babies. An obvious example occurs when one twin is a short napper and the other twin is a long napper – more about that later. At twenty-one months, the average nap duration is a little less than two and a half hours, but the range is wide: between one and four hours. At this age, some of the children who initially took brief naps are now taking longer naps, and some who had been long nappers are now taking briefer naps. My interpretation is that by twenty-one months, biology is no longer the primary influence on napping; social factors begin to play a role. For example, events such as the birth of a sibling, an older sibling starting preschool or the child herself now participating in organised and scheduled activities can cause children who have a biological need for longer naps to take shorter naps. Often, no problems occur if catch-up days are provided coupled with an extra-early bedtime.

The time of day when the nap occurs is also important. Some studies have suggested that an early nap, occurring in the mid-morning hours, is different in quality from a later nap, which occurs in the afternoon. As mentioned before, there is more active REM sleep than quiet sleep in the first nap, and this pattern is reversed in the second nap. So naps occurring at different times are different! Even for adults, a nap earlier in the day is lighter and less restorative than an afternoon nap, which consists of deeper sleep.

Long naps occurring at the right time make the child feel rested. Levels of cortisol, a hormone that increases with stress, dramatically fall during a nap, indicating a reduction of stress in the body. Not taking a needed nap means that the body remains stressed. Brief naps or naps that are out of synchrony with other biological rhythms are less restful, less restorative. But a short nap is better than no nap. It still has a positive effect on alertness.

Children can be taught how to take naps. A nap does not begin and end the way an electric light can be turned off and on. In fact, a nap or night sleep involves three periods of time:

the time required for the process called falling asleep, the sleep period itself and the time required to wake up. One father complained to me, 'I can't see the pre-Zs coming out of his head', meaning he had difficulty seeing the lull in activity or quieting that precedes sleep. In later chapters I will show you how to recognise the 'pre-Zs' and teach your children to fall asleep.

PRACTICAL POINT

Do not expect your baby to nap well outside his cot after four months of age. If you don't protect your baby's nap schedules, you can produce nap deprivation.

When children do not nap well, they pay a price. Infants between four and eight months who do not nap well have shorter attention spans or appear less persistent when engaged in activities. By three years of age, children who do not nap or who nap very little are often described as non-adaptable or even hyperactive. Adaptability is thought to be a very important trait for school success.

One mother of a non-adaptable child said with a laugh that every morning she prayed to the 'nap god' to give her a break. In contrast, another mother described her son as a very easy child as long as she had a bed around. He was such a 'nap-monster' that she decided he just liked his own company best. Another mother described her son, who napped well, as the 'snooze king'.

Sometimes it appears that the older toddler needs exactly one and a half naps. While one nap is insufficient, two are impossible to achieve. These children are rough around the edges in the late afternoon or early evening, but parents can temporarily and partially compensate by putting the child to bed earlier on some nights.

An *earlier bedtime* may become a necessity when your child develops a single-nap pattern, between fifteen and twenty-one months. Earlier bedtimes help prevent bedtime battles, deter night waking, discourage extremely early morning awakenings, and regularise and prolong naps. Why, then, do many parents resist the notion of putting their children to sleep when they first appear tired at night, even though it is clear that the brain is sleep-sensitive? First, parents naturally want to be with their children and play with them. Second, there is a powerful inhibitory fear that if their child is put to bed very early when tired, she will get up extra early the next day. Third, because I recommend that, along with an earlier bedtime, the parents not go to the child at night, except for feeding, parents are naturally frightened about the possibility of prolonged crying when they put the child to bed or in the middle of the night. This fear of possible crying discourages parents from trying for an earlier bedtime.

Here is an example of how a family started early, at eight weeks of age, to focus on an earlier bedtime. The baby was not overtired and did not have extreme fussiness/colic, so the transition went smoothly. For 20 per cent of babies with extreme fussiness/colic, this easy change to an earlier bedtime at eight weeks of age is not realistic.

Jaden's Story

When our daughter Jaden was born, we were anxious to start off on the right foot with her sleep habits. We immediately focused on no more than two hours of wakefulness with a bedtime around 10:00 or 11:00 P.M., which was very easy to accomplish. After a few weeks, though, we still weren't really seeing very long night-time stretches. When Jaden was eight weeks old, we visited Dr Weissbluth to discuss her sleeping pattern. Dr Weissbluth told us that at six weeks, we should have incorporated an early bedtime in addition to keeping shorter periods of wakefulness. We left wondering whether an early bedtime would really work for someone so young. We really expected that Jaden would be up within an hour or two after we put her down. We started off with a 7:00 P.M. bedtime. She still woke up in the late evening to eat, but we put her promptly back to bed. There were a few bumps in the road for the first couple of nights – sometimes she would wake up a few times and cry – but we kept at it. After a few days, Jaden went from sleeping a four- to five-hour stretch in the evening, to seven, then eight, then nine or ten hours a night. In fact, she seemed happy to be sleeping so much! If she woke up for a feed, she would eat and immediately fall back asleep as soon as we put her back in her cot. We couldn't believe how easy it was. The earlier we got her to bed, the better she slept. Her daytime naps even seemed longer and more restful. She is now seven months old. We now try to get her down between 6:00 and 6:30 each night, and she is extremely happy about it. (So are we!)

Over and over again I have seen children who are put to bed too late. It becomes a vicious circle: the child's nap schedule is messed up, and the child is fussy in the late afternoon or early evening. This fatigue-driven fussiness ends in a wired state at bedtime, which interferes with the ability to go to sleep easily. As a result, the parent keeps the child up until he crashes. The next day the child is still tired, the naps are messed up, and so on. The circle never ends.

The solution is obvious in Meg's story.

Meg's Early Bedtime

Our daughter Meg has been a good sleeper from the very beginning. Since she was six weeks old she has gone weeks when she would sleep through the night (from 10:00 to 6:00), and weeks when she would wake up twice for a feed.

At seven months, she began waking once a night for a bottle. This was fine until she turned eight months old. We had been told by a doctor that she should no longer need to be fed in the middle of the night, but we thought we would wait until Meg's nine-month appointment with Dr Weissbluth to address the problem.

We had never been very consistent with Meg's bedtime. We would put her to bed when she appeared tired (rubbing eyes, yawning), anywhere from 7:00 to 7:45, but occasionally even later. It usually took her between fifteen and thirty minutes of crying to fall asleep. I thought this was normal. She had always gone to bed rather late and she had always taken a while to fall asleep.

At Meg's nine-month appointment we asked Dr Weissbluth about her night waking. He made a very simple suggestion. He told us that we should put Meg to bed twenty minutes earlier at night. He said that her night waking would disappear and she would still wake up at a normal hour in the morning. I told him that we had been putting her to sleep when she appeared tired at around 7:30, give or take thirty minutes. He said that once she appears tired it is too late and she should already be in bed.

The first night we put her to bed at 6:45. We were very sceptical. We were sad to put her down so early when she seemed so wide awake and happy. She cried for about five minutes and then fell asleep, and with no night waking! The same thing happened the next night – about five minutes of crying and then asleep until morning. Sometimes she would wake up as early as 5:30, but we would give her a bottle and she would fall back to sleep, sometimes until almost 8:00!

It has been almost four weeks since our nine-month appointment. Bedtime is an absolute joy. Meg eats dinner, takes a bath, and is in bed about 6:30. Sometimes I hesitate to put her down so early when she seems to be in such good spirits, but she cuddles with her blanket and her doll, sucks her thumb, closes her eyes, and sleeps till morning. It's the sweetest thing I have ever seen.

As Meg's parents said about my recommendation for a much earlier bedtime, 'He made a very simple suggestion.' Sometimes simple approaches work better than complex solutions. Here's another example.

Jared's Sleep Story

When we met with Dr Weissbluth, Jared, now nineteen months old, was waking up every hour and a half to two hours during the night. He would have to fall asleep while we were walking and carrying him on our shoulder. When placed in the cot, Jared would awaken and abruptly 'pop up'. He would only sleep in the bed 'nest' we created for him on the floor of our family room. We endured three months of the night waking before we consulted Dr Weissbluth.

We were instructed to place Jared in bed in an awake state between 6:00 and 7:00 in the evening and that we should leave him there until 6:00 in the morning. Our initial reaction was that Jared would carry on relentlessly when placed in his cot so early, and that the recommended approach was too strict and would never work. Much to our shock and delight, the first night we tried the new routine, Jared was asleep after five minutes of crying, and remained asleep for eleven hours, not waking until 5:30 the next morning. During the next two nights, Jared went to sleep on his own, with no episodes of crying. On the fourth night, he lay down in the bed with his favourite stuffed animal under his arm, as he has done since. Our baby was clearly overtired from going to bed at 8:30 and not being allowed to relax and go to sleep without interference. We never expected it to be so simple and provide such an immediate result. Jared wakes up happy, energised, and ready for a day full of adventures. Now, several months later, Jared is most happy when going to bed at 6:30, and will go to his bed himself if he is tired.

Probably the most common worry is that the earlier bedtime will produce an earlier wake-up time, as expressed by Anna's story.

Anna's Transition from Two Naps to One

At eighteen months it became apparent that Anna was ready to make the transition from two naps to one, but would need some help because she fought the morning nap. We began, as Dr Weissbluth suggested in his book, by gradually delaying the morning nap till 11:00 A.M. or so. Over a two-week window we were able to continue to push back the nap to sometime between noon and 1:00 P.M.

In his book, Dr Weissbluth suggested an earlier bedtime to help prevent night waking or early-morning waking. Anna was going to

> bed at 6:30 P.M. and sleeping until 7:00 A.M., so we really questioned this theory. My husband and I agreed that Dr Weissbluth's advice has always been right on the mark, so we decided to put her down an hour earlier. We feared that she would wake up at 5:30 or 6:00 A.M. after her usual twelve or thirteen hours of sleep. To our surprise, she awoke at 9:00 A.M., and she was in the most cheerful mood to date!
>
> Family, friends, even strangers constantly tell us what a happy, cheerful child we have. The reality is that she is a very well-rested child.

Not napping means lost sleep. Over an extended period of time, children do not sleep longer at night when their naps are brief. Of course, once in a while – when relatives visit or when a painful ear infection keeps the child awake – a child will make up lost daytime sleep with longer night sleep. But day in and day out, you should not expect to satisfy your child's need to sleep by cutting corners on naps and then trying to compensate by putting your child to sleep for the night at an earlier hour. What you wind up with is a bad-tempered or demanding brat in the late afternoon or early evening. Your child pays a price for nap deprivation, and so do you.

Spending hours holding your child in your arms or in a rocking chair while he is in a light, twilight sleep also is lost sleep because you have delayed the time when he will fall into a deep slumber. It is similar to having a bedtime that is too late. It's a waste of your time as well. Brief catnaps during the day, 'motion' sleep in cars or baby swings, light sleep in the pushchair at the pool, and naps at the wrong time are all poor-quality sleep.

> **PRACTICAL POINT**
>
> **When your child does not nap well and you keep him up in the evening, he suffers.**

Here is an example of how one family learned to appreciate napping.

How Charley's Parents Became Nap Zealots

I am aware that the practice of toting your baby along with you on every occasion is the new social thing. No doubt it stems from the 'me' generation's philosophy that a baby should not be allowed to interfere with your lifestyle. So parents everywhere are seen with their infants: in supermarkets, restaurants, the homes of friends . . . and for the unflappable, at cocktail parties, dinner occasions, even cross-country trips. Although some of these examples may appear to be extreme, be advised, new mothers, that the pressure is on to be a '*nouvelle*' mum.

As with anything in vogue, you need the appropriate raw material to make it work. And the fact is, my husband, Tom, and I simply do not have the baby to make this new 'porta-kid' trend work for us. Oh, we tried. But it was, and continues to be, completely futile. So we gave it up when Charley was three months old.

Charley is now seven months into his life. From the beginning, there has been only one of life's necessities that he requires as much as milk and oxygen, and that is sleep. In fact, we used to shake him when we first brought him home to make sure he was alive. The baby slept . . . serious sleep.

In the beginning he would sleep anywhere. After his second month, he would sleep only in his cot. And that's another subject. I maintain that the person(s) who decreed that a child's bed should be 'stimulating' and full of coloured linens and mobiles did not have a child of his/her own! If I had to do it all over again, I would buy a solid, dark-coloured comforter and pads. After Charley's second month, he would spend hours on end trying to pick the red, white and blue flowers off the sheet. This is no lie. And he would scream unmercifully for us to remove this distraction, which was preventing him from needed slumber!

Since his second month, Charley has slept through the night and half of the day. If we disallowed him this necessity, he became a different baby. 'Grumpy' did not do justice to his fatigue condition. Without this sleep, our peaceful, alert, sweet and cuddly baby turned into a raging beast. We did this to him when we denied him sleep – not according to our expectations but according to his own internal requirements.

Charley gives us his cues, simply and clearly. He doesn't cry at first. He mumbles, then grumbles and, finally, if his unaware parents or sitters persist, he wails.

At first we couldn't believe he was tired so often. We changed his nappies a thousand times and force-fed bottles. We took him on endless trips in the buggy and walked him around incessantly trying to calm our 'miserable' baby with the rhythm of our heartbeats. Nothing worked. Nothing, that is, until we finally, out of sheer nervous exhaustion, laid him in his bed to sleep.

Charley still naps four to five times during the course of a day. He's also a very happy child. When Tom and I go anywhere, we go alone, leaving our contented, sleeping son in the hands of a competent baby-sitter. Our friends, especially our childless friends, think we're overprotective. Well, thank God, Charley is not their baby. We are no longer concerned about our parental image; un-educated criticism doesn't count. If we cannot find a baby-sitter, we don't go. We simply would have a better time watching television . . . anything, even doing the washing, beats the hell out of driving your baby and yourselves crazy. And our family is now harmonious, having discovered the secret of sleep.

PRACTICAL POINT

When you maintain a healthy nap schedule and your child sleeps well during the day, jealous friends will accuse you of being overprotective. They'll say, 'It's not real life' or 'Bring her along so she'll learn to play with other children' or 'You're really spoiling her'. Suggestion: Change friends, or keep your baby's long naps a family secret.

Sleep Consolidation

Consolidated sleep means uninterrupted sleep, sleep that is continuous and not disrupted by awakenings. When awakenings or complete arousals break our slumber, we call it disrupted sleep or sleep fragmentation. Abnormal shifts of sleep rhythms towards lighter sleep, even if we do not awaken completely, also cause sleep fragmentation. Ten hours of consolidated sleep is not the same as ten hours of fragmented sleep. Doctors, firefighters and mothers of newborns or sick children who have their sleep interrupted frequently know this very well.

The effects of sleep fragmentation are similar to the effects of reduced total sleep: daytime sleepiness increases and performance measurably decreases. Among healthy adults, even one night of sleep fragmentation will produce decreases in mental flexibility and sustained attention, as well as impairment of mood. Adults with fragmented sleep often fight the ill effects of fragmented sleep with extra caffeine. Alcohol unmasks or uncovers the hidden fatigue and makes them 'feel tired'. However, well-rested pre-teens who are given the same amount of alcohol, during research studies, do not 'feel tired'.

PRACTICAL POINT

Let sleeping babies lie!
Never awaken a sleeping baby.
Destroying sleep continuity is unhealthy.

Protective Arousals

Sometimes our brains awaken us in order to prevent asphyxiation in our sleep. These awakenings, or protective arousals, occur when we have difficulty breathing during sleep, which can be caused by large tonsils or adenoids obstructing the air passage. (I will discuss this problem in detail in Chapter 10.)

Arousals may also prevent cot deaths, or sudden infant death syndrome (SIDS), which kills young infants. This tragedy might be caused by a failure to maintain breathing during sleep or a failure to awaken when breathing starts to become difficult.

Sleep Fragmentation

MAJOR POINT

Some arousals from sleep are normal.

After several months of age – beyond the age when cot death is most common – frequent arousals are usually harmful, because they destroy sleep continuity. Arousals are complete awakening from either a light, deep, or REM sleep. Arousals can also be thought of as a quick shift from deep sleep to light sleep without a complete awakening.

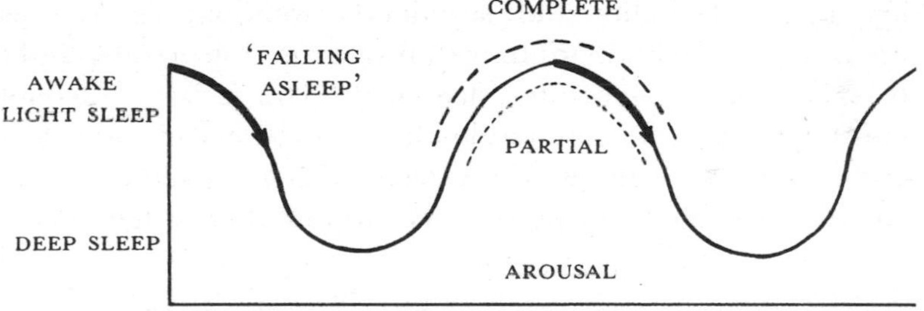

FIGURE 4: AROUSALS DURING SLEEP

Figure 4 is a simplified illustration of the cycling from deep sleep to light sleep that normally occurs after about four months of age. During partial arousals, we stay in a light sleep state and do not awaken. But during complete arousals, or awakenings, we might become aware that we are looking at the clock, rolling over, changing arm positions or scratching a leg. This awareness is dim and brief, and we return to sleep promptly.

As we can see, arousals come in several forms, and depending on which types occur, how many times they happen, and how long they last, we pay a price: increased daytime sleepiness and decreased performance. Some arousals, however, always occur naturally during healthy sleep. The brain, not the stomach, makes arousals. Please don't confuse arousals from sleep with hunger.

It's not just night sleep that can be fragmented. I believe naps can also be fragmented when parents rely on 'motion' sleep in a baby swing or car, or when they allow catnaps in the pushchair. Holding your dozing child in your arms in a rocking chair during the day also probably prevents good-quality day sleep. These naps are too brief or too light to be restorative. Stationary sleep is best. If you use a swing for soothing, turn it off once your baby falls asleep.

PRACTICAL POINT

After four months, naps of less than one hour cannot count as 'real' naps. Sometimes a nap of forty-five minutes may be all your child needs, but naps of less than thirty minutes don't help.

By four to eight months of age, infants should have at least a midmorning nap and one in the early afternoon, and the total nap duration should be two to four hours. Night sleep is ten to twelve hours, with one, two, or no interruptions for bottle-feeding. If you are breast-feeding and using a family bed, you might feed your baby at night many times. In this situation, both mother and baby are often more asleep than awake during the feeding and neither suffer from sleep fragmentation. When children do not get healthy, consolidated sleep, we call the problem 'night waking'. As I will discuss later, night waking itself is usually due to normally occurring arousals. The real problem is the child's inability or difficulty returning to sleep unassisted.

PRACTICAL POINT

Some arousals from sleep are normal. Problems occur when children have difficulty returning to sleep by themselves. They have not learned the process of 'falling asleep'.

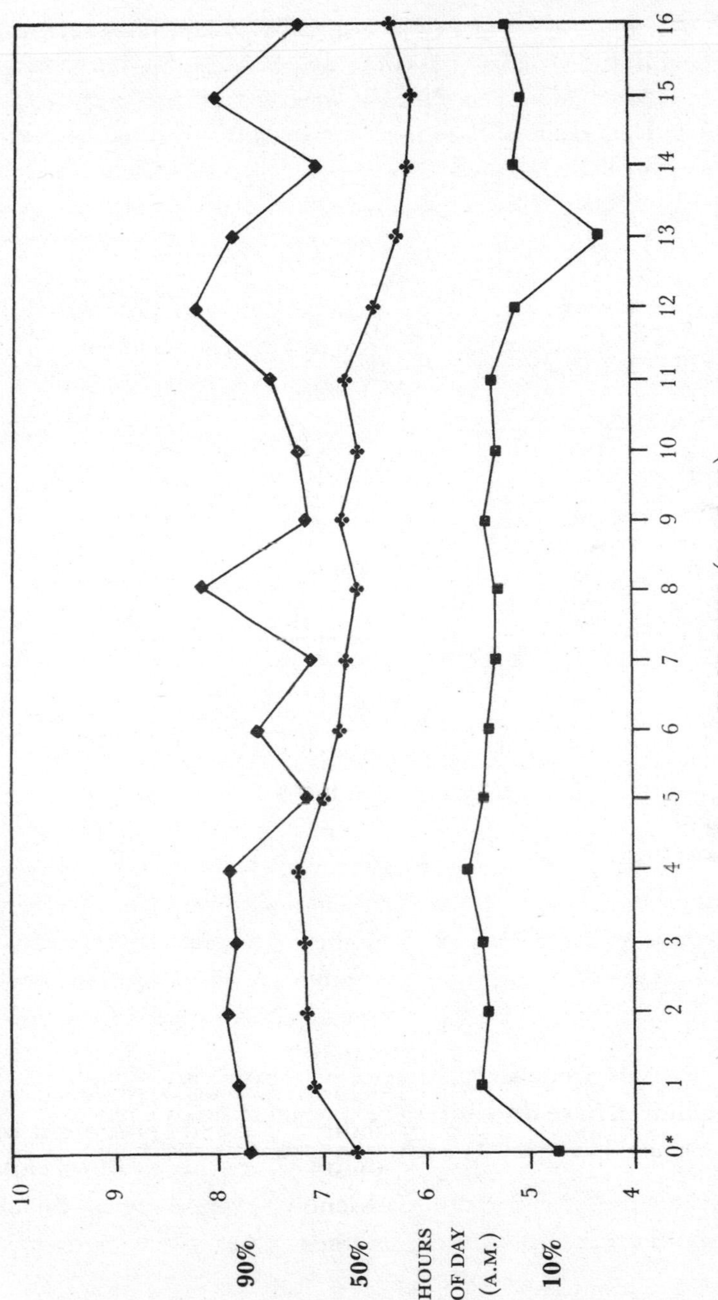

FIGURE 5: HOUR AT WHICH CHILDREN ARE AWAKE FOR GIVEN AGES

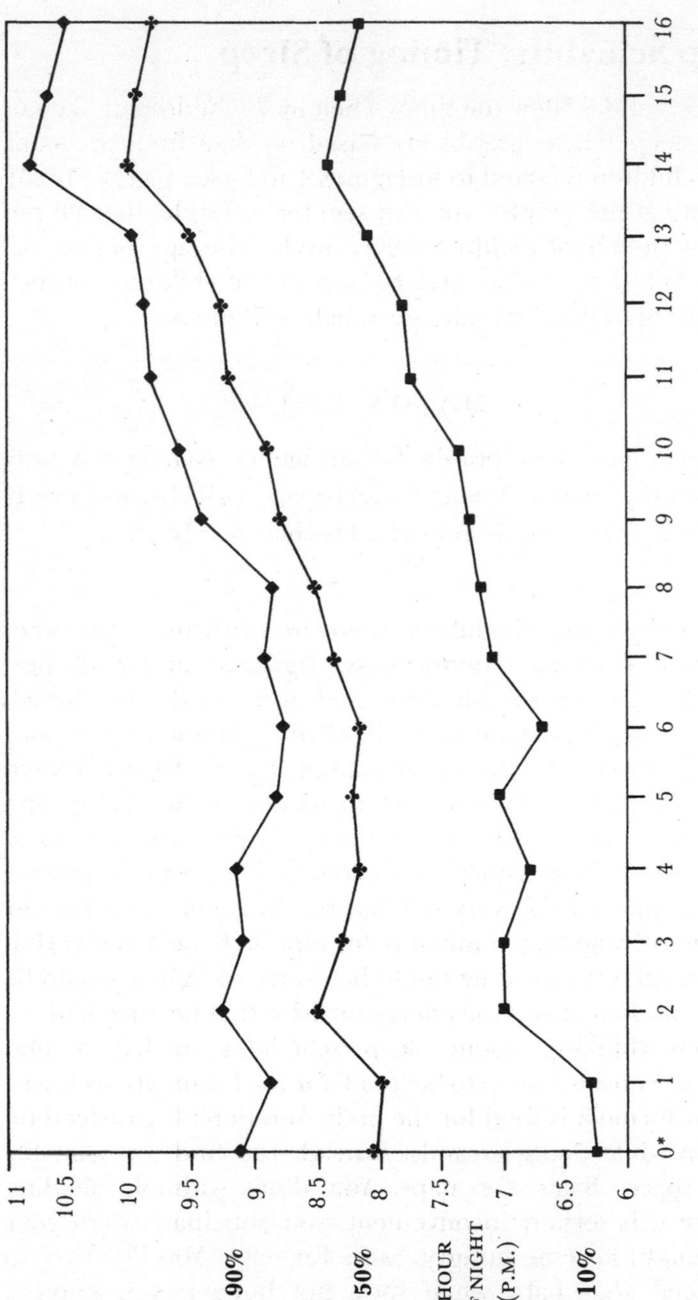

FIGURE 6: HOUR AT WHICH CHILDREN ARE ASLEEP FOR GIVEN AGES

Sleep Schedule, Timing of Sleep

Figures 5 and 6 show the times when most children awaken or go to sleep. These graphs are based on data from the same 2,019 children referred to in Figures 1 to 3 (see pages 21–23). Looking at the graphs, you can see, for example, that 90 per cent of preschool children (those under the age of six) fall asleep before 9:00 P.M., and 10 per cent of children between the ages of two and six fall asleep before 7:00 P.M.

> **MAJOR POINT**
>
> **Junk food is not healthy for our bodies. Neither is a 'junk sleep' schedule. You try not to let your child become overly hungry, so don't let your child become overly tired.**

When sleep/wake schedules are not in synchrony with other biological rhythms, attentiveness, vigilance and task performance are measurably decreased and moods are altered. Jet-lag syndrome is one example of this. Another is the poor sleep quality some shift workers suffer due to abnormal sleep schedules. Shift workers complain mainly of headaches and stomach aches. These are the most common complaints of older children with unhealthy sleep schedules. So if your child doesn't appear to be very sick but has frequent headaches or episodes of vague abdominal pain, especially near the end of the day, ask yourself if he might be overtired. A clue would be that he no longer has the energy or drive that he once had.

When thinking about sleep schedules in babies and toddlers, consider sleep to be 'food' for the brain, just as breast milk or formula is food for the body. You don't breast-feed on the run while doing errands; instead, you find a reasonably quiet space. Same for naps. You don't withhold feeding because it is socially inconvenient; you anticipate when your child might become hungry. Same for naps. You don't try to force-feed your baby when she's not hungry; you know a hungry period will naturally come. Same for naps. A parent coming home late from work would not starve his baby by withholding food until he arrived and could feed the child. Same for the bedtime hour; don't 'sleep starve' your baby's brain by keeping her up too late.

Night Sleep Organisation

Before six weeks of age, the longest single sleep period, unfortunately, is randomly distributed around the clock. In some babies, this longest sleep may actually be only two to three hours! But by six weeks of age (or six weeks after the due date, for babies born early), the longest single sleep period will predictably occur in the evening hours and last three to five hours.

PRACTICAL POINT

During these early weeks, you may find breast-feeding too demanding or too frequent, and think that you might want to stop so that you can get some rest. On the other hand, you also may want to continue nursing. See it through until your baby is past six weeks of age. Then you, too, will get more night sleep.

After six weeks of age, babies sleep longer at night. So do mums! Also, babies start social smiling at their parents, and they then become less fussy or irritable. Life in the family definitely changes after six weeks. One exception is the premature baby, whose parents might have to wait until about six weeks after the expected date of delivery. Another exception is the extremely fussy/colicky baby, whose parents might have to wait until their child is three or four months old.

Daytime Sleep Organisation

At about three to four months of age, daytime sleep is organised into two or three long naps instead of many brief, irregular ones. Mothers, especially nursing mothers, should learn to nap when their baby naps. You never know what the night will bring; you might be up a lot holding, walking, or feeding.

Abnormal sleep schedules usually evolve in infants and young children when parents keep them up too late at night. Parents do this because they (1) enjoy playing with their baby, (2) cannot put the child to sleep, but wait for their child to crash from total exhaustion, or (3) both. Some parents leave work late, have a long commute to the day-care site to pick up their child and then arrive home even later. This lifestyle is extremely difficult for the child if naps are not regular at the day-care centre and he is put down too late to sleep at night. Unfortunately, if both parents are working outside the home, then naps may suffer at weekends because the parents do too many errands with the child or attempt to spend too much time playing with their child to make up for the minimal time together during the week. Sleeping well during the day may also suffer when parents skip naps in favour of organised, scheduled preschool activities. These baby classes are usually fun for both child and parent, but if they take up too much time, the child becomes overtired.

One common mistake is keeping bedtime at *exactly* the same hour every night. Usually this hour is too late and is based more on the parents' wishes than the child's sleep needs. It is important to have a fairly regular routine of soothing events before putting your child to sleep, but it makes biological sense to vary the bedtime a little. The time when your child needs to go to sleep at night depends on his age, how long his previous nap lasted and how long his wakeful period was just before the bedtime hour. The time when he wants to go to sleep may be altogether different! Obviously, the bedtime hour is not fixed or unchanging. If your child is unusually active in the afternoon or if she misses a good afternoon nap, then she should be put to sleep earlier.

This is true even if a parent, returning home late from work, does not get to see her child. If one parent is arriving home late, then she or he might walk in the house and immediately begin a twenty- to thirty-minute soothing-to-sleep routine without playtime. If the parent returns very late, the child should be put to bed as usual; keeping a tired child up to play with a tired parent does no one any good. At the cost to the parent of having less time with his child, the benefit is no bedtime battles, no night-waking habits, no early-morning arousals, good-quality naps, a well-rested child, a well-rested spouse and relaxed private time for the parents in the evening. Usually under these circumstances there is morning time to spend together and relaxed weekends for the family because everyone is well rested.

The completely opposite scenario occurs when one parent, usually the father, demands that the other parent, usually the mother, keep their child up late so that he can play with him or her. Not only does the child suffer, but it is the mother who is the unappreciated victim, because she is trying to maintain marital harmony and trying to keep her child well rested – and she can't do both. Obviously this is not simply a child's sleep problem but a family problem.

PRACTICAL POINT

To establish healthy sleep schedules at four to eight months of age, become your infant's timekeeper. Set his clock on healthy time.

Allowing brief naps in the early evening or long late-afternoon naps in order to keep a child up late at night will eventually ruin healthy sleep schedules. If your child misses his early-afternoon nap, in order for him to be able to fall asleep close to his biological bedtime hour and avoid the overtired state, it is better to have no nap and an early bedtime than a late nap and a late bedtime. Similarly, you may occasionally need to wake your baby in the morning in order to establish an age-appropriate mid-morning nap that is needed to set the sleep schedule for the rest of the day.

Sleep Regularity

The best time for your child to fall asleep at night is when she is just starting to become drowsy, before she becomes overtired. For young children in day care, dual-career families with long commutes, older children with scheduled activities or teenagers with tremendous amounts of homework, it may be impossible to catch that magical drowsy state. These children will be better off if the bedtime is occurring at approximately the same time every night. For teenagers, this might mean consistent bedtimes throughout the week with later times at the weekends. In one study, regularity of the bedtime schedule was assessed in 3,119 teenage school students. They discovered that a more irregular sleep schedule was associated with more daytime sleepiness. These teenagers had lower grades, more injuries associated with alcohol or drugs and more days missed from school. Going to bed around 11:00 P.M. compared to sometimes 10:00 P.M. or midnight might produce the same amount of sleep, but the more regular schedule is probably better.

Another report examined the sleep of 202 children between four and five years of age. Here, too, variability in bedtime was associated with daytime problems described as 'less optimal' behavioural adjustments in preschool. For example, these children did not 'comply with teacher's urging to join an activity', 'show enthusiasm for learning something', and they argued and fought more than other children. The authors thought these children with chronically variable sleep schedules might experience states similar to jet-lag syndrome characterised as nagging fatigue and cognitive disorientation. This particular study examined the role of family functioning as well as school behaviour and concluded that the link between sleep behaviour and school adjustment was not a common by-product of family stress.

A bedtime that never varies, for example, always putting your preschool child to sleep at exactly 7:00 P.M., does not take into account the biologic variability, from day to day, of activity levels or lengths of naps. So it makes sense to vary the bedtime by thirty to sixty minutes based on how your child looks and behaves during the late afternoon. On the other hand, for older children who are not napping, having bedtimes that are hours earlier or later from day to day has been shown to be unhealthy.

PRACTICAL POINT

Even if the bedtime is too late, a regular bedtime is better than an irregular bedtime.

Biological Rhythms

To better understand the importance of maintaining sleep schedules, let's look at how four distinctive biological rhythms develop. First, immediately after birth, babies are wakeful, then fall asleep, awaken and fall asleep a second time over a ten-hour period. These periods of wakefulness are predictable and not due to hunger, although what causes them is unknown. Thus a partial sleep/wake pattern or rhythm emerges immediately after birth. Second, body temperature rhythms appear and influence sleep/wake cycles. Body temperature typically rises during the day and drops to lower levels at night. At six weeks of age, temperature at bedtime is significantly higher than later in the night. After six weeks of age, as temperatures fall more with sleep, the sleep periods get longer. By twelve to sixteen weeks, all babies show consistent temperature rhythms. It is exactly at six weeks of age when evening fussiness or crying begins to decrease from peak levels and night sleep becomes organised, and it is at twelve to sixteen weeks when day sleep patterns become established.

A third pattern is added by three to six months of age, when the hormone cortisol also shows a similar characteristic rhythm, with peak concentrations in the early morning and lowest levels around midnight. (This hormone is related to both mood and performance and will be discussed further in Chapter 3.) Interestingly, a part of the cortisol secretion rhythm is related to the sleep/wake rhythm and another part is coupled to the body temperature rhythm. I wish Mother Nature were simpler!

Melatonin rhythmicity is a fourth pattern to consider. Initially, a newborn has high levels of circulating melatonin, which is secreted by the mother's pineal gland and crosses the placenta. Within about one week, the melatonin that came from the mother has disappeared. At about six weeks of age, melatonin begins to reappear as the baby's pineal gland matures. But the levels are extremely low until twelve to sixteen weeks of age. Then melatonin begins to surge at night, and the hormone appears to be associated with evolving sleep/wake rhythms by about six months of age. (Melatonin supplements should not be given to babies or young children to make them sleep better; there is no evidence that it is safe.)

Even at only a few months of age, then, interrelated, internal rhythms are already well developed: sleep/wake pattern, body temperature, and cortisol and melatonin levels. In adults, it appears that a long night's sleep is most dependent on going to sleep at or just after the peak of the temperature cycle. Bedtimes occurring near the lower portion of the temperature cycle result in shorter sleep durations.

Shift work or jet travel in adults, or parental mismanagement in children, might cause disorganised sleep. What is 'disorganised sleep'? When you are awake but your body clock is in the sleep mode or when you crash from exhaustion when your body clock is in the awake mode, then your wakefulness or sleep is occurring out of phase with many biological rhythms. The result is poor-quality sleep or poor-quality wakefulness. Imagine the sound from an orchestra if the violin section started to play their part after the woodwinds had already started!

Many studies have been conducted with shift workers and in sleep labs on the internal desynchronisation of circadian rhythms, the uncoupling of rhythms that are normally closely linked and shifting rhythms that are out of phase with one another. The most common complaints in these adults are headaches and abdominal pain. Such people appear healthy and can function reasonably well except for the fact that they have pain in their head and/or stomach.

REMINDER

Never wake a sleeping baby.

There is a large paediatric literature on headaches and recurrent abdominal pains; also, this is very familiar territory to parents of school-age children who have highly scheduled, busy lifestyles. Additional consequences of disorganised sleep include fatigue, stress, and perhaps chronically elevated cortisol levels. Once in place, a pattern of disorganised sleep sets in motion other specific sleep disturbances, such as night waking or an inability to fall asleep easily. Furthermore, recent research has shown that the hormones that are important to regulate sleep are also involved with the immune system, which helps us to fight infections. And research has shown that even modest sleep loss can impair cellular immune function. An article published in *Science News* in 2002, 'Missed ZZZ's, More Disease: Skimping on sleep may be bad for your health', describes how 'poor sleep habits are as important as poor nutrition and physical inactivity in the development of chronic illness'. They specifically cite obesity, diabetes, and cardiovascular disease. Although this article addressed adult health concerns, there is a growing concern that too many of our children are becoming more overweight or obese. So remember what our grandmothers used to say: 'Early to bed, early to rise, makes you healthy . . .'

I often tell parents to become sensitive to their child's personal sleep signals. This means that you should capture that magic moment when the child is tired, ready to sleep and easily falls asleep. The magic moment is a slight quieting, a lull in being busy, a slight staring ahead, and a hint of calmness. If you catch this wave of tiredness and put the child to sleep then, there will be no crying. I like the analogy of surfing, because timing is so important there, too – you have to catch the wave after it rises enough to be recognised but before it crashes. But if you allow a child to crash into an overtired state, it will be harder for him to fall asleep, because he is trying to fall asleep out of phase with other biological rhythms. His ride to sleep then will not be easy or pleasant. Timing is most important! Remember, not every sleep wave is the same, and not every child learns quickly how to ride his sleep wave. But as with everything else, after practice it occurs effortlessly.

Cumulative Sleepiness

It's been known for many years that the effect of lost sleep accumulates over time. When you constantly have insufficient sleep, the sensation of sleepiness when you should be awake increases progressively. Let me explain what this means by giving an example. When adult volunteers have their sleep shortened by a constant amount, impairments in their mood and performance can be measured during the day. If the sleep disruption is repeated night after night, the actual measured impairments do not remain constant. Instead, there is an escalating accumulation of sleepiness that produces in adults continuing increases in headaches, gastrointestinal complaints, forgetfulness, reduced concentration, fatigue, emotional ups and downs, difficulty in staying awake during the daytime, irritability and difficulty awakening. Not only do the adults describe themselves as more sleepy and mentally exhausted, they also feel more stressed. The stress may be a direct consequence of partial sleep deprivation or it may result from the challenge of coping with increasing amounts of daytime sleepiness. Think how hard it would be to concentrate or be motivated if you were struggling every day to stay awake.

If children have constant amounts of sleep deficits, do they show these same escalating problems during the day? Yes! I believe the young child's brain is as sleep-sensitive as, if not more so than, an adult's. It is also possible that severe or chronic sleep deficits occurring early during the period of rapid brain growth might hard-wire circuits to produce permanent effects. This would be difficult to prove, because young children cannot report how they feel and we assume it is 'natural' for them to have difficult temperaments, have tantrums, get frustrated, become easily angry and so forth. In addition, in older children we have learned to accept as 'normal' vague neurological differences – learning difficulties or attention deficit hyperactivity disorder (which, oddly enough, we treat with stimulant medications).

The problem with concluding that constant sleep deficits are associated with these problems is that early night-time sleep deficits may be mild and masked by long naps. If the brain has been permanently changed due to severe or chronic sleep loss, then, when the naps disappear and school requires more mental vigilance and focused attention, pre-existing problems may appear. It is not simply academics that might suffer. We do not know the contribution of healthy childhood sleep towards creativity, empathy, a sense of humour or adult mental health. Part of the problem is, of course, that we don't have yardsticks to measure items such as creativity or empathy, so we do not yet have a way to measure the contribution that healthy sleep during childhood might make.

I do know that many parents keep their child up an extra twenty or thirty minutes at night to have fun, and notice no problems in the beginning. Later they call and ask why their 'good sleeper' is now resisting bedtime or is irritable in the morning for 'no obvious reason'. Because the change in routine was small and in the past, they don't even think about it. But during our conversation they will recall that because of the longer spring and summer days, or because 'it didn't seem to cause any problems', they pushed the child's bedtime back. The interval between allowing the too-late bedtime and the emergence of sleep-related problems was months in young children who had always in the past been well rested and were taking good naps, or weeks in children who were always on the edge of being overtired anyway. When such parents were asked if they thought their child appeared able to go to sleep twenty or thirty minutes earlier, the answer was almost always yes.

> **MAJOR POINT**
>
> **Small but constant deficits in sleep over time tend to have escalating and perhaps long-term effects on brain function.**

In older children who have outgrown naps, the interval before the effects of cumulative sleepiness show themselves may be very long because of high motivation in the child and many exciting parent-directed events such as classes, lessons or excursions, which help mask impaired vigilance or performance. The right bedtime is based on your child's age (see previous graphs on pages 43 and 44 for age-appropriate norms) and your child's behaviour, mood and performance, especially in the late afternoon.

Twenty-five-Hour Cycles

Although harmonious biological rhythms promote healthy sleep, random bad days are bound to occur. One explanation for 'off' days, when the child's sleep is irregular for no apparent reason, is that our basic biological clocks have about twenty-five hours in their cycle, not twenty-four. In other words, without time cues, our free-running sleep/wake rhythms appear to complete one full cycle every twenty-five hours. As long as we train our children to match sleep/wake rhythms to night and day, problems are usually avoided. Other babies appear to get off schedule every few weeks and parents then must work to keep them well rested. I suspect that babies, like adults, differ in their individual ability to adjust their twenty-five-hour biological rhythms to society's twenty-four-hour clocks. Most parents, however, find that the effort to reset a baby's clock is worth it, because otherwise the child becomes increasingly tired and irritable.

When parents make the effort to help the child get needed sleep, the child becomes better rested, and it becomes easier for her to accept sleep, to expect to sleep, to take long naps and to go to sleep by herself. Some parents always have to endure days of disruption following trips, illnesses or immunisations because any irregularity of schedule upsets sleep rhythms.

Here is one family's account.

Susan's Night Waking

Last summer, Susan's night waking had become so frequent that she was basically awake more than she was asleep. We had been instructed by a paediatrician at the parenting class we attend to 'meet our child's needs'. So we were getting up as frequently as she asked and rocking her back to sleep. This happened three or four times a night and often took thirty to sixty minutes. A part of me wanted to do this. Needless to say, however, after months of this night-time routine, my husband and I became quite exhausted and began to resent our child. I knew I was in trouble when I would get up and go into the baby's room and yell at her and then begin crying myself. The point I'm trying to make is simple: when a problem like a child's sleep habit gets out of hand, the parents are partially responsible.

Finally, on our own, we decided to let her cry it out. By the way, my husband had a much easier time psychologically with letting her cry. He knew it was in her best interest and was able to remain unemotional about it. It took about a week, and she cried for about two hours for quite a few of those nights. Finally it seemed that she got the idea.

Unfortunately, the next week we were scheduled to go on our summer holiday. We didn't want to cancel the trip, but we knew we were taking a chance on destroying the results of our hard work. We stayed at a place where there were no cots, so we made a sleeping area for Susan in the corner of the room. She'd wake up in the middle of the night and think it was playtime.

When we got back from the trip we tried to get into the routine of letting her cry it out, but by that time we didn't have the energy to go through a week of crying again. So we fell back into a poor night-time routine. Another month went by, and we knew we could not go on. We discussed it with the teacher at our parenting class, and she finally recommended the process of just letting Susan cry it out. This time it took about five days before she was back to sleeping through the night. The improvement lasted about a month.

Susan received a vaccination shortly after that. I went into her room for only a moment to check on her one night. Then she began waking each night, and we were into our old routine. We repeated the process yet one more time. I think it took about five nights to get her to sleep through the night again. After that, Susan slept through the night regularly for months. She eventually asked to be put down before she was asleep at night rather than being rocked to sleep. She began taking long naps this spring, which seemed slightly strange.

This summer when we went on holiday Susan slept in a cot in our room. She'd awaken in the night and again think it was playtime. It didn't take long for her to get back into her old bad habits. We had hoped we were beyond that, since she had been sleeping through the night for so many months . . . but since our trip she's been up at night practising long dialogues, and it looks as though we'll have to go through this one more time.

This sounds like the story of a child who is always on the edge of being overtired and in whom natural disruptions are not easily tolerated. Slightly overtired children are more easily thrown off balance and take longer to recover. Well-rested children tend to be more adaptable and take occasional changes of routine in their stride.

PRACTICAL POINT

A well-rested baby with a healthy sleep habit wakes with a cheerful, happy attitude. A tired baby wakes up grumpy.

Sleep Positions, SIDS

A common misconception held by Western parents is that all children sleep better on their stomachs. Yet a Chinese mother whose baby preferred to sleep on her stomach said she knew something was very wrong with her infant, because all Chinese babies sleep on their backs! She truly worried that stomach sleeping was unhealthy.

The truth is that some babies seem to sleep better and fuss or cry less when asleep on their backs. Contrary to many parents' fears, sleeping on the back does not cause a misshapen skull. In the past, tradition and social circumstances dictated which sleeping position most parents selected. Now it appears that *sleeping on the back is safer because it helps prevent sudden infant death syndrome.* Fortunately, most babies sleep equally well on their backs as on their stomachs.

A variant of the myth that babies sleep better on their stomachs is that when the child at five months rolls over, away from the sleeping position selected by the parents, the parent has to intervene and roll the child back. Actually, leaving the child alone allows the child to learn to sleep in different positions. If you roll your child back and he instantaneously returns to sleep, obviously there is no problem. On the other hand, going to your child to roll him back can become a game for the infant by five months of age. Games should occur at playtime, not when it's time to sleep. Remember, not going to your baby allows him to learn to roll back alone, learn to sleep in the new position and learn to remember the next night not to roll in the first place.

Likewise, when the older child pulls herself to a standing position in her cot, parents do not need to help her get down. A child might fall down in an awkward heap, but she will not hurt herself. Next time she will think twice about standing up and shaking the cot railings, or she'll be more careful when letting go.

Parents who rush in to roll the baby over or to help a child down run the risk of reinforcing this behaviour, encouraging it to be repeated night after night. Children are very crafty and learn quickly how to get parents to give them extra attention. Don't deprive your child of the opportunity to learn how to roll over or sit down unassisted at night.

The Benefits of Healthy Sleep: Sleep Patterns, Intelligence, Learning and School Performance

Do sleep patterns really affect learning in children? Yes! Different studies of children at different ages all agree on this point. Focusing on perfectly normal, healthy children, let's consider the data by age groups: infants, preschoolers and school-age children.

Infants

A study at the University of Connecticut showed that there was a strong association between the amount of time infants were in REM sleep and the amount of time they spent when awake in the behavioural state called 'quiet alert'. In the quiet alert state, babies have open, bright eyes, they appear alert, their eyes are scanning, their faces are relaxed and they do not smile or frown. Their bodies are relatively quiet and inactive. One mother described her four-month-old, who was frequently in this quiet alert state, as 'a looker and a thinker'. She's right! These infants don't miss a thing. A study of sleep development at Stanford University showed that environmental factors, not simply brain maturation, are responsible for the proportion of time infants spend in REM sleep. Unfortunately, the exact environmental factors were not identified, but presumably parental handling could influence all of these items: sleep patterns, the proportion of REM sleep and the amount of time the child is in the quiet alert state.

Infants who are notoriously *not* quiet alert are those with colic or a difficult temperament. Their fussy behaviour may be due to imbalances of internal chemicals such as progesterone or even cortisol. High cortisol concentrations in infants have been shown to be associated with decreased duration of non-REM sleep. So, even in infants, as in adults, there seem to be connections between internal chemicals, sleep patterns and behaviour when awake. Also, these fussy children tend to have irregular schedules and short attention spans. Among two- to three-month-old infants, one study showed that the more irregular and impersistent the child was, the slower the rates of learning. Looking ahead to Figure 9 (see page 395), you can see how colicky or difficult-temperament children, who sleep for brief durations and have irregular schedules and short attention spans, might not learn quickly to fall asleep unassisted. Thus they easily could become sleep-deprived, fatigued and hyperactive older children. (This concept of increased alertness, wakefulness and irritability due to chemical imbalances will be discussed in Chapter 3.)

I think naps are especially important for infants. In my own studies, I've found that how long the infant sleeps during the day is strongly associated with persistence or attention span. Infants who take long naps have longer attention spans. They spend more time in the quiet alert state and seem to learn faster. Infants who do not nap well are either drowsy or fitfully fussy, and in either case they do not learn well.

PRACTICAL POINT

Naps promote optimal alertness for children. Children who nap well spend relatively more time in the quiet alert state when awake.

It is a myth that long naps interfere with acquiring socialisation skills or infant stimulation. While it's true that 'nap-monsters' are less available for all the classes or activities that abound today – swim-gym, parent-and-toddler groups, or infant-stimulating groups – is that so bad? Do infants suffer because they don't participate in so many activities? Are they less likely to get into the right preschool, which feeds to the right nursery school, which feeds to the right junior school? No.

Please do not confuse the quantity of time spent in these organised activities with the high-quality social awareness that well-rested children exhibit. The truth is that these infant-stimulation groups are often not important for infants but instead serve legitimate parental needs by allowing mothers and fathers to meet other parents and escape from their isolation at home.

Preschool Children

Three-year-old children who nap well are more adaptable. (Adaptability means the ease with which children adjust to new circumstances.) *Adaptability is the single most important trait for school success.* The briefer the naps, the less adaptable the child. In fact, the major temperament feature of three-year-olds who do not nap at all is nonadaptability. It is exactly these non-napping, nonadaptable children who also have more night wakings!

My research has shown that when infants who are easy at five months of age develop into grumpier, more difficult three-year-olds, it is because they have developed a pattern of brief sleeps. In contrast, difficult infants who mellow into easier three-year-olds have developed a pattern of long sleeps. I think that parents' helping or hindering regular sleep patterns caused these shifts to occur.

School-Age Children

In 1925, the father of the Stanford-Binet Intelligence Test, Dr Lewis M. Terman, published his landmark book, *Genetic Studies of Genius.* He compared approximately 600 children with IQ scores over 140 to a group of almost 2,700 children with IQ scores below 140. For every age examined, the gifted children slept longer!

Two years later, about 5,500 Japanese schoolchildren were studied, and those with better grades slept longer!

Even seventy-nine years later, Dr Terman's study stands apart in design, execution and thoroughness. A 1983 scientific sleep laboratory study from Canada has provided objective evidence confirming Terman's result, that children of superior IQ had greater total sleep time. Both studies agreed that brighter children slept about *thirty to forty minutes longer each night* than average children of similar ages.

Another study from the University of Louisville School of Medicine examined a group of identical twins that were selected because one twin slept less than the other. At about ten years of age, the twin with the longer sleep pattern had higher total reading, vocabulary and comprehension scores than the twin with the shorter sleep pattern.

PRACTICAL POINT

Please don't think that it has no lasting effect when you routinely keep your child up too late – for your own pleasure after work or because you want to avoid bedtime confrontations – or when you cut corners on naps in order to run errands or visit friends. Once in a while, for a special occasion or reason, it's okay. But day-in, day-out sleep deprivation at night or for naps, as a matter of habit, could be very damaging to your child. ***Cumulative, chronic sleep losses, even of brief duration, may be harmful for learning.***

Children diagnosed with attention deficit hyperactivity disorder or learning disabilities have been shown to have sleep-related difficulties, though we don't know which came first. Nevertheless, one careful intervention study showed that improvements in sleep dramatically improved peer relations and classroom performance.

Research on creative adults supports the concept that originality of ideas and the quality of experiences suffer when you cut back on sleep. What you lose in waking time is made up in terms of a richer life. Have you ever nodded off at an evening event that you really wanted to attend but were too tired to fully enjoy?

There are many other studies that show an association between sleeping and school performance, but these involve children with allergies or large adenoids. (These problems are discussed in Chapter 10.)

SLEEP STRATEGIES

Drowsy Signs

As your baby shows signs of becoming drowsy, you should begin a soothing-to-sleep routine. These signs usually start within one or two hours of wakefulness at a few weeks of age. About 20 per cent of babies have colic and they may not show these drowsy signs, so you have to watch the clock more carefully. If your child often shows signs of fatigue, note how long she has been awake and next time begin the soothing process about twenty minutes earlier.

It is not necessary for your child to be drowsy and awake when you put him down or you lie down with him in your bed. Sometimes your baby goes from drowsy to sleepy very quickly, and there is no good reason why some books suggest that you should then wake up your baby before you put him down or lie down with him.

DROWSY SIGNS, SLEEPY CUES, SLEEP SIGNALS

Moving into the sleep zone

Becoming Drowsy
Decreased activity
Slower motions
Less vocal
Sucking is weaker or slower
Quieter
Calmer
Appears disinterested in surroundings
Eyes are less focused
Eyelids drooping
Yawning

FATIGUE SIGNS

Entering overtired zone

Becoming Overtired
Fussing
Rubbing eyes
Irritable
Grumpy

Soothing to Sleep

What exactly is soothing? Soothing is restoring a peaceful state. To soothe your newborn is to render her calm or quiet, to bring her to a composed condition. You are attempting to establish a peaceful state of tranquillity by reducing the force or intensity of fussiness. Your goal is to soften, tone down or render less harsh fussiness or crying. Soothing is pacifying or calming. You want to bring comfort to your baby and a cessation of agitation. Snuggling her close to your body, she feels your warmth and senses your affection and protection. Cuddling is the close embrace you do with someone you love. Sometimes you just want to nestle with her as you take a cosy position and press her close to you or lie down close to her. At best, when a child is tired, we hope to lull her into a relaxed sleepy state.

Bodily contact, sucking and gentle rhythmic motions over long periods of time seem to work best. Sometimes loud mechanical sounds like the waste disposal or hair dryer seem to help. Be careful, however, not to bombard your baby with stimuli. Initially, try to appeal to one sense at a time: tactile (massaging, rubbing, kissing, rocking, patting, changing from hip to shoulder), auditory (singing, humming, playing music, running the vacuum cleaner), sight (bright lights, mobiles, television), dim light or darkness when drowsy or rhythmic motion (swings, cradles, car rides, going for a walk). Sometimes, doing too many of these things simultaneously or with too much force has a stimulating rather than a relaxing effect. However, if your baby remains fussy, try combinations of these different modalities.

Try to synchronise your actions with your baby's rhythms. If he is tense, taut, with deep exhausted heaving sobs and little physical movement, try rubbing his back ever so gently or moving your cheek over his in a slow rhythm that coincides with his breathing pattern. If he is boxing with his fists, jerking his legs and arching his back, maybe a ride on your shoulders will grab his attention and arrest the spell. You will find that after a while you become attuned to nuances within your baby's rhythms and respond accordingly.

Father Care: Our Secret Weapon for Soothing

Before your baby is born, fathers should make the decision to become involved in caring for the baby from the very beginning. Some fathers hold back initially, afraid they might 'do the wrong thing' when holding, burping, bathing, changing,or feeding the baby. After mothers get their strength back, they should deliberately leave the house at a weekend for a few hours to visit a friend, spend time with the older kids, get their hair done or go shopping at a time when they expect the baby to go through a cycle of feeding, changing, bathing and putting to sleep. Guess who has to do the work then? Often a father will feel more comfortable doing these things when the 'expert' is not looking over his shoulder. So the first point is for fathers to start early in practising baby care.

Second, fathers should plan ahead for the six-week peak of fussing/crying that occurs in all babies. They should come home early or take a few days off work if they are able. Make adjustments if your baby is born before or after the expected date of delivery, because the six-week peak is counted from this due date. At six weeks of age, babies fuss/cry more and sleep less. Less sleep for the baby means less sleep for the mother. All mothers need help in caring for their six-week-old and themselves. Fathers should give mothers a well-deserved break at this time by taking the baby out for long walks or car rides in the evening or night. The baby might not sleep well during these outings, but at least the mother gets a break.

The third point is that fathers can practice and learn how to help their baby fall asleep. For example, after nursing her baby, the mother could pass her son to the father, who then rocks his baby gently for a while and puts him down to sleep or lies down with him in their bed and they both snooze. (This may only occur at weekends when the father is around.) The participation of fathers in putting their babies to sleep will help them gain confidence in becoming a parent. If the mother is giving expressed breast milk in a bottle, fathers and babies may have an easier time accomplishing the feeding if the mother actually leaves the house. This is because the baby can smell the mother's presence and might resist taking the bottle if he knows his mother is home. So, maybe at weekends, when it's time for the baby's nap, mum leaves the house and has fun while dad gives the bottle and puts his baby down to sleep.

Fourth, fathers can learn how to soothe baby fussiness and crying and spend lots of time doing the soothing. For example, fathers can learn infant massage. Classes are offered everywhere; call your local maternity hospital or go on-line. Fathers can learn lullabies (your baby will not care how well you sing). A baby bath might be especially soothing, and fathers can spend time letting the warm water calm the baby. A father can learn to do everything a mother does to soothe the baby except breast-feed. For babies six months of age or older, fathers can attempt to help lengthen naps by responding immediately as a mini-nap nears its end (baby just begins to whimper or cry) by attempting to soothe the baby back to sleep for a nap extension. If mothers do this, it might be more stimulating than soothing.

Lastly, a father can request to help feed or soothe the baby in the middle of the night when the mother needs extra sleep. This is a little bit tricky because many mothers have the attitude that nobody can do the soothing as well as they can, and also that dads need their rest so they can go out to work well rested in the morning. With this attitude, the mother rejects or resists the idea that baby care in the middle of the night should be a shared experience. For some families, this might be the right course of action. But if the mother is distressed, exhausted, sleep-deprived or going through baby blues, then extra help at night from the father is absolutely needed to give the mother a little more sleep. After all, no matter how stressful his job might be, the father at work always gets some breaks. A mother with a baby might not get any breaks during the day. In one study of children one to three years of age, sleep problems were solved when fathers took over the management of the bedtime routine and night awakenings. Dr Klaus Minde observed that the fathers were 'more forthright and authoritative' and the mothers felt tired in the evening and perceived their toddlers as particularly difficult at that time. In this study, the fathers used the 'graduated extinction' or 'controlled crying' method.

Fathers need to understand that when children are overtired and not sleeping well, it is sometimes useful to go to a *temporarily* ultra-early bedtime to repay the sleep debt. The child awakens better rested, then learns to nap better, and later is able to have a later bedtime. If fathers refuse to help prevent and solve sleep problems, then they have to accept responsibility for their overtired child's behaviour – and not blame the mother!

Sucking Is Soothing

Anything you can do to encourage your baby to suck will help soothe her. Offering the breast, bottle, pacifier, finger or wrist usually helps calm your baby. If you are breast-feeding, one way to help distinguish between sucking for soothing and sucking for hunger is that the sucking for soothing is often rapid, repeated sucks with very little swallowing. In addition, the fussy baby does not suck in a rhythmic steady fashion; instead, she starts and stops, twists and turns. If she is hungry, the pattern is usually a rhythmic suck-swallow, suck-swallow, and so forth. If you are bottle-feeding, do not assume that when your baby eagerly takes several ounces that this means she is hungry. Many babies with extreme fussiness/colic suck more than they need and spit up a lot.

Because sucking is such a powerful way to calm a baby and babies often fall asleep with sucking, I think it is unnatural and unhealthy for parents to deliberately do things that interfere with sucking. One popular book that promotes 'no-cry sleep solutions' tells parents to remove the breast while he is sucking, before he falls asleep, and if the baby continues to want to suck after the removal, it tells parents to hold the baby's mouth closed to prevent the sucking. Another popular book describes sucking as one of the major ways that babies can calm themselves, but then goes on to recommend that you wake your baby up during sucking if he falls asleep at the breast. Furthermore, the author instructs you to begin this practice at one month of age! Both books make the assumption that if the baby falls asleep while sucking, you will be creating a sleeping problem. There is no good evidence to support this assumption. Mothers in my practice do not deliberately interfere with sucking at the time of soothing to sleep, and their babies sleep well. Both books also incorrectly assume that feeding and sleeping are tightly linked. So they both encourage you to force-feed your baby in order to help him sleep longer. Phrases like 'cluster feed' or 'top off the tank' to help him sleep or 'He's awake when he's hungry and asleep when he's full' reveal a profound ignorance about how the developing brain, not the stomach, controls sleep/wake rhythms. I believe it is much more natural to follow your baby's needs. If your baby is hungry, feed him. If your baby is fussy, soothe him. If your baby is tired, put him to sleep. If you're not sure what he needs, encourage sucking at the breast or bottle until he seems satisfied because he is full or calm or asleep.

Rhythmic Rocking Motions

Rhythmic motions are one of the most effective methods of soothing your infant. Use a cradle, rocking chair, baby swing, or sling; take the baby for car rides, dance with her, or simply walk with her. Rocking motions may be gentle movements or vigorous swinging, depending on what your child responds to. Gently jiggling or bouncing may calm your baby. Some parents claim that raising and lowering the baby like an elevator is effective. Perhaps these rhythmic movements are comforting because they are similar to what a baby feels in the womb.

Swaddling

Gentle pressure, such as that experienced when embraced or hugged, makes us feel good. Swaddling or gentle wrapping, sleeping in a car seat or being held in a soft baby carrier or sling are other ways to exert gentle pressure. Here, too, perhaps the sensation of gentle pressure resembles a state of comfort that the baby feels before he is born. Both rhythmic motions and gentle pressure may be effective because perhaps human babies are born too early. The theory is that human babies are born earlier compared to other primate babies because as the pelvic bones developed to support an upright posture, they became narrower. So human babies had to be smaller at the time of birth. If correct, then it is likely that rhythmic motions and gentle pressure exert their soothing effects because they partially re-create the sensations that the baby felt in the womb.

Massage

Massaging babies has been observed in many different cultures and has a long history. It is not just a new fad. One particular benefit from massaging your newborn is that the mother or father directly benefits from this activity. While lovingly stroking your baby, you smile at your baby, talk softly or you might sing or hum. These efforts, while focused on your baby, also relax you! Since fathers cannot breast-feed their babies, I encourage them to develop an intimate bond with their newborn by practising baby massage right away – even before any fussiness begins. Using a natural cold-pressed fruit or vegetable oil, gently stroke the skin and gently knead your baby's muscles. All the movements are performed gently – books with pictures and videos are available to assist you. Baby massage is not a gimmick or a cure for extreme fussiness. However, it does soothe babies. Equally important, it provides you with a singular opportunity to be completely focused on your baby – turn off the phones and pagers. You are doing something quite different from feeding, changing and bathing. Comforting your baby this way will give you an inner calmness that will help you get through possible rough times when your baby is extremely fussy and not very soothable.

Respect Your Baby's Need to Sleep: The One- to Two-Hour Window of Wakefulness

Immediately after the baby is born, you will see what people mean when they say 'sleeping like a baby'. For a few days, babies sleep almost all the time. They barely suck and normally lose weight during this time. If your baby was born early, this very drowsy time might last longer; if your baby was born past the expected date of delivery, the drowsy period might be brief or nonexistent. A few days later, babies begin to wake up more. This increased wakefulness reflects the normal maturation of your baby's nervous system. I tell families that the brain wakes up after three or four days just in time to catch the breast milk that is just now available in ample amounts. He looks around more with wider eyes and is able to suck with more strength and for longer periods. Within days, the weight loss stops and a dramatic growth in weight, height and head circumference begins. Also, longer periods of wakefulness begin to appear after a few days. Although your baby is intently interested in you and is quickly able to recognise your face and voice, he is not yet curious about objects such as toys or mobiles. He does not appear to care about the general buzz or noises, colours or other activities surrounding him, and therefore, he falls asleep almost anywhere. The extremely fussy/colicky baby is not like this and appears to have difficulty falling asleep and staying asleep even at only several days of age. All babies gradually seem to become more aware of action, motion, voices, noises, vibrations, lights, wind and so forth as they become more curious. Now they often do not 'sleep like a baby'.

During the day, within a one- to two-hour time 'window' of wakefulness, your baby will become drowsy and want to go to sleep. I discovered this window during my research on naps. If you soothe a baby during the beginning of drowsiness, most will easily fall asleep. The exception is the extremely fussy/colicky baby who might fall asleep but not easily; these babies need longer and more complex soothing efforts to help them fall asleep. The other exception is during the evening fussy periods and especially around six weeks of age.

Here are some ways to note that your baby is becoming drowsy. Watch for the drowsy signs – quieting of activity, less movement of the arms and legs, eyes that are not as sparkling, eyelids that droop a little, less-intense staring at you and sucking that may be weaker or slower. If your baby is over six weeks old, you may notice less socially responsive smiling or your baby may be less engaging. This is the time to begin soothing to sleep. All babies become this way within one to two hours of wakefulness.

What happens if you miss this one- to two-hour window? Your baby will become overtired if she cannot fall asleep because of too much stimulation around her. When you or your baby becomes overtired, the body is stressed. There are chemical changes that then occur to fight the fatigue, and this interferes with the ability to easily fall asleep and stay asleep. Babies vary in their ability to self-soothe and deal with this stress, and parents vary in their ability to soothe their babies. So not all babies go bonkers if they are kept up a little too long. But you will have a more peaceful and better-sleeping baby if you respect his need to sleep within one to two hours of wakefulness. I consider this to be the beginning of sleep training for babies.

Sleep training begins with developing a sense of timing so that you are trying to soothe your baby at the time when your baby is naturally getting drowsy before falling asleep. Some young babies will need dark and quiet environments to sleep well and others will appear to be less sensitive to what is going on around them. Respect your baby's individuality and do not try to force him to meet your lifestyle. I like the analogy with feeding: we do not withhold food when our baby is hungry. We try to anticipate when he will be hungry, so he will be somewhere calm where we can feed him. We do not feed him on the run. The same applies for sleeping.

If your young baby does not sleep, continue trying to soothe. Do not let him cry or ignore him. You cannot spoil a baby. You cannot teach a baby a crying habit.

Other Soothing Methods

Be sceptical about the supposed miracles accomplished with hot-water bottles, herbal teas or recordings of heartbeat or womb sounds. There has been a great deal of nonsense written about burping techniques, nipple sizes and shapes, baby bottle straws, feeding and sleeping positions, lamb's wool pads, diets for nursing mothers, special formulas, pacifiers, and solid food. There is no good evidence that chiropractic spinal manipulation helps babies. These items have nothing to do with extreme fussiness, crying, temperament or sleeping habits.

Many useless remedies can be purchased without a prescription. Anti-wind drops, such as simethicone, have not been shown to be more effective than a placebo in well-conducted studies. One popular pellet contains chamomile, calcium phosphate, caffeine and a very small amount of active belladonna chemicals (0.0000095 per cent). Another remedy contains natural blackberry flavour, Jamaica ginger, oil of anise, oil of nutmeg, and 2 per cent alcohol. Maybe enough alcohol will sedate some infants! Please read labels carefully – any natural substance, flavouring agent or herb can have pharmacological effects. Call a school of pharmacy or a medical school to find experts in the study of natural herbs and plants, to find out if a particular plant or herb is dangerous.

Beware of gimmicks. Newborns have been drowned in rocking waterbeds, strangulated by having their necks overhang a trampoline-like cot platform and suffocated by burying their heads into pillows. Beware of prescribed drugs. *The Times* headline of 22 May 1998, screamed, 'Baby died after drop of medicine for wind.' A midwife had 'diagnosed trapped wind' and prescribed what was thought to be peppermint water.

Also be cautious in using home remedies. One mother almost killed her baby by giving a mixture of Morton Salt Substitute with lactobacillus acidophilus culture, as prescribed in a popular book.

Everything Works . . . for a While

When you believe that something is going to calm your baby – herbal tea, womb recordings, lamb's wool blankets, you name it – often it appears to work, for a while. You are emotionally expecting relief because you trust the advice of an authority. Your fatigue may breed inflated hopes for a cure, and the day-by-day variability in infant crying creates the illusion that a particular remedy works. What is really happening is a placebo effect, the emotional equivalent of an optical illusion.

Mothers may fool themselves into believing their babies are better because of a new formula or special tea. Of course, reality sets in after a few days and shatters the illusion. Some mothers sincerely believe that their babies habituate to, or become accustomed to, the benefits from the new formula or tea much like a drug addict needs increased doses to produce the desired feeling. Some doctors believe the mothers' reports and agree that the babies really did improve for a day or two because the babies received novel stimulation.

Novelty is unlikely to be important because parents report that upon reintroduction, weeks after the special tea or gimmick was discarded, they see no improvement. In other words, there was no placebo effect the second time around. Naturally, if the baby coincidentally outgrows extreme fussiness/colic when a useless remedy is introduced, the mother, the family, and even the doctor might become convinced that the useless remedy actually cured the extreme fussiness/colic!

Resources for Soothing

Some families have vast resources to invest in soothing their babies, but other families are not so fortunate. Twenty per cent of babies have colic and require much more soothing, and families with a colicky baby and limited resources to soothe might easily become overwhelmed and frustrated. The other 80 per cent of babies are more easily soothed and usually do not overly stress their parents. So you want to pay attention to whether your child has colic or not, and take some time to reflect on how able you will be to enlist help to soothe your baby. It is often more than a one-woman job! If you have a baby who fusses and cries a lot and is difficult to console, and your available resources for soothing are limited, you might modify some of the plans you made before your child was born regarding a family bed or cot.

Consider a balance between the baby's disposition to express distress and the parents' capability to soothe their baby. Not only do babies vary in their expression but parents also vary in their capability to soothe. The resources for parents' ability to soothe fussiness and crying and promote sleep in their baby include the following.

RESOURCES FOR PARENTS' ABILITY TO SOOTHE

- **Father involvement versus absent father**
- **Agreements or disagreements between parents regarding child-rearing such as breast- versus bottle-feeding or cot versus family bed**
- **Absence or presence of marital discord**
- **Absence or presence of intimacy between wife and husband**
- **Absence or presence of baby blues or postpartum depression**
- **Absence or presence of other children requiring attention**
- **Ease or difficulty in breast-feeding**
- **Absence or presence of medical problems in child, mother, father or other children**
- **Number of bedrooms in the home**
- **Absence or presence of relatives, friends or neighbours to help out**
- **Help or interference with sleep routines from grandparents**
- **Ability or inability to afford housekeeping help**
- **Ability or inability to afford child care help**
- **Absence or presence of financial pressures such as mother having to return to work soon**

Bedtime Routines

Just as soothing helps your child feel safe and secure, bedtime routines help all children calm down before falling asleep, because both are associated with the natural state of relaxed drowsiness. As with soothing, bedtime routines should be started early, before sleepy signs change into overtired fussy signs. Older children and more regular babies will develop predictable sleep times, and these children might be 'slept by the clock'. Pick and choose from the following list based on your child's age and your personal preference. Try to follow the same sequence at all sleep times.

BEDTIME ROUTINES

Before sleep times, reduce the amount of stimulation: less noise, dimmer lights, less handling, playing and activity
Bedroom should be quiet, dark (use room-darkening shades) and warm, but not too warm
Bathe
Massage after bath with smooth, gentle motions
Dress for sleep
Swaddle if it comforts and relaxes your baby, use a warm blanket from the clothes dryer
Lullaby, quiet singing or humming – be consistent
Favourite words, sounds or phrases – be consistent
Feed
May put down drowsy but awake, but do not deliberately awaken before sleeping. This often fails for colicky babies and all six-week-olds in the evening
Do not rush in at the first sound your baby makes

In addition to being consistent in your bedtime routines, you must cultivate patience, because it may take time for your child to get the message that this is not the time to be playing. I would also add that, except for premature babies and trying to correct a sleep problem, you should never wake a sleeping baby.

Breast-feeding versus Bottle-feeding and Family Bed versus Cot

How you feed your baby and where you sleep with your baby might depend on many factors, including whether the baby is easy or difficult to soothe and whether you and your baby are well rested or not. Ask yourself these questions:

Do you spend a total of more than three hours per day soothing your baby to prevent crying? That is, when you add up the total amount of minutes spent walking, rocking, driving around in the car, swaddling, singing, humming, running water, offering the breast or bottle even when not hungry, using a pacifier, and so forth, does the total exceed three hours?

Do you behave this way more than three days per week?

Have you been doing this for more than three weeks?

If you answered 'yes' to all three questions, then your baby has colic. There may be **no** crying because of your soothing effort, just endless fussing. Or, she might sometimes cry anyway despite your soothing efforts. If you answered 'no' to some of the questions but your baby fusses often, especially in the evening and especially around six weeks of age, then your baby has common fussiness. If you answered 'yes' to all three questions, please stop here and skip ahead to Chapter 4 to better understand the challenges you will be up against.

Breast-feeding versus Bottle-feeding

Breast-feeding is considered best for baby and mother. The decision on how to feed your baby may be influenced by the support or lack thereof from your husband, your mother or other family members. However, many babies are bottle-fed because of adoption, prematurity or medical problems with the baby or mother. Bottles can contain expressed breast milk or formula, so 'bottle-feeding' may include feeding breast milk. Formula-fed babies grow up to be just as healthy as breast-fed babies. Many studies have shown that breast-feeding does not prevent extreme fussiness/colic, does not prevent sudden infant death syndrome, and does not prevent or cause sleeping problems. At night, breast-fed babies are often fed more frequently than formula-fed babies, but it is not known whether this is caused by the breast-feeding mother responding more promptly to her baby's quiet sounds or whether breast milk digestion causes the baby to wake up more often. In general, research has shown that sleep/wake rhythms evolve at the same pace whether the baby is breast-fed, formula-fed, demand-fed, schedule-fed or whether cereal is given in the bottle or by spoon. Some babies with a birth defect of the digestive system are fed continuously by vein or tube in the stomach. Because of the constant feeding, they are never hungry. These babies develop the same sleep/wake rhythms as all other babies. This is why I tell parents that 'Sleep comes from the brain, not the stomach'. Although there are rare medical exceptions, changing formulas will not reduce fussiness/crying or promote better sleeping.

Of course, if your baby is not being fed enough, then she might be too hungry and fuss/cry or not sleep well. In this situation, the child will not be gaining weight and some help will be needed to establish a better breast milk supply or evaluation for medical problems that are causing poor weight gain. In my practice, I encourage first-time mothers to give a bottle of expressed breast milk or formula once per twenty-four hours when their baby is two to three weeks old. This allows fathers and other family members to have the pleasure of feeding the baby, as well as giving the mother a mini-break once a day to rest and allow for the healing of cracked or painful nipples. It also gives the parents the chance to have a date to recharge their energy. Fathers can be more helpful during fussy/crying periods or middle of the night feedings to allow mothers a little more sleep. Some experienced mothers, who have previously breast-fed successfully, give the single bottle sooner. They have confidence in their ability to breast-feed and either give formula in the hospital or start pumping sooner. They know that the single bottle does not confuse the child or interfere with breast-feeding. The reason the bottle is given every twenty-four hours is to keep the baby adapted to taking the bottle. Some babies do well with less frequent bottles, but others will reject all bottles if days go by without having had one.

Family Bed versus Cot

Our goal is a well-rested family, and a family bed – sometimes described as co-sleeping or bed sharing – may be right for your family. The decision to sleep with your baby might be made before the child is born because this is what you want for your family. You might decide that unrestricted breast-feeding day and night, always caring for your baby and sleeping with your baby at night or day and night will promote a tighter or more sensitive bond between you and your baby. Parents then begin the practice of co-sleeping as soon as the baby is born. Researchers use the term *early co-sleepers* to describe these children. Alternatively, you might not have thought about or not really wanted to have a family bed, but you discovered that because your baby was so fussy/colicky, or when your child was older and not sleeping well, that the only way anyone got any rest was to sleep with your baby in your bed. Researchers use the term *reactive co-sleepers* to describe these children. Scientific studies have shown that co-sleeping in infancy is often associated with the later development of sleep problems. I suspect that the majority of these problems occur among the formerly 'reactive co-sleepers'. In other words, some parents find that the family bed is a short-term and partial solution to sleeping problems, and that the sleeping problem continues long after the child has been moved to his own cot or bed.

About a third of white urban families frequently sleep together in a family bed for all or part of the night. By itself, this is neither good nor bad. Studies in the United States suggest that the family bed might encourage or lead to a variety of emotional stresses within the child; opposite results were found in studies conducted in Sweden. This probably reflects differences in social attitudes towards nudity, bathing and sexuality. Think of it as a family style, one that does not necessarily reflect or cause emotional or psychological problems in parents and children.

But when someone is not getting enough sleep, either

parent or child, the family bed can cause potential problems. I suspect this often develops in older toddlers because by the age of one to two years, sleeping together is often associated with night waking. Once there is a well-established habit, the child is unwilling to go to or return to his own bed.

So if you want to enjoy a family bed, fine. But understand that your cuddling in bed together may make any future changes in sleep arrangements difficult to execute. Remember, while it sounds like an easy solution to baby's sleep problems, you may wind up with a twenty-four-hour child even when he gets older.

In contrast, many families use a family bed overnight only during the first few months, and then shift baby to her own bed for overnight sleep. Then at 5:00 or 6:00 A.M., parents might bring their older infant or child into their bed for a limited period of warm cuddling.

Sleeping with your baby might include day and night or just night, all night or part of the night, in your bed or using a small cot attached to your bed, with other children in your bed or other children in your bedroom but not in your bed. All of these variations are collectively called 'family bed'. In many cultures, families sleep together because of tradition or a limited number of bedrooms. It is rare in Japan or in traditional or tribal societies for children to sleep apart from their parents. There is a great appeal for sleeping together. A powerful word to describe soothing is 'nestling', and this easily brings forth the image of creating a nest for your baby in your bed.

Both the U.S. Consumer Product Safety Commission and the American Academy of Pediatrics actively discourage the family bed because of the risk of entrapment between the mattress and the structures of the bed (headboard, footboard, side rails and frame), the wall or adjacent furniture. There is the hazard of suffocation or overlying by an adult who is in an unusually deep sleep caused by alcohol or mind-altering drugs. Also, soft surfaces or loose covers can cause suffocation. They point out that there is no evidence that bed-sharing protects against sudden infant death syndrome. Also, there is no evidence that bed-sharing prevents extreme fussiness/colic.

So, if you want to use a family bed, try to make it a safe environment by not drinking or taking drugs at night and making sure your baby is always sleeping on his back. Also, fill in the spaces between the bed and any walls or furniture and eliminate loose bedding.

Different Decisions for Different Babies

Research – both my own and others' – has shown that about 80 per cent of babies have common fussiness and 20 per cent have extreme fussiness, also called 'colic'. What happens to these babies over the first four months? At four months of age, some children are super-calm, regular, smiling all the time and good sleepers, while other babies are the opposite. The good sleepers are described as having an 'easy' temperament; the opposite have a 'difficult' temperament. Some children are more in-between and are described as having an 'intermediate' temperament. How you care for your baby influences the temperament at four months of age.

These temperaments are explained in detail in Chapter 4. For now, I will just lead you through a numerical exercise involving a hypothetical group of a hundred babies. The reason this exercise is useful is because it might:

1. **Help you set your expectations on what you will need to do with your baby, both during the first several weeks (for soothing) and the following several months (to prevent sleep problems).**
2. **Help you decide whether you will breast-feed or bottle-feed.**
3. **Help you decide whether you will use a family bed or cot.**

Out of a group of one hundred babies, 80 per cent (eighty babies) will have common fussiness, and 20 per cent (twenty) will have extreme fussiness/colic. My research has shown that these two groups of babies differ in how their temperaments develop.

Consider the eighty common fussy babies at four months of age:

A. 49 per cent, or thirty-nine babies, are temperamentally easy
B. 46 per cent, or thirty-seven babies, are temperamentally intermediate
C. 5 per cent, or four babies, are temperamentally difficult

Consider the twenty extremely fussy/colicky babies at four months of age:

D. 14 per cent, or three babies, are temperamentally easy
E. 59 per cent, or twelve babies, are temperamentally intermediate
F. 27 per cent, or five babies, are temperamentally difficult

Of the original hundred babies, the largest temperament group is 'intermediate'. Forty-nine babies (49 per cent) are in the temperamental category of intermediate. Temperament measurements form a gradation and the temperament categories represent arbitrary cut-off points. So it is possible that the thirty-seven babies in group B, who had common fussiness, tend towards being temperamentally easier and the twelve babies in group E, who had extreme fussiness/colic, tend towards being more difficult. I suspect that the parents of the twelve babies in group E had to put forth much more soothing effort into this intermediate temperament group than the parents of the thirty-seven babies in group B.

Of the original hundred babies, the next largest temperament group is 'easy'. Forty-two babies (42 per cent) are in the temperamental category of easy. Of these, thirty-nine babies in group A were born mellow, self-soothing and calm, and/or their parents were unusually skilful in soothing and/or their parents had vast resources to help them soothe their babies. Not so with the three babies in group D. These babies had extreme fussiness/colic at birth. They were not born mellow, self-soothing or calm. I think these lucky three babies had super-hero parents who put forth enormous effort to soothe and probably also had lots of other resources to help them maintain this effort over four months.

The smallest temperament group is 'difficult'. Only nine babies (9 per cent) of the original hundred are in this temperament category. The four babies in group C had common fussiness, but they may have been almost, but not quite, extremely fussy/colicky. Remember, the measurements used to determine whether a baby has common fussiness or extreme fussiness/colic are graded, and arbitrary cut-off points are used to make the determination. Alternatively, for these four common fussy babies, maybe *something went wrong* with the parents' ability to soothe. Why might parents be unable to really soothe their baby? Some reasons may include maternal depression, an unsupportive husband, too many other children to care for, illness, financial problems, stress from the extended family, and marital problems between husband and wife. The five babies in group F may have overwhelmed all the resources that the parents could bring to bear on soothing their baby. This implies that factors within the baby were so powerful that no matter what the parents did, the baby's extreme fussiness/colic led to a difficult temperament at four months of age. It is also possible that the difficult temperament evolved because there was a combination of factors within the baby in addition to the problems within the parents or family that conspired to create an overtired child. Pre-existing problems such as marital discord only get worse when parents are trying to cope with an extremely fussy/colicky baby. Parents' inability to soothe may grow out of, or be a response to, the fatigue, frustration and exhaustion of trying, without much success, to soothe an extremely fussy/colicky baby.

I believe that how babies sleep influences the development of temperament at four months of age. And how babies sleep during the first few months is a combination of both factors within the child and the parents' ability and skill at soothing. It is also my belief that at four months of age, the difficult temperament represents an overtired baby and the easy temperament represents a well-rested baby. The temperament that your baby has at four months of age is **not** permanent. Temperament changes over time as babies develop and parents change how they soothe their children. Stability of individual temperament measures does appear to develop during the second year of life or shortly after the second birthday. If you are reading this book before you have had your baby, be prepared to invest enormous efforts in soothing and consider yourself unlucky if your child is among the 20 per cent of extremely fussy/colicky babies. However, if you have already had your baby and you are in the midst of suffering through four months of extreme fussiness/colic, re-evaluate some of your decisions, if necessary, regarding how you soothe your baby and what is best for your baby and family. Be optimistic because everything settles down at about four months. Everyone gets a second chance at about four months to help their child sleep better.

Common Fussiness

Eighty per cent of babies have common fussiness, and the parents of these babies are lucky. These babies do not require a lot of parental soothing. They tend to be self-soothing, mild and calm; they fall asleep easily and sleep for long periods.

Breast-feeding these babies is relatively easy because the mothers tend to be better rested and the babies tend to be more regular. The duration of a breast-feeding, how long you nurse, may be relatively short and infrequent because nursing is mainly for satisfying thirst and hunger. When these babies are fussy, methods of soothing other than breast-feeding often work. In fact, the popularity of many techniques or strategies for soothing babies is due to the fact that, for these babies, most everything works well!

Bottle-feeding these babies either formula or expressed breast milk with or without breast-feeding is a family decision that is usually easily made. Some considerations are to allow the father or other children the pleasure of feeding the baby, thus enabling the mother to get some needed extra sleep at night, to return to work by continuing to pump her breasts at work, or to make it easier for the parents to arrange an evening for an old-fashioned date.

Before your baby is born, you might decide that you want to sleep with your baby or that you want to use a cot or bassinet. For 80 per cent of all babies, those with common fussiness, it doesn't matter, they are fairly adaptable and self-soothing. You can sleep with your baby at both naps and at night, or only at night. Or, you might sleep with your baby when she first falls asleep, put her down in her cot, and then at the first night feeding, bring her into bed with you. Or, you might have a co-sleeper attached to your bed and use it for part or all of the night. You can put your baby to sleep within one to two hours of wakefulness. Watch for drowsy cues that are usually obvious in these babies, then any soothing-to-sleep method is likely to work and the baby and parents usually sleep well. Parents are at a low risk for feeling distressed, and I think maternal depression is not very likely. Some of these common fussy babies, however, will occasionally behave like the extremely fussy/colicky baby and your plans might have to be altered. Only about 5 per cent of these babies seem to develop into overtired four-month-olds.

During the first four weeks, your baby is really 'sleeping like a baby'. Elliot, my first son, described his first son as having a look on his face like 'I didn't do it', or seeming almost intoxicated during this time. Sleeping with your baby in your bed or placing your baby in the cot is usually a piece of cake. During weeks four to eight, your baby will become more wakeful and alert and have more evening fussiness. Elliot said that his son now had a more quizzical look, like 'Who are you?' and 'Give me back my pacifier'.

Extreme Fussiness/Colic

Twenty per cent of babies have extreme fussiness/colic, and the parents of these babies are unlucky. These babies require a lot of parental soothing. They tend not to be self-soothing and they often appear intense, agitated, and have difficulty falling asleep and staying asleep.

Breast-feeding these babies is often difficult because the mothers tend to be exhausted or fatigued from sleep deprivation and the babies tend to be irregular. The duration of the breast-feeding, how long you nurse, may be long and frequent because in addition to satisfying thirst and hunger, much of the nursing is for reducing fussiness. When these babies are extremely fussy, methods of soothing other than breast-feeding often do not work. Frustration or despair is common because many of the popular techniques or strategies for soothing babies fail, even though many other mothers (80 per cent) swear by them.

Some considerations going through the mind of the mother are whether something is wrong with her breast milk, whether her breast milk is sufficient, or whether her diet or the current formula is causing the extreme fussiness/colic. Because soothing at the breast often seems to work when other soothing methods fail, the mother does not want to give it up. But painfully dry or cracked skin around the nipple may make breast-feeding an ordeal. The discomfort and pain associated with breast-feeding, plus unrelenting exhaustion from sleep deprivation, may conspire to cause so much stress that the breast milk supply becomes insufficient. Mothers who have enormous support – a dedicated husband who spends a lot of time soothing, housekeeping help or baby care help – can get through this difficult time much more easily than mothers who lack a support system. Mothers who have other children to care for, pressure to return to work, medical problems, baby blues or postpartum depression may find the additional stresses associated with breast-feeding these extremely fussy/colicky babies to be overwhelming.

Bottle-feeding these babies either formula or expressed breast milk can be a benefit to some mothers or create more stress in others. The benefits of complete or partial bottle-feeding is that the mother might get more rest because others can feed her baby, and the parents are calmer because they know for certain that their baby is not hungry because they can see how much the baby is swallowing. In other mothers, giving bottles can create the feeling of having failed as a mother. Recognising that bottles are not as soothing as the breast, these mothers feel guilty because they think they are causing their babies to fuss/cry more, and they worry that something in the formula is causing the fussiness/crying. If you want to breast-feed, a compromise position is to have someone else give a single bottle of expressed breast once per twenty-four hours. This will not cause 'nipple confusion' or interfere with lactation. It will give the mother a mini-break, will allow her to get a little more sleep, and it will allow the parents a night out.

Before your baby is born, you might decide that you want to sleep with your baby or that you want to use a cot or bassinet. But for 20 per cent of babies, those with extreme fussiness/colic, the plans that you made for sleeping with your baby might have to be altered because these babies tend to be difficult to soothe and have difficulty falling asleep and staying asleep. Watching for drowsy cues is usually frustrating in these babies because they are not obvious, and even if you keep the intervals of wakefulness less than one to two hours, it is still difficult to soothe them. When they finally do fall asleep, they do not stay asleep for long. As a result, parents are often sleep deprived. Parents are at a high risk of feeling distressed and I think that maternal depression is more likely to occur.

Because these babies are difficult to soothe, breast-feeding in the family bed may be the best or only strategy that works. Although the mother's sleep may be fragmented by frequent feeding for both nutrition and soothing, this is probably the most powerful soothing method for these babies. During the first four weeks, your baby is not really 'sleeping like a baby'. Placing your baby in the cot is usually stressful. During weeks four through eight, your baby will become even more wakeful and alert and have more evening fussiness, causing the parents to be at an even greater risk for distress. About 27 per cent of these infants are at risk for becoming overtired four-month-olds.

There is some research to suggest that parents who made the commitment to use the family bed from day one, and stick with it, will wind up with better-rested babies than those families who initially wanted to use the cot but later brought their baby into their bed because it was the only way the parents could get any sleep. In the former group, sleep problems are less likely to develop as the children get older. But in the group where it was used only in response to soothing or sleeping difficulties, the family bed appears to be a short-term solution, but in reality it creates a long-term sleep problem. What really is happening is that parents who are overwhelmed by the fussy/crying behaviour and have limited resources for soothing their baby, reluctantly use the family bed to gain some relief, but the limited resources for soothing persist and may often cause sleeping problems in older children. (This will be discussed more in Chapter 5.)

Breast-feeding the Fussy Baby

by Nancy Nelson, RN, IBCLC

One of the most difficult things for many breast-feeding mothers is not knowing how much milk your baby is getting. When you are the mother of a 'fussy baby' it can be even more of a concern. When a baby is crying, most well-meaning observers will comment that the baby must be hungry. As the mother, these comments may cause you to feel frustrated and guilty. After all, you are responsible for feeding the baby! To allay your fears, keep track of the baby's output of urine and stool. After the sixth day of life, your baby should be producing six or more wet nappies and one or more stools in a twenty-four-hour period as a sign of adequate intake of breast milk. Babies usually need to feed eight to twelve times in a twenty-four-hour period during the first few weeks of life. In the beginning they may cluster feed. This means they may want to feed very frequently for a few hours and then go into a sleep stretch of four or five hours. As they become more efficient, they decrease the number of feedings. The baby should be back to birth weight by two weeks of age and should gain a minimum of five ounces a week for the next two to three months.

If you are concerned that your baby is fussy because you have a **low milk supply**, it would be helpful to see a lactation consultant who will do a feeding observation. This includes a study of your baby's ability to transfer milk from your breast by a strong nutritive suck followed by audible swallows. A pre- and postfeeding weight should be included in order to get an idea of how much milk the baby is taking in during the feeding. The baby should be weighed both before and after the feeding with a nappy on so as not to lose the weight of urine or stool that may have been produced during the feeding. This can be reassuring if the baby gains between two and four ounces during the feeding. If the baby gains less, it might alert you to a problem with either the baby's method of transferring the milk or your milk supply. If the milk supply is low or the flow is too slow, a supplemental feeding system may help to improve the suck and give the baby the additional calories he needs. Use of a hospital-grade electric breast pump can augment the breast milk supply as well. Some mothers may decide to feed the baby additional pumped breast milk by bottle or feed formula if they are unable to pump enough milk to meet the baby's needs.

Occasionally **breast engorgement** may cause the baby to be fussy at the breast. To deal with engorgement, use warm compresses or take a warm shower prior to feeding the baby. Use breast massage as well. You may be able to express some milk by hand or with a good-quality breast pump to take out a little milk and make the breast softer and easier for the baby to latch on to. Do not pump too much milk because it could continue an oversupply problem and prolong the engorgement. In between feedings, use cold compresses on your breasts to decrease the swelling and give pain relief. Engorgement may occur within the first week after your baby is born or later when the baby begins to skip feedings as he gets older.

A baby can be fussy at the breast if the mother has **flat or inverted nipples**. Breast shells may be worn in between the feedings in order to evert the nipples. Using a breast pump for a few minutes prior to putting the baby to the breast will help to pull the nipples out and also start the flow of milk so the baby will get milk right away and be more likely to continue sucking instead of pulling off the breast and crying. Occasionally, nipple shields may help to keep the baby at the breast until the nipples are more everted. This should happen after about two to four weeks of breast-feeding. Seek the help of a lactation consultant as soon as possible if you are having difficulty with the feedings because of flat or inverted nipples.

A baby may be fussy at the breast because of **poor positioning**. Both mother and baby may be uncomfortable, which can lead to inadequate letdown and poor milk production. With a fussy baby, the rugby hold (where the baby is held on the side of the body and tucked close to the chest, so the baby is breastfeeding at the breast closest to that side) or the cradle-hold (holding the baby horizontally over the chest while breastfeeding) work best because you have more control over the baby's head. You can direct him to the breast and keep him there with these two positions. The baby's nose and chin should indent the breast. Babies usually nurse better when they are held more firmly by the mother. A firm pillow that supports the baby at the level of the breast is preferable to a soft pillow. A chair that gives good support is better than a soft couch. I cannot emphasise enough that a fussy baby will respond better to being held tightly and close in to the breast. Contact a lactation consultant if you are uncomfortable during breast-feeding. This may be the reason why your baby is fussy.

Almost all babies have some degree of **gastro-oesophageal reflux**. This is a medical term and simply means that the sphincter muscle, which leads to the stomach, is immature and may not close completely all the time. This allows some milk, along with stomach acid, to come back up into the oesophagus, leading to a feeling we call 'heartburn'. As anyone who has experienced this can attest, it is quite uncomfortable. Just as sitting upright can help an adult with heartburn feel better, holding the baby upright usually helps the baby feel better, too. Sometimes these episodes can occur during breast-feeding. Holding the baby more upright during the feeding or interrupting the feeding for a short time to comfort the baby by holding him in an upright position should help. Using a swing or a car seat may also help. As the baby matures, so does the muscle, and the episodes become less frequent. Sometimes a baby has a severe problem with reflux and is unable to feed well at all. This may be a case where prescription medication will be needed. Your health care provider should be consulted.

All new babies experience **wind**. When the baby begins to feed, it sets off a reflex that produces wind so that the baby will be able to pass whatever waste products are produced during the feeding more quickly. This avoids problems with constipation. Because breast milk needs little digestion it moves through the baby's system very quickly. You can often hear the sounds while the baby is still feeding. Although all babies are windy, some babies are not as upset by it as others seem to be. The time of day may be a factor as well. It often seems as if this wind problem becomes worse at the end of the day. This is often called the traditional 'fussy' time of the day. Babies seem to want to stay at the breast constantly and this may exacerbate the wind problem. The baby may need comforting or some cluster feeding. It is a good idea to pump a bottle of breast milk in the morning when the baby is calmer and not feeding so often. Have this milk available during this fussy time to allow another family member to feed the baby so you can get a break. As babies mature this problem resolves.

The milk at the beginning of the feeding from the breast is higher in lactose. This is called the 'foremilk'. The milk that comes after ten to fifteen minutes of nursing from that same breast is called the 'hindmilk'. It is higher in fat and balances out the lactose so as not to produce so much wind. If the baby takes in too much foremilk and no hindmilk, it may result in **lactose overload** and more wind production. Try to keep the baby on one breast for at least twelve to fifteen minutes in order to get the hindmilk. As the baby gets older and becomes more efficient at nursing, he will be able to get to the hindmilk in a shorter period of time. Hindmilk can have a sedating effect on the baby and help a fussy baby to fall asleep. Most new babies will naturally fall asleep at the end of a feeding because of the sedating effects of the hindmilk. Recently there has been advice given to awaken the baby at the end of the feeding in order to allow them to fall asleep in the cot on their own. I feel that as babies get to be three or four months old, they will remain more awake at the end of the feeding. This is the time for them to learn how to put themselves to sleep. This pattern should be allowed to develop naturally.

When the baby is just learning how to breast-feed, the **let-down reflex may be overwhelming** and lead to gagging and choking. This may cause the baby to pull off the breast and become fussy. Put firm pressure over the breast for a minute to stop the rapid flow and put the baby back to the breast. Try to pump a little milk prior to the feeding to see if you can elicit the letdown before the baby goes to the breast. This may not help too much because usually the baby will elicit a more forceful letdown, but it is worth a try. The rugby hold (see page 89) or holding the baby in a sitting position on your lap might help. The baby straddles your body with his legs and faces you directly. As the baby gets older, he will be able to handle the letdown reflex without a problem in any feeding position.

Allergic reactions to foods in the mother's diet are rare but sometimes occur. The most common cause of allergy is cow's milk. Besides extreme fussiness with feeding, there is frequent spitting up, blood in the stool and poor weight gain. The baby's GP should be contacted if these symptoms occur. If you must go on an elimination diet, make sure that you get information about how to supplement your diet so that you remain in good health and can continue to produce enough breast milk for your baby. It usually takes at least two weeks to see results from an elimination diet.

Rarely will **soaps or creams being used on the breast or nipples** cause the baby to fuss and pull off the breast. If you have started using something new on your skin and the baby fusses, clean it off and start over.

Yeast infections can occur in the baby's mouth or on the mother's nipples. You might see white patches in the baby's mouth. The baby may also develop a nappy rash. Your nipples could be very red or itchy. There is a burning sensation of the nipples following the feeding. Your baby may be fussier during his feedings. See your GP. If a yeast infection is diagnosed, both you and the baby should be treated. If the baby is using bottle teats or dummies, these should be replaced with new ones. They should be washed daily with hot soapy water and allowed to air dry. Change your diet by eating more yogurt or taking an acidophilus supplement daily.

Some babies become fussy if they are **overstimulated**. They may have better breast-feeding sessions if the lights are dim and they are allowed to feed with only ambient sounds.

If you have implemented these suggested techniques and you still have a **fussy baby**, it may be that the baby is not hungry. She may be drawn to the breast for comfort, but once she starts to nurse does not really need to feed at that time. Remember, a baby under twelve weeks of age does not have much ability to self-soothe. As parents, we need to meet these needs just as much as we need to provide them with the other necessities of life. Many of the things that seem to help soothe them are measures that imitate the in utero environment. Make sure that the baby is comfortable – not too warm or too cold. A clean nappy should be provided. The baby may be comforted by being held tightly and cuddled or rocked. Besides cuddling and rocking, swaddling, or ongoing sounds like music, dryers, or fans may help. Perhaps a dummy will give your baby some additional soothing. The use of a soft side or front sling will give you the chance to get other things done while you are providing comfort for your baby. Another person – the father or a grandparent – may be enlisted to calm the baby without the baby being stimulated by the smell of the breast milk that envelops the mother. This also gives the mother a chance to get a little time for herself. Try to take a nap or get some exercise. These activities will help you feel refreshed.

Later, after the baby has been calmed by other methods, the mother will be ready to breast-feed more calmly.

It takes time and the trying of different techniques to find out what your baby needs and how best to meet those needs. Feel free to experiment. The baby may respond to certain things at one time and to other things at another time. Remember, it is a learning process, so don't expect you or the baby to be perfect.

Take good care of yourself during this time. Eat well. Take your prenatal vitamins. Stay well hydrated and get some outdoor exercise, if not daily at least five days per week. Try to use relaxation techniques – yoga, meditation, massage or a warm bath – to help you get through the difficult times. Share your feelings with the baby's father or other family members and let them take turns walking, rocking and cuddling the baby. Set small goals for yourself – like reading one chapter in a book or taking a fifteen-minute walk.

New-mother support groups help a lot because you learn that other mothers and babies are going through the same adjustment period that you are. Most reasons for infant fussiness will be worked out within the first six weeks of life. A few may take a little longer, but by three months of age it is usually resolved. Remember, overall, this is a very short time in the life of you and your baby. Try to hug and cuddle your baby as much as you can in order to help him get through this rough time. Together you can do it.

As discussed by Nancy Nelson, lactation consultants can be very helpful and I would encourage you to seek one who has been certified by the International Board of Lactation Consultant Examiners (IBLCE) and is entitled to use the title International Board Certified Lactation Consultant (IBCLC). In general, successful breast-feeding will require the family to make adjustments to fit the needs of the baby, and breast-feeding may not work well if the parents attempt to force the baby to fit into the family's schedule, especially if the baby has extreme fussiness/colic.

Keep reminding yourself that extreme fussiness/colic is not indigestion. It is not caused by formula or breast milk. Switching from one formula to another will not stop the crying. Some manufacturers of infant formula try to sell their product by claiming that their product will reduce fussiness. The so-called research they cite to support their claims is weak, unconvincing and has not been reproduced.

Do not let extreme fussiness make you give up breast-feeding if you want to continue. Your baby is still getting all the benefits of breast milk, even if she seems at times not to appreciate them. If you stick with it, you can look forward to many calm, pleasant months of nursing once the extreme fussiness has run its course.

Still, nursing an extremely fussy baby is undeniably a challenge. When feeding, infants with extreme fussiness/colic tend to be gulpers, twisters and forceful suckers. Sometimes they seem to reject the breast entirely. The determined nursing mother is in a fix; it is difficult to nurse a tense, twisting infant, but nursing is one of the few manoeuvres that appear to calm such a child (at least temporarily). Non-nutritive nursing, using your breasts as a dummy, may calm baby, but it is no picnic for mother! Here is a description of the nursing predicament by the mother of one of my young patients.

The first three weeks of Michael's life led me to believe that having a baby would be a breeze. His behaviour was almost identical from day to day. He was very calm, and so were my husband and I. Michael would eat – breast-feeding about eight to ten minutes on each side. He had no problems burping after each meal. Then I'd either hold him for a while, lay him on his back, and talk or play with him. The usual schedule, from the time he got up until he went to sleep, would be one to one and a half hours. He would usually sleep anywhere from two and a half to four hours. Everyone said to me, 'You're so lucky to have such a good baby.'

As the fourth week approached, Michael's behaviour changed dramatically. He no longer wanted to sleep during the day. I felt

> as though all he wanted was my breast. I concluded that he either was continually hungry or had strong sucking needs.
>
> By the middle of each afternoon, I was exhausted. Almost every hour I found myself breast-feeding. Sometimes I could put him off for two hours, but he'd cry a lot. I'd change his nappy, walk him, hold him, tilt him, sing to him, change his position and so on. Nothing would please him except my breast, which was terribly tiring, to say the least. The thing that saved our lives is that he slept long hours through the night – probably from exhaustion after being up all day. The worst times were mid-afternoon, and again between 5:00 and 10:00 P.M., after which he would sleep for around five hours straight. He would fuss and cry and nothing would calm him except when he was nursing.

If your situation is similar to this mother's, give yourself some relief by trying the following suggestions:

1. Space feedings a few hours apart. One mother said, 'I must have Chinese breast milk; he gets hungry just one hour after nursing.' If you last nursed your baby well less than two hours ago (not a snack or a sip), there is no room in his stomach for more milk and your breasts contain little or no milk for him. Nursing too frequently is pointless, and if it causes you pain or exhaustion, it is destructive. See if the baby will accept a dummy instead.
2. Ask your doctor about hydrocortisone ointment. A famous paediatric dermatologist who nursed her own children suggests treating cracked nipples with 1 per cent hydrocortisone ointment. It is safe for both mother and baby, and seems to work better than any other treatment. Many of my patients' mothers have reported rapid healing of sore nipples by using this treatment. After nursing, allow your breasts to air dry. Then apply a thin film of the 1 per cent hydrocortisone ointment to the dry or cracked areas. Make sure you use ointment, not cream; the cream might cause a painful burning sensation. When you are about to nurse again, do not

wipe or wash off any of the ointment. Most of it will have been absorbed into your breast skin and the small amount the baby absorbs will cause no harm. Basically, the skin of the breast can become very dry, cracked or fissured from being wet or damp for prolonged periods of time.

3. Don't exhaust yourself. The mother of an extreme fussy infant stored breast milk so her husband could feed the baby once during the night and her mother could handle a similar daytime feeding. In this way, she was able to get some extra rest. When the baby was several weeks old, the baby's grandmother went home and the father returned to work. Now, all alone and very busy, the mother saw her previously ample supply of breast milk dwindle to almost nothing. We discussed how she had decreased her fluid intake, how she was worried about her mother's departure, and how she was generally under strain. I reassured her that while it was important to continue having the child suck at her breasts to stimulate milk production, a single bottle of formula for one or two days would not harm the baby or inhibit lactation. She increased her fluid intake, rested more, and after four to five days was again nursing with more than ample milk production. Throughout this period, the child continued to have extreme fussiness/ colic spells with periods of inconsolable crying. But this mother now knew that the crying was not related to nursing.

Another mother of one of my patients felt especially bad when nursing failed to calm her baby.

> It's early evening and my daughter is screaming and restless. Nothing seems to calm her, not even nursing. I didn't think Chelsea was colicky, but she really was fussy. Although her fussiness wasn't an everyday occurrence, it persisted from her second or third week of life until about two months of age.

At first I thought something I was eating was giving her wind. Then I thought her behaviour was due to my inexperience as a mother. As these episodes continued, I began to feel desperate, sad and exhausted.

I felt inadequate as a parent. I didn't know how to comfort my child, or whether what I was doing was right. I especially felt inadequate when Chelsea rejected my breast. It seemed as if nothing could console and comfort her.

We had visions of a child who could be comforted at the touch of her mum or dad. Soon all the sleepless nights and exaggerated feelings of incompetency led to exhaustion. Would this cycle ever end? Well, it finally did. With the help of our paediatrician, we soon began to realise that this behaviour was normal and would not last indefinitely. I also found that her fussiness was neither caused nor enhanced by my behaviour. Along with this realisation came the light at the end of the tunnel. I then knew her fussiness would not last forever.

I became aware of certain behavioural changes that manifested themselves either before or after each fussy period. She would startle easily, have difficulty falling asleep and then sleep for shorter periods of time. Also, during her fussy periods, she exhibited different behavioural characteristics. She was restless and would scream with a quivering chin. She would become stiff or have rigid movements. She would not nurse, and when she did she would suck frantically. She would become overtired but would not sleep. Sometimes she would be wide awake one moment and sound asleep a second later.

Chelsea is now three months old. Her fussy periods have ceased and she wakes in the morning with a smile that lasts all day. We really love our 'perfect' child.

Sometimes a nursing mother notices that the baby seems calmer in her husband's arms than in her own. She may feel that her husband does a better job of soothing the baby, that perhaps the baby 'prefers' him to her. What is really happening is quite simple. The baby recognises that his mother is the source of milk. When she holds him, he quite naturally squirms and twists, rooting around, looking to suck, even when he's not hungry.

I want to encourage every mother's desire to nurse her extreme fussy/colicky baby. It is an important accomplishment for both of them. One mother called me when her extremely fussy/colicky baby was exactly three months old. She was determined to continue nursing and to start working part-time. Her husband was a fireman and found it very difficult to be around a crying baby on his days off. She was under enormous stress. All her friends claimed that if she would feed her baby formula, the crying would disappear. She wanted to – and did – keep on nursing after the extreme fussiness/colic disappeared to show them, and herself, that nursing was not the cause of the crying. Here is a report from the mother of another one of my patients; persevering with nursing helped her maintain her confidence and self-esteem.

> Both my husband and I questioned our best judgements and our ability to care for Lisa. At one point I questioned my ability to nurse and felt that I was literally poisoning my baby. Her screaming episodes came a predictable ten minutes after every feeding. At times I felt tortured. I consider myself a rational and caring person, yet often found myself crying in the shower or praying that my husband could somehow relieve the tension, anger and helplessness that I felt.
>
> At six weeks, Lisa seemed to be easing into patterns and appeared to be getting good, deep sleep. Her smiling times were numerous, but she still had hours of screaming. I overcame my fear of nursing and decided to continue weeks after I had planned to stop. Nursing became the one pleasurable experience the baby and I had together. When I finally did wean Lisa, it was a sad time; we were separate after being together for so long.

Six weeks of age or *six weeks after the due date* is truly a magic turning point for many babies.

Solid Foods and Feeding Habits

Do you remember how drowsy you feel after eating a huge celebration dinner? Big meals make us sleepy, so shouldn't solids make babies sleep better? Wrong. Feeding rhythms do not alter the pattern of waking and sleeping.

Sleeping for long periods at night is not related to the method of feeding, whether it be breast or bottle. This is a fact; look at some of the studies cited at the end of this book (see page 458). The studies I think are the most convincing involve comparing the development of sleep/wake rhythms of infants fed on demand with those who are continuously fed intravenously because of birth defects involving their stomachs or intestines. The babies who were fed on demand cycled between being hungry and being full. The other babies were never allowed to become hungry. The objective recordings in sleep laboratories show that there were no sleep differences between these groups of infants. Other studies involve the introduction of solid foods; they all show that solid food, such as cereal, does not influence night-time sleeping patterns. No published studies have ever shown that the method of feeding (breast milk versus formula, or scheduled feedings versus demand feedings) or the introduction of solids affects sleep.

Some studies, however, do indicate that formula-feeding is more popular than breast-feeding among mothers who are more restrictive. Mothers who feed their babies formula tend to be more interested in controlling their infant's behaviour and like being able to see the number of ounces of formula given at each feeding. These parents are more likely to perceive night waking in a problem/solution framework and consider the social wants of the child instead of nutritional needs. In contrast, the nursing mother, perhaps more sensitive to the health benefits of breast-feeding, might respond to night waking more often or more rapidly because she perceives herself as primarily responding to her infant's need for nourishment. After a while, of course, the child learns to enjoy this nocturnal social contact. Over time, the baby learns to expect attention when he awakens.

This explains why there is no difference in night waking between breast- and formula-fed infants at four months, but by six to twelve months, night waking is more of an issue among breast-fed babies.

The bottom line is that cereal does not make babies sleep better. Formula may appear thicker than breast milk, but both contain the same twenty calories per 28 grams. Giving formula to breast-fed babies or weaning them also will not directly cause longer sleeping at night, although it is possible that attitudes toward breast-feeding may indirectly foster a night-waking habit. Here is one family's account of how breast-feeding led to a night-waking habit.

Maren's Wake-up for Breast-feeding

Maren was born on 18 July 1984, after an uneventful pregnancy and an easy delivery, three days past term.

We were committed to breast-feeding, with no preconceived expectations of its duration. Maren behaved as a normal infant for about two weeks, at which point persistent crying spells began to occur daily. Though we were assured real colic was worse, we came to refer to these spells as 'Maren's colic'. We endured the inconsolable crying without much complaint. Although her crying mostly lasted one to two hours, the worst individual days would include unabated crying spells lasting for eight to ten hours. Various experiments were tried to ease the colic suffering, including having Maren sleep with us, having her sleep on a hot-water bottle, and so on. Predictably, none worked. At two months, the colic ended relatively abruptly.

From two months on, a very happy, trusting relationship developed between Maren and me. For about seven months, Maren was fed virtually exclusively on breast milk. From seven to ten months, increasing amounts of solid food were introduced at breakfast and lunch. Maren has always been a happy, bubbly, joyful child. The breast-feeding seemed to contribute to this sunny disposition. Maren's nap patterns were completely normal. Generally, I would sleep with her in the morning. Part of the feeding ritual for these ten months included twice-nightly breast-feeds for Maren, interrupting my sleep.

Massive campaigns were mounted by both sets of grandparents to convince me that breast-feeding needed to end. These began at two months and reached fever pitch around seven months. We listened politely. Except for a brief experimental period at around eight months, I didn't attempt to pump my breasts to permit me extra sleep. This was a conscious decision; direct feeding was easier and more satisfying for both of us.

Breast-feeding, in addition to the satisfaction it provided, was an indispensable part of the sleeping ritual. From birth to eleven months, Maren expected to be held, fed and gently rocked or lulled to sleep in the pleasant company of her mother. At around nine months, Maren's rapid growth was taking its toll. There was more solid food in the daytime now. After nearly a year without a full night's sleep, I was beginning to reach a whole new level of fatigue.

New attempts were begun to get Maren to sleep without my direct attention. Her father would give her a bottle, rock her and sing to her. Female friends of the family, familiar to Maren, would do the same. Maren was a good sport about these experiments but preferred my attention. At eleven months, we agreed it was time to wean Maren to a bottle.

Maren didn't like the plan much. She obviously disliked formula as much as I disliked feeding it to her. For nearly a week she rejected cow's milk. I ended the morning nap breast-feeding ritual first. Juices (orange, apple, pear) in the morning or during car rides helped to improve Maren's familiarity with bottles. They also allowed my husband, Larry, to feed her while I rested later in the mornings. Putting cow's milk in a special bottle (formed and painted to look like a dog) allowed this unpleasant white stuff to become gradually more acceptable. After a few days, Maren started to respond more favourably to her 'pooch juice' and the games I created and associated with it.

I experienced some depression with the cessation of breast-feeding. As that special link came to an end, my contribution to Maren's development suddenly seemed more mundane, repetitive and less satisfying. This depression came on and off for two months. It was a strange feeling, since it was offset at all times by the joy that comes from having a developing child.

Maren was fully weaned at eleven months. The last feeding to change over was at bedtime. But even if she was given milk at bedtime, Maren continued to wake up once or twice per evening, crying to be fed. The next step was to get her to sleep through the night. We were repeatedly advised to let her cry herself to sleep. The phrase 'even for five or six hours' was used, a reminder of colic days. We considered this proposition, but continued to feed Maren warm milk, sing lullabies and rock her to sleep, once or twice per night. The big question: what was waking her up?

We decided it was mostly habit, and that she just wanted the comfort of our company. A new go-to-sleep ritual was introduced: after much playing and affection, Maren was put to bed with her favourite doll, not rocked to sleep. If she woke, warm milk was provided, but Maren was purposely not picked up. Maren cried ten minutes when left alone the first night, then rested her head on top of her favourite doll and drifted off to sleep. After expecting possibly an hour or more of crying, this was an unbelievable, almost anticlimactic relief to us. After two or three nights of feeding without picking her up, Maren began sleeping through the night.

At the end of month eleven, the go-to-sleep is routine. Maren rarely cries at all. Key elements: a big dinner, a bath, gentle play, 225 ml of warm milk, hugs and her favourite doll. Even a babysitter can do it. At one year, Maren had finally learned to sleep eight hours straight.

We did a few things we are sure were right. For us, especially me, we sensed Maren's needs and delivered them unasked. This created an extraordinary self-assurance in her, and led to a happy household. Maren seemed to cry less than other children and to be a bright, curious, quick learner. Other things we are happy about: lots of new games all the time; plenty of visual stimulation; boisterous motions and playing; exposure to music, texture, any stimulation we could dream up. It all seemed to add to her alertness, her trust in us, and the regularity of her sleeping.

There are also some things we may not have done so well. We may have gone too long before we tried to put her to sleep alone.

Our parents continuously warned us we were being too indulgent. They may have been right. But then, first-time parents are like that.

Solutions to Help Your Child Sleep Better: 'No Cry', 'Maybe Cry', or 'Let Cry'

There are many ways to help your child sleep. You should choose the solution that works best for you and your child. Some do not work well for the extremely fussy or colicky baby, some will be difficult to use because of limited resources for soothing and some are appropriate only for older children. Also, one method may be more powerful in the hands of some families than in others. Often I will refer to ignoring all crying or extinction as the preferred solution to help your child sleep better because I think this works best for the 20 per cent of babies who have extreme fussiness/colic; after four months of age, I think they represent the largest group of children with sleep problems or have more severe sleep problems. However, I understand that this is probably the hardest sleep solution for parents and you should always first consider trying other sleep solutions that involve less crying. This is especially true if your child does not have extreme fussiness/colic.

'NO CRY' SLEEP SOLUTIONS

Start early, when you come home from the hospital, to avoid the overtired state by trying to soothe your baby to sleep within *one to two hours of wakefulness*
Always hold your baby, always respond and soothe your baby as long as needed to induce sleep; sleep with your baby
Always respect 'drowsy signs' so your baby never becomes overtired
Always try to put your child to sleep drowsy but awake
Motionless sleep
Establish and consistently practise bedtime routines
Practise scheduled awakening, also known as focal feeding
Get fresh air in between naps, go for a walk

Control the wake-up time
Slowly and gradually give your child less attention around falling asleep or during the night
White noise
Room-darkening window shades
Relaxation
Stimulus control

'MAYBE CRY' SLEEP SOLUTIONS

Father puts baby to sleep
Make bedtime earlier
Focus on the morning nap
Sleep rules
Silent return to sleep
Day correction of bedtime problems

'LET CRY' SLEEP SOLUTIONS

Ignoring all crying or extinction
Ignoring some crying, also known as controlled crying or graduated extinction
Check and console
Cot tent

Parents have told me the first solution needs to be emphasised because it is not intuitively obvious that babies, who sleep so much, need to return to sleep after only one to two hours of wakefulness. In addition, this pattern of brief intervals of wakefulness appears to help many babies avoid sleep problems throughout the first four months.

> **MAJOR POINT**
>
> **Babies need to sleep after one to two hours of wakefulness.**

Prevention versus Treatment of Sleep Problems

There sometimes appears to be a contradiction between whether or not to let your child cry. For 80 per cent of babies who have common fussiness, if the parents have ample resources for soothing, sleep solutions that involve no crying, such as the 'one- to two-hour rule', should work to *prevent* sleep problems. A few, about 5 per cent, of common fussy babies do become very overtired four-month-olds. To *treat* or correct the sleep problem, some crying might occur. However, in this group, improvement in sleep patterns and improvement in the child is often dramatic and rapid.

For 20 per cent of babies with extreme fussiness or colic, however, if the parents have enormous resources for soothing, sleep solutions that involve no crying, such as 'Always hold your baby, always respond and soothe your baby as long as needed to induce sleep; sleep with your baby', might work to *prevent* sleep problems. But about 27 per cent of these extremely fussy/colicky babies do become very overtired four-month-olds. *Treatment* to correct the sleep problem might involve more crying, and improvement in sleep patterns and inprovement in the child is often slow and not dramatic. This is especially hard for parents because they have already endured four months of sleep deprivation associated with the child's constant fussiness, crying and not sleeping.

Rarely, some parents want to let their child cry to help him sleep after the peak of fussiness and crying has passed at six weeks of age, but he is under four months of age. One example is the mother who has to return to work and desperately wants to see if her child will sleep better at night with less attention. Another example is the exhausted and overwhelmed mother who is becoming depressed or getting angry or resentful towards her baby. Under these and similar circumstances, I usually try to enlist the assistance of the father to help his wife put the baby to sleep, to feed and soothe the baby at night, and to try to give the mother a well-earned break by making her go somewhere for several hours or a night to get some uninterrupted sleep. Obviously, these suggestions are impractical for some families. Nevertheless, the instructions are to give the child less attention at night, perhaps feeding only twice at night, and ignoring crying for either brief or long periods of time and to do this for only four or five nights. Sometimes the crying quickly diminishes, especially in the child who had common fussiness. Sometimes the crying does not decrease, especially in the child who had extreme fussiness or colic, and the plan is abandoned. Parents then resort to whatever method maximises sleep and minimises crying until the child is older.

Action Plan for Exhausted Parents

Healthy Sleep

Think of 'healthy' sleep as a collection or group of several related elements grouped together to form a 'package'. All must be present to ensure good-quality or healthy sleep. The five elements of healthy sleep are:

1. Sleep Duration: Night and Day

Does your child sleep as long as she needs at night and for naps?

How long your child needs to sleep depends on her age and temperament. Restricted sleep impairs mood, performance, development and cognitive ability.

2. Naps

Is your child taking naps or do you sometimes skip naps?

If a nap has been missed, try to keep your child up until the next sleep period in order to maintain the timeliness of the sleep rhythm. Move the next sleep period a little earlier before your child becomes extremely overtired. If the naps are too long because your child has become overtired; you might have to wake him from a nap in order to maintain the timeliness of the sleep rhythm at night. The morning nap develops before the afternoon nap and disappears before the afternoon nap. Not all naps are created equal. Babies are born to be short or long nappers. An earlier bedtime may be required when two naps are needed but you can get only one.

3. Sleep Consolidation

Is the sleep interrupted (fragmented) or uninterrupted (consolidated)?

Some arousals from sleep normally occur. Some arousals are protective. Too many arousals fragment sleep and this causes impairments in mood and performance.

4. Sleep Schedule, Timing of Sleep

Do naps start and bedtimes begin just when your child is becoming drowsy?

A bedtime that is too late will produce an abnormal daytime sleep schedule. Variability in activity and length of naps causes some variability in the bedtime. Watch your child more than the clock.

5. Sleep Regularity

Do naps or bedtimes occur at approximately the same times?

Even if the bedtime is a little too late, regular bedtimes are better than irregular bedtimes.

Resources for Soothing

Learn to recognise *drowsy signs* – study the box on page 63.

If your baby is colicky, begin the soothing to sleep after one to two hours of wakefulness. Soothing to sleep involves:

Getting dad to help out
Encouraging sucking – do not worry if your baby falls asleep while sucking
Rhythmic rocking motions
Swaddling
Massage

Consider a balance between the baby's disposition to express distress and the parents' capability to soothe their baby.

HEALTHY SLEEP IMPROVES

Mood, temperament, cognitive development and performance.

Never wake a sleeping baby.

Not only do babies vary in their expression of fussiness/crying, but parents also vary in their ability to soothe. The resources for parents' ability to soothe fussiness and crying and promote sleep in their baby include those shown in the box on page 74.

Bedtime Routines

Study the list on page 75.

Breast-feeding versus Bottle-feeding and Family Bed versus Cot

- **Breast-feeding: All the time, part time (expressed breast milk versus formula), never.**
  For about 80 per cent of babies, the common fussy babies, mothers are better rested and feeding is mostly for nutrition. Breast-feeding is usually easy.

  For about 20 per cent of babies, those with extreme fussiness/colic, mothers are fatigued from sleep deprivation. The stress from loss of sleep might inhibit lactation. Breast-feeding may be difficult because it is used for nutrition and soothing. Nursing more frequently and for longer durations might cause more discomfort or pain if the skin of the breast becomes cracked or dry. The mother might worry that there is not enough breast milk or her diet is causing the breast milk to upset the baby because of the extreme fussiness/crying. Consider a single bottle of expressed breast milk given once per twenty-four hours by someone else.
- **Family Bed: All the time, part time, never, with or without a co-sleeper.**
  For about 80 per cent of babies, those who have common fussiness, an early commitment to a family bed usually works well. Sleep problems later are unlikely.

  For about 20 per cent of babies, those with extreme

fussiness/colic, an early commitment to a family bed may be associated with sleep-deprived parents for several weeks, but the strong soothing power of bodily warmth, close physical contact, sounds of breathing, or hearing a heartbeat when sucking at the breast, or the smell of breast milk may make the effort worth it. Sleep problems might occur later if the child is allowed to stay up too late when about four months old.

During the day some parents with extremely fussy/colicky or common fussy babies are overwhelmed because they may have limited resources for soothing. For parents who initially did not want to have a family bed but later made that decision because of its soothing power, sleep problems are more likely to occur. The sleep problems are more likely to occur and persist not because of the family bed but because of the limited resources for soothing to continue.

Solutions to Help Your Child Sleep Better: 'No Cry', 'Maybe Cry', or 'Let Cry'

Start early, when you come home from the hospital, to put your child to sleep within one to two hours of wakefulness.

Study the list of sleep solutions on pages 103–104.

Different solutions are needed for different babies.

Does your baby require soothing more than three hours a day because he fusses or cries?
Does this occur more than three days a week?
Has this been going on for more than three weeks?

If you answered 'yes' to all three questions, your child has extreme fussiness or colic. Enlist all the soothing resources you can to help soothe your baby. If you want to, or if you need to, consider sleeping with your baby day and night for several weeks or months. Always hold your baby and always respond to her. Drowsy signs may be absent, so try to soothe her to sleep after one to two hours of wakefulness. Soothe your baby as long as needed to induce sleep. Motion may be needed during sleep to help your baby sleep longer.

If you answered 'no' to any of the questions, your child has common fussiness. Watch for drowsy signs developing within one to two hours of wakefulness. Soothe your baby and put her down or lie down with her when she is drowsy but awake. Motionless sleep may work well.

CHAPTER 3

Sleep Problems and Solutions

Disturbed Sleep

We really do not know how young children feel because they cannot talk to us; all we can do is observe them and guess their feelings. When they do not sleep well, their behaviour changes and presumably they feel worse. I think we should carefully consider how we feel and behave when our sleep is disturbed, so that we can better understand and sympathise with our children.

Daytime sleepiness resulting from disturbed sleep typically causes us to feel a mild itching or burning in the eyes. Our eyelids feel heavy. Our limbs feel heavy, too, and we tend to be lethargic. We are less motivated, lose interest easily and have difficulty concentrating. Our speech slows; we yawn and rub our eyes. As we get sleepier, our eyes begin to close and we may even find our head nodding.

But this familiar picture of adult sleep is not usually seen in infants and young children who suffer from disturbed sleep. While it is true that infants who are usually well rested yawn on occasions when they are overtired, it seems that chronically tired infants do not yawn much or nod off. Instead, when most tired young kids get sleepy, they get grumpy and excitable. My first son at age three coined the perfect word to describe this turned-on state: *upcited*, a combination of *upset* and *excited*, as in

'Don't make me upcited!' when we admonished him for behaving like a monster.

Mood and Performance

Before we look at common sleep problems, let's review how disturbed sleep affects mood and performance.

> **REMEMBER**
>
> **When your infant or young child appears wired, he may be tired.**

Two very interesting Australian studies on adults have helped to shed light on childhood 'upcited' behaviour. One study showed that the level of activation of the nervous system was associated with certain personality traits, sleep habits, and activity of the adrenal gland. Poor sleepers were more anxious and had higher levels of the hormone cortisol, which typically rises during stressful situations.

The second study was complex, but I think its results will better help you to understand your child's behaviours.

Adult volunteers report their moods on four scales:

1. **Tired to rested**
2. **Sluggish to alert**
3. **Irritable to calm**
4. **Tense to relaxed**

The first two scales reflect degrees of *arousal*, while the third and fourth scales reflect degrees of *stress*.

The researchers measured four different chemicals (cortisol, noradrenaline, adrenaline and dopamine) that our bodies make naturally. These powerful chemicals affect our brain and how we feel, and they are related to the four scales in different ways.

For example, fatigue produces an increase in adrenaline concentrations. That is, when we are tired, our body chemically responds with a burst of adrenaline to give us more drive or energy. We become more aroused, alert and excitable. Concentrations of cortisol, a stress-related hormone, also increase with increasing alertness. In children, cortisol concentrations remain high when they do not nap. Perhaps the nap allows the brain to be alert without needing the added boost cortisol would provide. Increasing irritability and tenseness – stress factors – are both associated with increasing concentrations of adrenaline, noradrenaline and dopamine. Yet the specific chemical patterns or biochemical fingerprints for irritability and tenseness are not the same.

These studies support the notion that when an overtired child appears wired, wild, edgy, excitable or unable to fall asleep easily or stay asleep, he is this way precisely because of his body's response to being overtired. Think of how you feel when you work hard and lose sleep in order to finish a major project. You are highly motivated and fight the daytime sleepiness. The impairments of performance and discomfort of sleepiness increase. After a while, you feel keyed up. This hyperalert state is a natural, protective, biologically adaptive response that enabled Neanderthal man to fight, flee or hunt prey even when tired. Thankfully, modern man is able to get out of this state by taking holidays. But have you noticed how, at the start of a holiday, it takes a few days to unwind?

It's a vicious circle: sleep begets sleep, but sleeplessness also begets sleeplessness. When babies miss the sleep they *need*, the fatigue causes a physical or chemical change in their bodies. These chemical changes directly affect their behaviour and interfere with maintaining either the quiet alert wakeful state or blissful sleep. The children are fractious because they are overtired.

> **IMPORTANT POINT**
>
> **Some chronically tired children are always keyed up and never unwind.**

Other studies also have proven that adults who sleep for only brief durations are more anxious. When we study adults who are irritable, feel tense, are poor sleepers and have high concentrations of these hormones, we find the old chicken-or-egg dilemma: which came first?

I think an experience familiar to all of us can help resolve the dilemma. As previously described, if we work hard to get an important job done, we can push our bodies with lots of caffeine-laden coffee and cola and very little sleep. At the end of the project, though, if we suddenly stop and take a holiday, it takes a few days to get rid of our accumulated nervous energy. We really cannot enjoy low-intensity pleasures, like walking barefoot on the grass or playing quietly with children, because we are all keyed up. After a few days, we eventually calm down, unwind and relax, and then we can enjoy recreational reading and quiet activities. This tells me that our lifestyle and sleep habits can affect our internal chemical machinery, which in turn causes us to feel certain ways. In a study at Dartmouth College, coronary-prone type A students had more night wakings than type B students. A vicious circle could develop whereby the fragmented sleep causes increased arousal, the student feels more energised, and, sensing this greater level of energy, works even harder late into the night to achieve more, but at the same time loses more sleep.

IMPORTANT POINT

Loss of sleep produces central nervous system hyperarousal.

Babies only two or three days old also have elevated cortisol levels during the period of behavioural distress following circumcision. Infants over four months of age as well as older children can push themselves hard fighting sleep in order to enjoy the pleasure of their parents' company and play. The resulting sleep disturbances might produce fatigue, and the body would naturally respond by turning up production of those chemicals, such as cortisol, responsible for maintaining alertness and arousal. Perhaps researchers may someday find that different patterns of sleep deprivation (total sleep loss, abnormal schedules, nap deprivation or sleep fragmentation) produce different patterns of chemical imbalances.

Here are some terms used by professionals to describe the behaviour of hyperalert, or 'wired', children with disturbed sleep:

Physiological activation
Neurological arousal
Excessive wakefulness
Emotional reactivity
Heightened sensitivity

Obviously we all get slightly irritable, short-tempered and grumpy when we do not get the sleep we need. Jokes and cartoons don't seem very funny when we're tired. But children might be even more sensitive to mild sleep loss, and yet simply appear to be wilder or more unmanageable. Perhaps off-the-wall behaviour in children is due to sleep loss that is severe, chronic and prolonged but not recognised as such by parents.

So often I have heard comments like, 'She's so tired, she's running around in circles.' This is not a new observation; a classic paper published in 1922 described the 'increased reflex-irritability of a sleepy child'. In dramatic contrast, over and over again I have seen well-rested children in my practice who spend enormous amounts of time in a state of quiet alertness. They take in everything with wide-open eyes, never missing a thing. They find simple little toys amusing or curious. They never appear bored, although the toy they pick up is one they have played with many times. Parents of children four to twelve months of age can dramatically change their children's behaviour depending on how much sleep they allow their kids to get.

In a study published in 2002 of four- to five-year-olds, author John E. Bates stated, 'In clinical treatment of young, opposi-tional children, we have seen some spectacular improvements in manageability associated with the parents instituting a more adequate schedule of sleep for their children. Our clinical impression in these cases was that the changes were too rapid to be accounted for by other changes, such as parental discipline tactics.'

REMEMBER AGAIN

A sign of sleeping well is a calm and alert state. Upon awakening, well-rested children are in good cheer and are able to play by themselves.

I believe that in infants and young children, a cause-and-effect relationship exists between disturbed sleep and fitful, fussy behaviours. In addition, as described in Chapter 2, the harmful effects of excessive daytime sleepiness do not stay the same, but rather tend to accumulate. This means that there is a progressive worsening in a child's mood and performance even when the amount of lost sleep each day or night is constant. So a baby becomes increasingly grumpy even if her nightly sleep is constantly just a little too brief.

PRACTICAL POINT

A constant small deficit in sleep produces a cumulative reduction in daytime alertness.

As the child develops, the relationship between disturbed sleep and problems of mood and performance becomes less clear because of the increasing complexity of psychological and intellectual function. It is even possible that chronically disturbed sleep causes children to grow up experiencing excessive daytime sleepiness, low self-esteem or mild depression. In one study, about 13 per cent of teenagers with disturbed sleep were reported to be like this. They usually took longer than forty-five minutes to fall asleep or woke frequently at night. Some of these teenagers may simply have never learned self-soothing skills to fall asleep easily when they were much younger. As adults, they are described as insomniacs.

One theory of adult insomnia is that it is characterised by an internalisation of emotions associated with a heightened or constant state of emotional arousal plus physiological activation, which causes disturbed sleep. But distinct differences exist between adult insomniacs whose insomnia started in childhood and those whose insomnia started in adulthood. The childhood-onset insomniacs took longer to fall asleep and slept less than the adult-onset insomniacs. I think this kind of data tends to support the notion that the failure to establish good sleeping habits in infancy or early childhood may have long-term harmful effects, such as adult insomnia. And among psychologically unhealthy adults, the more severe the sleep difficulty, the more severe the degree of mental illness.

Let's now review some of the most common sleep problems that can disrupt our children's sleep and their solutions.

When you consider solutions for your child's sleep problems, it is important to think of healthy sleep as a collection or group of five related elements, described in Chapter 2, grouped together to form a 'package'.

FIVE ELEMENTS OF HEALTHY SLEEP

1. **Sleep duration: night and day sleep**
2. **Naps**
3. **Sleep consolidation**
4. **Sleep schedule**
5. **Sleep regularity**

All five elements must be present to ensure good-quality or healthy sleep. In the following discussions, I might emphasise one part of the 'package' as being especially important for solving a problem, but keep in mind that the solution might fail if other elements of healthy sleep are absent. Also, some sleep problems occur at specific ages. Here, I will provide a brief outline of the solution and I will refer you to the chapter appropriate for your child's age for more detailed instructions. It is best to first read here and then read the appropriate chapter for your child based on his age. Reading the preceding and following age-appropriate chapters will also help.

For any particular problem, there may be more than one cause or solution. Your child's age and temperament might influence which solution you will want to try first. Also, not all solutions are practical for all families. So please read the entire section for any particular problem before trying to help your child. Also, because many of these problems are interrelated, it might be worthwhile to browse through this entire chapter; you might discover some additional solutions. One important principle for solving sleep problems is to execute a schedule or behavioural change for several days to determine whether the change helps before making another change in routine. Be patient and keep a sleep log.

Sleep Log

A sleep log is a series of bar graphs showing on each day when your child was awake, asleep, quiet in bed or cot, and crying in bed or cot. On the horizontal axis, show the day of the week and on the vertical axis, the time of day. Each bar represents a twenty-four-hour snapshot of a day and the graphic view of all the bars allows you to see trends in sleeping patterns. A detailed diary makes it hard to see the wood for the trees.

REMEMBER, SLEEP BEGETS SLEEP

The more rested you are, the easier it is to fall asleep and stay asleep. The more tired you are, the harder it is.

Excessive Daytime Sleepiness

Superficially, we tend to think of being either awake or asleep. But just as there are gradations between light sleep and deep sleep, there are gradations of wakefulness. Task performance, attentiveness, vigilance and mood may be influenced by the degree of daytime wakefulness. When we do not feel very awake during the day, we say that we feel 'sleepy'. Excessive daytime sleepiness or impaired daytime alertness is a result of disturbed sleep.

The Stanford Sleepiness Scale is a self-rating instrument developed at Stanford University to describe the different states or levels of daytime sleepiness. Obviously, children who are depressed or irritable due to sleep deprivation will have high numerical ratings.

LEVEL	DESCRIPTION
1	**Feeling active and vital; alert; wide awake**
2	**Functioning at a high level, but not at peak; still able to concentrate**
3	**Relaxed; awake; not at full alertness; responsive**
4	**A little foggy; not at peak; slowing down**
5	**Fogginess; beginning to lose interest in remaining awake; slowed down**
6	**Sleepiness; preferring to be lying down; fighting sleep; woozy**
7	**Almost in reverie; sleep onset soon; lost struggle to remain awake**

Morning Wake-up Time Is Too Early

Make sure that the bedroom is dark and quiet in the morning. Window-darkening shades and noise from such as a humidifier will help reduce the startling effect of street noises. Keep a sleep log to help find the best bedtime.

The most common cause for waking up too early before four months of age is extreme fussiness/colic (see Chapter 4). The most common cause, after four months, is a too-late bedtime.

If you suspect the bedtime is too late, slowly make the bedtime earlier. Try twenty minutes earlier for four nights to see whether your child will fall asleep at the earlier time and sleep in later. Do everything you currently are doing at bedtime but simply start the bedtime ritual at an earlier time. If this seems to help a little, repeat the process with an additional twenty-minute earlier bedtime for four more nights.

You can again repeat this process until it is clear that you have reached a too-early bedtime because your child no longer easily and promptly falls asleep. Now you might want to return to the last step and let your child stay up an additional twenty minutes. This gradual shift in bedtime may produce no protest crying.

If you think the bedtime is too late because your child appears tired much earlier, then move the bedtime much earlier right away. The abrupt shift may or may not produce protest crying. For young children, at night, use Ignoring, discussed on page 211; Partial Ignoring, discussed on page 214; or Check and Console, discussed on page 215. For older children, use Sleep Rules, discussed on page 325 and 353, or Silent Return to Sleep, discussed on page 320. Ignoring your child until 6:00 to 7:00 A.M. will probably be needed. For younger children, the option of bringing them to your bed for soothing may produce extra ZZZs in the morning.

Sometimes, after four months, a child is already going to bed very early, around 5:30 or 6:00 P.M. The entire schedule becomes shifted: too early a wake-up time causes too-early or poorly timed naps and a very tired child in the late afternoon who goes to sleep easily very early in the evening. For young children, it should help to simultaneously move their bedtime a little later, maybe twenty to thirty minutes every four nights, and ignoring them until about 6:00 A.M. For older children, use the fifth Sleep Rule, discussed on page 353, with a clock radio to tell them when they can leave their room. If you move the bedtime too late, your child might become so overtired that the wake-up time does not become later, instead he simply wakes up more overtired. However, for some older, persistent children, I have temporarily pushed the bedtime to a very late hour and it caused them to sleep in later. They receive lavish praise and token rewards (such as a small treat, stickers or stars) for sleeping in later. Then the bedtime is slowly and gradually moved to an earlier time but the later wake-up time is preserved because the child continues to receive the praise and rewards.

Finding the bedtime that is just right for your child might require some back-and-forth adjustments; make one change and then wait four days to see whether it helps. And be patient.

Morning Nap Is Absent, Too Short, Too Long or at the Wrong Time

The morning nap develops at three to four months of age in 80 per cent of children and a few months later in 20 per cent of children who had colic. Correcting a too-early wake-up time or a too-late bedtime might be needed.

Sometimes the morning nap is short because that is all the sleep your child can get at that time – that is, your child is a short napper. About 20 per cent of children between about six and twenty-one months always have short naps in the morning and afternoon, no matter what parents do. Between six and nine months of age, they may appear to be too short because the child requires many short naps, or 'snaps', throughout the day and often appears tired. As long as the bedtime is early, by nine or twelve months, most of these children are taking fewer and longer naps and no longer appear tired. I think that most of these short nappers are those who had colic when younger.

The most common cause of an absent or a too-short morning nap is an interval of wakefulness that is too long between the wake-up time and the beginning of the nap. For the child under four months of age, sometimes starting the morning nap after only one hour of wakefulness allows the child to be soothed back to sleep before she becomes overtired. In an older child, starting the nap at the wrong biological time may either shorten the nap or make it less restorative; either too early or too late, it messes up the rest of the day. Use the morning nap rhythm that is well developed, 9:00 to 10:00 A.M., as an aid to help the child sleep. If needed, stretch the interval of wakefulness using 9:00 A.M. as your target time. You might only get to 8:30 or 8:45 A.M. because your child is becoming overtired. It's a balancing act: you want to start the nap when the biological nap time begins, but you also want to avoid the overtired state. You are willing to allow the child to become a little overtired but not become so worn-out that he has great difficulty falling asleep.

Sometimes an older brother or sister has a scheduled activity that interferes with the morning nap. Some options are to try to get relatives or a neighbour to watch your younger child at home while you drive your older child to the activity, or try to carpool to reduce the number of days per week your younger child misses out on a good morning nap. Often the young child might fall asleep in the car seat during the drive and the parent allows the child to continue to nap in the car seat, either in the car or when the car seat is placed in the cot. It looks awkward to us, but many young children appear to sleep well in the cosy car seat.

Sometimes the wake-up time is too late because the bedtime is too late and the child cannot fall asleep at 9:00 or 10:00 A.M. ***'Control the Wake-up Time'*** simply means waking your child around 7:00 A.M. in order to get a good-quality nap to begin around 9:00 A.M. To avoid an overtired child, the bedtime will have to be moved earlier. Parents or a parent may not like this solution because they like to play with their child late at night and/or they like to sleep in later in the morning.

If the morning nap is too long or too late in the morning, it may interfere with your child's ability to fall asleep easily around 12:00 to 2:00 P.M. for the second nap, and the result is an overtired child by late afternoon. The reason the morning nap is too long or too late is usually because the bedtime is too late. Limiting the morning nap to one to two hours by waking your child is necessary because it is important to protect the second nap. At the same time, moving the bedtime earlier will cause your child to awaken in the morning better rested, and this will then automatically shorten the morning nap.

NAP HINTS

Before the morning or afternoon nap, go outside in order to, briefly but intensely, stimulate your child with physical activity at the park or in the sandbox; expose your child to light, wind, clouds, voices, music, traffic sounds; go for rides in the pushchair. Then tone it down as you get near nap time. Now spend an extra long time soothing; include a bath if it is soothing in the nap time routine. Make the room dark and quiet.

Afternoon Nap Is Absent, Too Short, Too Long or at the Wrong Time

The afternoon nap usually lasts until about three years of age and gradually disappears after the third birthday. If the afternoon nap disappears too soon, your child may become overtired in the late afternoon and have difficulty falling asleep at night. Either re-establishing the afternoon nap (if your child is substantially under age three) or moving the bedtime earlier (if your child is substantially over age three) should help. If the afternoon nap persists in much older children the bedtime might progressively get later and later, causing bedtime battles to develop. Eliminating the afternoon nap will permit an earlier bedtime and help erase bedtime battles.

Bad timing is a common cause of problems associated with the afternoon nap. If the afternoon nap is too early, well before noon, because of a too-short morning nap, it will not be as restorative and your child might be well overtired by late afternoon. One mother said her son was a 'French fry' by the end of the day because he was crispy. Under nine months of age, this might lead to a late or long third nap that causes the bedtime to become too late. If the afternoon nap is too late, well after 2:00 P.M., it may interfere with an early bedtime.

Sometimes the afternoon nap conflicts with scheduled

activities, such as preschool for the child or scheduled activities for the older brothers and sisters. Try to minimise these conflicts regarding the older children by using baby-sitters, car pools or skipping some, but not all, of the classes for your infant. An earlier bedtime might be essential when the afternoon nap is shortened or skipped.

Day care may be associated with poor-quality naps because there is bad timing, too much noise, not enough help for long soothing, or crying from other children. The morning nap usually disappears more easily in day care because the child is already better rested in the morning from the previous night's sleep. Sometimes there are no alternatives available to the family in their choice of day care, and although it is especially hard on these families, an earlier bedtime will help these children.

IMPORTANT POINT

If the morning or afternoon nap is sometimes far too short or skipped, try to keep the child up and go to the next scheduled sleep time, but move it a little earlier. Protect the sleep schedule.

Third Nap Is Absent, Too Short, Too Long or at the Wrong Time

The third nap, around 3:00 to 5:00 P.M., is variable: it may be short, long or absent. It usually disappears by nine months of age. If it is a long nap, your child might be able to go to bed later at night. But if it is too long, the very late bedtime might become associated with bedtime battles because your child is way past his biological time for evening sleep. So either shorten (if your child is way under nine months) or eliminate (if your child is nine months or older) the third nap. Even a brief, baby power nap lasting twenty to forty minutes late in the afternoon or early in the evening might interfere with an early bedtime.

So if you are struggling with bedtimes, consider eliminating this third mini-nap and try for an earlier bedtime.

Sometimes, around nine to twelve months of age, a child falls asleep around 5:30 P.M. and is up around 7:30 or 8:00 P.M., then is up playing with parents for a few hours until 10:00 P.M., and finally goes back to sleep but does not sleep well at night. The parents think the child is taking a third nap at 5:30 P.M. But in reality the child needs a very early bedtime, maybe around 6:00 P.M., and no playing between 7:30 and 10:00 P.M.

REAL LIFE

Special events often result in skipped or shortened naps for children. Do not become a slave to your child's nap schedule. The more you protect the sleep routine for regular days, the less disruptive those special days will be.

Needs Two but Can Get Only One

The bedtime might be too late and/or the wake-up time too early, causing your child to be very tired in the morning. This morning fatigue causes him to take a mega-nap in the morning that interferes with his ability to take an afternoon nap. As a result, he is not well rested in the late afternoon or early evening. Or, scheduled morning activities might conflict with a nap around 9:00 to 10:00 A.M., resulting in a very late morning nap around 10:30 or 11:00 A.M. Even if this is a brief nap, it may recharge your child's battery and interfere with a long afternoon nap. During the transition between two naps and one nap, roughly twelve to twenty-one months, there may be some days when one nap works well and other days when your child takes two naps. This transition time, however, might be associated with an inability to get in two naps when he clearly needs them. The solution here is a twenty- or thirty-minute earlier bedtime.

Needs a Nap but Refuses to Nap

Holidays, trips, illnesses or other changes in routine might cause your two- to three-year-old child to give up napping and be very tired during the day. Another common cause of no napping occurs when the child drops the morning nap but the parents do not make the bedtime a little earlier. Over many weeks or months, your child develops 'cumulative sleepiness' until he hits a wall and becomes well overtired. In this state, it is difficult for him to nap because his body is geared up to fight the fatigue. When you try to re-establish the nap, he either just plays in his cot, or cries, or a combination of both.

If your child is substantially under three years old, try a temporarily super-early bedtime to help him wake up better rested. In other words, for four or five nights, put him to sleep when he is drowsy at 5:00 or 5:30 P.M. This might backfire and cause him to wake up too early. If this happens, for those four or five mornings, ignore him until 6:00 A.M. Often, the early bedtime will help erase his sleep debt so he is more able to relax and take a nap. To help re-establish the nap habit, you might want to have intense morning stimulation and an extra long and soothing nap time ritual. Leaving him alone in his cot for no more than one hour, even if he cries, often will allow the nap to occur because he is tired and not receiving any stimulation from his parents. Or, you might have to lie down with him in your bed to help induce sleep. If successful, then you would very slowly and gradually transition him back to his cot. (See page 177 for transitioning children from parent's bed to child's cot.) Once the nap has been re-established, the bedtime can be made a little later. Children who slip in and out of good sleeping patterns are usually the ones who are always going to bed slightly too late. They don't usually have major problems, but they are always on the edge of becoming overtired and they easily and quickly become overtired whenever there is a disruption of sleep routines.

If your child is substantially past his third birthday, trying to re-establish the nap may not make sense, and trying to establish an earlier bedtime will help your child sleep better. Here is a report of how a *temporarily* super-early bedtime and the use of the 'nap hints' on page 123 helped create long and regular naps.

A 5:30 P.M. BEDTIME UNTIL HENRIK'S NAPPING GOT BETTER

When our pastor asked us if our eight-month-old son, Henrik, was a 'serious, sullen' boy, I knew we had a problem. Just one month before, my friend had sent us a note saying how Henrik was the happiest baby she'd ever seen. She could elicit a belly laugh from him with just a sideways glance. Now, our pastor, an experienced grandfather, was pulling out all the stops – goofy faces and exaggerated sneezing – and Henrik wouldn't crack a smile. But it wasn't because he was suddenly sullen or serious; he was exhausted.

What I had hoped was just a napless phase that he'd outgrow was catching up with him and choking his vibrant personality. We needed help.

I called our paediatrician's office and explained our predicament: while Henrik was sleeping better at night, his daytime naps were becoming history. Over the past two months, his decent, if erratic, nap schedule had faded into two brief naps and then disappeared altogether.

Getting my son to fall asleep was never a problem; nursing or rocking soothed him easily. It was getting him to stay asleep once I set him down where the trouble began. As soon as I'd set him in his cot, his back would arch and he'd be choked up before he touched the mattress. 'Nap time' had come to mean Henrik crying in his cot until my nerves couldn't take it any more, or him sleeping soundly on me.

I knew he needed to learn to soothe himself to sleep, but crying it out just didn't seem to work. The longer I'd let him cry, the more he would work himself up. I knew sleeping on me wasn't a good solution, but when I'd see the dark circles under his eyes and hear his voice husky from crying – and especially when he got his first cold – I just couldn't let him cry any more. He needed sleep.

So I'd get comfortable with him on the sofa and hope a good film was on TV.

When the nurse at our paediatrician's office suggested Dr Weissbluth's *Healthy Sleep Habits, Happy Child* (a book I had already devoured and loved), I decided to take it a step further and make an appointment to see Dr Weissbluth himself, since his office was near our home.

Eight days later, armed with a copy of his book and a sleep journal, we set off for our consultation with Dr Weissbluth. As soon as he walked into the room, I knew we'd find help. Dr Weissbluth listened to, empathised with, instructed and encouraged us in a manner that assured us we would get back on track.

After studying our son's erratic sleep patterns, he recommended an earlier bedtime and regular wake-up times for my son. Dr Weissbluth explained that Henrik was going to bed too late and wasn't getting enough sleep at night. (Henrik usually fell asleep between 8:00 and 9:00 P.M. and woke up around 7:00 A.M.) This lack of sleep and a consistent schedule – as odd as it may seem – is what was keeping him from being able to cry himself to sleep during the day. He was too overtired to sleep! Dr Weissbluth suggested a 7:00 P.M. bedtime and a 7:00 A.M. wake-up for the long-term goal, but said that we'd probably be looking at a 5:30 P.M. bedtime until Henrik's napping got better.

Once Henrik was up in the morning, we were to stimulate him through walks, outings and vigorous play. After that, a soothing period would precede his attempt at a 9:00 A.M. nap. I was to continue putting Henrik to sleep in my normal way (nursing and rocking) and then set him down in his cot. I was then to leave him alone for one hour either to sleep, cry or a combination of the two.

Then, after his morning nap, we were to repeat the process for his attempt at a 1:00 P.M. nap (or earlier if no morning nap was taken). And then we'd go about our afternoon until it was time for the evening soothe. He asked us to chart our sleep data so we could clearly see Henrik's progress.

After a round of handshakes and encouraging words, we left the office equipped to help our son become the sleeper he needed to – and could – become. We were to report back to Dr Weissbluth in a week. His confidence that we'd see improvement by then rubbed off on us. We couldn't wait to get going.

When we got home, we played and played, and then I soothed Henrik to sleep. When I set him down for his afternoon nap, he cried. I said a quick prayer, told him I loved him, walked out and closed the door on my wailing son.

As I walked down the stairs, I breathed in slowly, reminded myself that I was doing this for my son's well-being and hit the pause button on my emotions. I spent fifty-nine minutes e-mailing friends with one ear to the monitor to see if and when he'd stop crying. 'Didn't work today,' I was telling myself on the way back up the stairs. But by the time I got to his door I realised he was quiet. He fell asleep after fifty-nine and a half minutes of crying. If I had gone up one minute sooner, I would've cheated him out of this accomplishment. We were on our way.

The afternoon nap was the first to get back on track. It took about a week for him to be able to go down at all without crying, and he was still only sleeping for a half hour at a time. But he was sleeping – and on a schedule! I used to think that because Henrik was an erratic sleeper, a sleep schedule wouldn't work for him. Now I know that Henrik was an erratic sleeper because he lacked that schedule. (While the idea of a schedule sounds limiting, establishing a schedule was the most freeing thing for our family. We are now able to make accurate plans instead of having to wait around and guess when our son would be ready to go.)

The morning nap was more of a challenge. For two weeks he cried through his entire morning nap. It was difficult to put him down each day knowing he would cry, but his success in the afternoons, along with the giant hug I'd receive when I came to get my teary son, gave me the strength to keep going. Then one day he cried himself to sleep after twenty minutes, and from then on he would stay sleeping after we put him down. It took two weeks for Henrik to get back to two naps a day, but he did it.

Despite sleeping for only thirty to forty-five minutes at a time, Dr Weissbluth told us we should get him as soon as he woke up. He suggested we keep the 5:30 P.M. bedtime, which would naturally help lengthen his naps. Our days are now virtually tear-free.

My son is thriving on his new schedule. He's back to his giggly, healthy, and well-rested self. Instead of being the sullen boy in church, he's now the lively angel who sings out loud with joy – with or without the rest of the congregation.

Bedtime Is Too Late: Sometimes or Always a Battle

Past six weeks of age, biologically driven bedtimes tend to become earlier. If you are unable or unwilling to allow these early bedtimes, your child will become overtired. Common problems occur (1) in the post-colic child who is dependent on the family bed and breast-feeding to sleep but now wants to sleep much earlier than the parents do, (2) parents who have to use day care so extra time at night is required to bring the child home, or (3) dual-career families with long commute times from work. Solutions involve using others to help prepare the baby or child for bed (bathing, dressing for sleep, and feeding) and, as early as possible, the parents begin a *brief* bedtime routine. Although you will see your child less at night, you will have lovely morning time. To really enjoy the mornings, some parents will have to go to sleep earlier themselves! Other parents may be able to alter their work schedule to come home early on some days or do some of their work at home in the evenings after their child has gone to sleep. Obviously, not all parents can come up with a solution. Review the list of resources for soothing on page 74.

If circumstances cause your baby to go to bed too late, do the best you can but try for the earliest bedtime possible.

Night Waking, Difficulty Staying Asleep

Night waking occurs normally in all children, and the real problem is not developing the ability to return to sleep unassisted after the awakening. Night waking is the most common post-colic sleeping problem and is discussed in Chapter 4. All sleep problems eventually lead to night waking. The specific treatments depend on the child's age and are discussed in the appropriate chapter.

More Than One Child Creates Bedtime Problems

An older child, age about three years, might not nap and need to go to sleep around 6:00 or 6:30 P.M., especially if he has a very active day. His younger sister, age about six months, might be taking three naps and be able to stay up later. A parent cannot ignore the baby and attend to the three-year-old's bedtime routine. A solution is to eliminate the third nap for the baby so she goes down earlier, around 6:00 or 6:15 P.M., while the three-year-old is playing by himself. Twins who have different sleeping schedules, causing different bedtimes, are challenging to parents and sometimes there is no solution except putting them down at about the same time and if there is any crying associated with falling asleep, then temporarily separate them.

Unable to Fall Asleep

Young babies or children may have difficulty falling asleep except when they are in bed with their parents or in their arms. Most of these are children who had colic (see Chapter 4) or whose parents had used the family bed from the beginning. Read the sections on the Family Bed in Chapter 6, and 'Transition from Family Bed to Cot' on page 177. Older children and adolescents may have difficulty falling asleep and these are discussed in Chapter 9.

Afraid of the Dark or Being Alone

Fears are very common between the ages of two and four years. Thunder, lightning, barking dogs, shadows and many other scary items over which we have no control can frighten children. A light on in the hall or even a conventional low-wattage night-light might keep a sensitive baby from sleeping well. A dim guide light that produces a faint glow will usually be sufficient illumination. Extra long and soothing bedtimes will help. A new protecting teddy bear might help fight off fears and protect your child. A father might walk around the room and capture the 'monsters' and put them into a bag or box to remove them from the room. Guardian angels, charms, and the like may help make your child feel more secure. An older child might be given a bell to summon his mother or father with the understanding that he can use it only once. The parent will then come to soothe him, once, for a predetermined period of time, using a kitchen timer placed under a pillow or cushion to control the duration of the soothing time. Knowing that he can have some attention at night gives the child confidence and he will sleep better. The goal is to provide extra attention at night without it becoming open-ended and a ploy to fight sleep.

Will Not Stay in His Cot or Bed

One- or two-year-olds who climb out of their bed may receive too much social interaction from parents and therefore may continue the behaviour because they are curious and social. To protect their sleep and prevent the development of sleep problems, buy a crib tent. You may have to use strong sticky tape to keep the child from getting to the zipper. Parents are often reluctant to use a crib tent because they imagine their child will feel like a caged zoo animal, restricted or abandoned. Of course, there might be some protest crying for a few days. However, many children quickly seem to enjoy the comfort zone like a teepee or fort; they do not appear sad or angry. Some parents do not want to use a crib tent but feel more comfortable putting a latch lock on the door. If you stand at the door preventing your child from leaving the room, your child will fight sleep all the more because he is getting attention from you.

'Sleep Rules' (page 325) and 'silent return to sleep' (page 320) are used for the older child who will not stay in bed. Here, too, some parents know that they cannot be consistent at night, so they want to put a latch lock on the door. Whenever parents want to put a lock on the door, I ask that they have the child watch them put the lock on. One parent felt that the additional step of taking her three-year-old child along to the store where she purchased the lock for the door helped convince him that she was serious. The child is told that if he leaves the room, he will be put back in and the door will be locked. Almost all the time, the child picks up on her parents' serious demeanour and does not even attempt to leave the room in the first place. If, however, the child tests the rules and leaves the room, and the parents place her back into the room and lock the door, although there may be loud and long protest crying, it is usually only for one night, because the child is now highly motivated to prevent the door being locked.

Will Not Sleep Anywhere Else

Maybe your baby sleeps well in your home but does not sleep well at grandma's. Try to play the same music only at sleep times at both homes. Buy something soft and safe for your baby to feel or clutch and use it only at sleep times at both homes. Spray some fragrance or perfume around the cot or bed only at sleep times at both homes. Use the same sleep schedules and nap time and bedtime routines at both homes.

Only One Bedroom

When your baby becomes more curious and aware of the sounds and movements of people around him and you are using a cot, it might be time to move your baby to his own room. What do you do if you do not have an additional bedroom? Some families have their baby sleep at night in their bedroom and they use a sofa bed and convert their living room into their bedroom at night. In this way, the baby can go to bed early in a dark and quiet room and the parents know that their night-time sounds will not wake him.

Transition from Family Bed to Cot

Moving your baby from a family bed to a cot will be easy or difficult depending on whether the family bed was unwanted but occurred in reaction to extreme fussiness/colic or was wanted from the beginning. This will be discussed in detail on page 177.

Action Plan for Exhausted Parents

Young children and infants cannot tell us how they feel, so parents need to watch their behaviours. Does your child behave as though he were active, alert, vital and wide awake, or is he fighting sleep, woozy?

This chapter and the two previous chapters describe the terms *healthy sleep* and *disturbed sleep*. Obviously, sleeping is not an automatically regulated process such as the control of body temperature. Sleeping is more like feeding. We do not expect children to grow well if all they eat is junk food. Children need a well-balanced diet in order to grow. If the food that is provided is insufficient or unbalanced, this unhealthy diet will interfere with the child's growth and development. The same is true for unhealthy sleep patterns.

MAJOR POINT

Junk food is bad for the body. Junk sleep is bad for the brain.

REAL LIFE

If your child has a sleep problem that requires multiple changes, but you are only able to make some of the changes, go ahead and do the best you can.

Be consistent. Anytime you make a change, allow at least four to five days before making another change to see whether you have helped your child. Be patient.

1. Keep a sleep log as described on page 118.
2. Identify the main sleep problem as described in this chapter.
3. Read the brief solution outline and the age-appropriate section in later chapters or the action plan for that chapter.
4. Identify the elements of sleep that need improvement or correction for your child's sleep problem.
   Sleep duration: night and day sleep
   Naps

There are good naps and bad naps. Occasional nap strikes may not be harmful, but nap-stubborn kids are usually overtired.

   Sleep consolidation
   Sleep schedule
   Sleep regularity
5. Determine what you can and cannot do.
   Ignore morning crying that is too early versus bringing your baby to your bed
   Control the wake-up time
   Change the schedule for nap times
   Eliminate the third nap
   Change the schedule for bedtimes
   Change the nap time or bedtime routine
   Provide more soothing at sleep times
   Give less attention at night when your child is not hungry
   Use a crib tent or lock the door

IMPORTANT POINTS

Sleeping well is a 24/7 process. It's not just about how we get them to go to bed at night without crying.

Solving sleep problems may be a very tough prescription and demands a consistent approach.

There may be increased crying in the beginning, but the upside is that crying around sleep should be eliminated altogether.

CHAPTER 4

Sleep, Extreme Fussiness/Colic, and Temperament

How to Use This Chapter

I believe about 5 to 10 per cent of babies are at risk from developing 90 to 95 per cent of the severe sleeping problems that drive parents crazy. If your baby already has sleeping problems and you think you may have come down this path, this chapter will tell you the necessary corrections you need to make to solve the sleeping problem. However, you may be too exhausted to make it through the whole chapter, so you might benefit more by reading the summary and action plan at the end of the chapter. If you have not yet had your child, this chapter will help you later identify whether your baby is just starting on this path. Reading the entire chapter will enable you to prevent future sleeping problems.

This chapter is divided into four main sections. First, a detailed description of what is known about extreme fussiness/colic and its relation to difficulties in sleeping during the first three to four months; second, what is temperament; third, how the fussiness/crying during months three to four is connected to temperament at four months of age; and fourth, post-colic. I also present data that connects these two ages and tells you how likely it is that your baby will develop on one path or another. You can skip the data if your child already has or had colic and go directly to the management sections or the summary and action plan if you just want to decide what to do.

The section on post-colic is crucial to help prevent or solve any sleep problems in 20 per cent of children.

Introduction

If your child suffered from colic during infancy – and 20 per cent of all babies suffer from this mysterious condition – then you'll be most interested in learning how your child's colicky first months could have set the stage for unhealthy sleep habits and turned him into a 'crybaby'. This chapter will be of interest to you even if your baby never had colic, though, because all babies experience unexplained fussiness and crying in their first weeks of life, no matter what your ethnic group, no matter what birthing method brought your child into the world, no matter if your lifestyle is that of jet-setter or stay-at-home.

All parents, too, tend to use the same techniques and strategies to weather successfully those first few months of life with baby, whether it's fair sailing for the most part or they feel storm-tossed by colicky waves of crying. Sleep problems arise when some parents don't change their techniques for coping with crying and fussiness at bedtimes and nap times after about three to four months of age, after their babies have become more settled. That's when unhealthy sleep habits and their resulting problems begin.

Sleep and Extreme Fussiness/Colic

For 20 per cent of babies, I actually prefer the term 'extreme fussiness/colic' instead of colic because fussiness is a bigger problem than crying. All babies have some fussing and crying, and for 80 per cent of babies, I call this behaviour common fussiness/crying. My idea is that extreme fussiness/colic is a sleep disorder. I also suggest that post-colic sleep problems occur after three to four months of age because some parents experience difficulty in establishing age-appropriate sleep routines. Let us look at the facts.

What Is Extreme Fussiness/Colic?

Dr Wessel defined a colicky infant as 'one who, otherwise healthy and well fed, had paroxysms of irritability, fussing or crying lasting for a total of more than three hours a day and occurring on more than three days in any one week . . . and where the paroxysms continued to recur for more than three weeks'. He added the criterion 'more than three weeks' because nannies left families after about three weeks of crying. He thought nannies knew that if babies cried for more than three weeks, then the crying would continue. Because the mothers were now alone at night caring for their babies, they came to his office after three weeks complaining that their children were always crying. About 26 per cent of infants in his study had colic. Dr Illingworth defined colic as 'violent rhythmical, screaming attacks which did not stop when the infants were picked up, and for which no cause, such as underfeeding, could be found'. Together, they studied about 150 infants.

The *age of onset* of these behaviours is characteristic. Both Dr Wessel and Dr Illingworth found that the attacks were absent during the first few days but were present in 80 per cent of affected infants by two weeks and in about 100 per cent by three weeks. Premature babies also start their attacks shortly after the expected due date, independent of their gestational age at birth. The *time of day* when these behaviours occur is another characteristic. During the first month, crying appears at any time of the day or night, but later it occurs predominantly in the evening hours. In 80 per cent of infants, the attacks start between 5:00 and 8:00 P.M. and end by midnight. For 12 per cent of infants, the attacks start between 7:00 and 10:00 P.M. and end by 2:00 A.M. In only 8 per cent, the attacks are distributed anytime throughout the day and night. The *age of termination* of these spells is also characteristic. The attacks disappear by two months of age in 50 per cent of infants, by three months of age in 30 per cent and four months of age in 10 per cent of infants. The infant's *behavioural state* is associated with colicky behaviour. Among 84 per cent of colicky infants, the crying spells *begin when they are awake*, 8 per cent have spells start when asleep, and 8 per cent under variable conditions. For 83 per cent of infants, *when the crying spells end, they fall asleep*. It is now known that fussing as opposed to crying is the major feature of colicky behaviour, and parental distress over colic may be the major factor in producing post-colic sleep problems.

What Causes Extreme Fussiness/Colic?

A recent study showed that colicky infants had higher levels of serotonin, a chemical found in the brain and in the gut. This supported Linda Weissbluth's theory that some features of colic might be caused by an imbalance between serotonin and melatonin, another chemical found in the brain and in the gut. Concentrations of serotonin are high and present in infants during the first month of life and decline after three months. Immediately after delivery, concentrations of serotonin are higher at night and lower during the day. Melatonin, flowing across the placenta from the mother, causes high concentrations immediately after birth, but they rapidly fall to extremely low levels within several days. Melatonin increases slightly between one and three months, and only after three months is there an abrupt increase in melatonin levels with higher levels at night and lower levels during the day.

Serotonin and melatonin have opposite effects on the muscle around the gut – serotonin causes contraction, melatonin causes relaxation. Linda Weissbluth's theory is that in some infants, when serotonin concentrations are at the highest in the evening, they cause painful gastrointestinal cramps. The high night-time melatonin levels opposes the intestinal smooth muscle contraction caused by serotonin. On the other hand, melatonin and serotonin might be directly affecting the developing brain. For example, high levels of melatonin at night might cause night sleep to become longer.

Other hormones might be involved. In one study, extremely

fussy/colicky infants had a blunted rhythm in cortisol production while the control infants exhibited a clear and marked daily rhythm in cortisol that was not observed in the colicky infants. In addition, researchers in this study coded behavioural measures from videotapes and arrived at the same conclusion as have many other studies: the crying of these infants was not due to differences in handling by the mother; the colic was not simply a maternal perception.

Other studies have clearly shown that food hypersensitivity, gastro-oesophageal reflux, maternal anxiety and so forth are not linked to infantile colic.

Crying

Some degree of irritability, fussing or crying is universal – that is, crying for 'unknown reasons' occurs in all babies. Dr Brazelton reported that half of all babies cry for one and three quarter hours during the second week with a gradual increase to two and three quarter hours at six weeks, followed by a decrease in crying thereafter to one hour or less by twelve weeks of age. He called the fussiest infants 'colicky'. They cried two to four hours per day every day, and their crying also increased between six and eight weeks of age.

The distress caused to parents because of their inability to deal with this crying cannot be overstated. Recent government data has shown infant homicides to increase after the second week and peak at the eighth week, and the researchers concluded that the 'peak in risk in week eight might reflect the peak in the daily duration of crying among normal infants between weeks six and eight'.

There are no clear cut-off points in measurements of irritability, fussing or crying, whether by direct observation in hospital nurseries, voice-activated tape recordings in homes, or parent diaries. Thus, extreme fussiness/colic appears to represent an extreme amount of normally occurring, unexplained fussing or crying that is present in all healthy babies.

Because the spells of irritability, fussing or crying are universal, differing only in degree among infants; because the occurrence of spells peaks at forty-six weeks after conception and independent of parenting practices; and because the behaviours exhibit behavioural state specificity and a day-night rhythm, it is reasonable to believe that these behaviours reflect normal biological processes. One example is the normal biological process involving the development of wake/sleep control mechanisms. In all babies, the consolidation of night sleep develops during the second month (after the peak of crying occurs) and that periodic alternation of wake and sleep states is well developed by three to four months of age (when colic ends).

Fussing

Persistent low-intensity fussing, rather than intense crying, characterises infants diagnosed as having colic. In fact, to emphasise fussiness instead of crying, the title of Dr Wessel's paper was 'Paroxysmal fussing in infants sometimes called "colic" '. Fussing is not a well-defined behaviour, and although not defined in Wessel's paper, it is usually described as an unsettled, agitated, wakeful state that *would lead to crying if ignored by parents*. Because sucking is soothing to infants, some parents misattribute the 'fussing' state to hunger and vigorously attempt to feed their baby. These parents may misinterpret their infants as having a 'growth spurt' at six weeks because they were 'hungry' all the time, especially in the evening. They view their child as hungry, not fussy. Even if they spend more than three additional hours a day, more than three days a week, for more than three weeks 'feeding' them at night to prevent crying, these parents do not think their baby is colicky because there is so little crying. Over a thirty-four-month period, at newborn visits, I routinely questioned every new parent who joined my general paediatric practice whether their child fulfilled Dr Wessel's exact diagnostic criteria for colic. All families had been followed since the child's birth and received counselling regarding the normal development of crying or fussing. There were 118 extremely fussy/colicky infants out of 747 (16 per cent). However, *the vast majority of infants had little or no crying*. Instead, they fulfilled Dr Wessel's criteria because they had long and frequent bouts of fussing, which did not lead to crying because of *intensive parental intervention*.

Studies show that, between two to six weeks, there is an increase predominately in fussing, not crying. Furthermore, fussing and sleeping, but notably not crying, were found to be stable individual characteristics from six weeks to nine months of age. The amount of crying during the first three months did not predict crying behaviour at nine months. Crying alone is not a prediction of sleep problems. Two separate and well-designed studies agree with Dr St. James-Roberts that 'high amounts of early crying do not make it highly probable that an infant will . . . have sleeping problems at nine months of age'.

Colic-Sleep

Dr Kirjavainen asked parents to keep a daily diary and performed sleep recordings in the lab at night between 9:00 P.M. and 7:00 A.M. At about *four and a half weeks*, the total sleep time from the diary was significantly shorter in the colic group (12.7 versus 14.5 hours per day). The most dramatic decrease in sleep in the colicky babies occurred at night between 6:00 P.M. and 6:00 A.M. The diary data showed that by *six months* of age the extremely fussy/colicky infants slept slightly less than the non-colicky infants, but the group differences were small. The first sleep lab recording was performed when the infants were about *nine weeks* old. There were no differences in sleep characteristics between the groups in the night recordings. The second sleep lab recording was performed at about *thirty weeks* of age, and again, there were no differences in sleep characteristics between the infants formerly with and without extreme fussiness/colic.

Therefore, among infants with extreme fussiness/colic, parent diary data showed shorter total sleep times compared with the age-matched control group at *four and a half weeks*, but that by *nine weeks* there were no group differences in sleep lab data obtained during the night. Also, this report suggests that over time, between ages five and nine weeks, the sleep duration increased among extremely fussy/colicky infants. Based only on the sleep lab data, the authors concluded that infantile colic was not associated with a sleep disorder. However, Dr Kirjavainen told me that the lab data was questionable because all children slept poorly in the lab setting.

Dr St. James-Roberts used the term 'persistent criers' to describe extremely fussy/colicky infants. At *six weeks* of age, the extremely fussy/colicky infants slept significantly less than noncolicky infants (12.5 versus 13.8 hours per day). There were no group differences regarding time spent awake or time spent feeding. Extremely fussy/colicky infants slept less throughout the twenty-four-hour diary record. The clearest group differences for sleep were during the day. In fact, there were no group differences regarding sleep at night. In addition, at night, there were no group differences for cry/fuss behaviour. The clearest group differences for cry/fuss behaviour were in the daytime. The groups were similar in the timing and duration of the infant's longest sleep period. This analysis of sleep cycle maturation led to the conclusion that the 'chief difference between them lies in amounts of daytime fuss/crying and sleeping, rather than in the diurnal organisation of sleep and waking behaviour.' In addition, at *six weeks* of age, the less a baby slept, the more amounts of fuss/crying were observed. Because the authors observed no deficit in calm wakefulness, only sleeping, they felt that there was a specific trade-off between fuss/crying and sleep. In other words, more fuss/crying behaviour reduced sleep time only, not calm wakeful time. The researchers concluded that persistent crying is associated with a sleeping deficit.

Another study of extremely fussy/colicky infants using sensors embedded within a mattress to continuously monitor body movements and respiratory patterns showed that at *seven* and *thirteen weeks* of age, they slept less than common fussy infants. The extremely fussy/colicky infants had more difficulty falling asleep, were more easily disturbed and had less quiet, deep sleep.

At about *eight weeks* of age, it was noted that colicky infants slept significantly less (11.8 versus 14.0 hours per day). The colicky infants slept less during the day, evening and night; however, the big difference in sleeping was during the night-time. Again, crying more was associated with sleeping less. The authors concluded that extreme fussiness/colic might be associated with a disruption or delay in the establishment of the circadian rhythm of sleep/wake activity. At *four months* of age, my study showed that the average total sleep duration based on parental reports of forty-eight infants who had had extreme fussiness/colic, based on Dr Wessel's exact definition, was 13.9 plus or minus 2.2 hours, much less than those with common fussiness/crying.

In my general paediatric practice, where all parents receive anticipatory advice regarding sleep hygiene at every visit, parents of extremely fussy/colicky infants describe a late development of early bedtimes, self-soothing to fall asleep at night, longer night sleep periods, fewer night wakings and regular, longer naps compared to common fussy/crying infants. This suggests that while extreme fussiness/colic may be associated with a delay in maturation of sleep/wake control mechanisms, the data shows that by *six*, *eight* and *twelve months* there are no differences in **duration of night sleep** between extreme fussiness/colic and common fussy/crying groups.

However, **night waking** has been reported to be more common following extreme fussiness/colic at *four*, *eight* and *twelve months*. This might be interpreted as a persistent impairment of the learned ability to return to sleep unassisted during a naturally occurring night-time arousal from sleep.

Colic-Wakefulness

Parents of extremely fussy/colicky infants often report that daytime sleep periods are extremely irregular and brief. Also, some parents of extremely fussy/colicky infants describe a dramatic increase in daytime wakefulness and sometimes a temporary but complete cessation of napping when their infants approach their peak fussiness at age six weeks. It has been suggested that, before three to four months of age, the period of inconsolability in the evening hours, when the infant cannot sleep and cries, may reflect periods of high arousal similar to the circadian 'forbidden zone'. In adults, the forbidden zone is a time period during which sleep onset and prolonged, consolidated and restorative sleep states do not easily occur. In this context, it might be more appropriate to describe colic not as a disorder of impaired sleep but as a disorder of excessive wakefulness in the evening. This view is supported by recent sleep lab investigations showing that, in infants, a circadian forbidden zone does exist between 5:00 and 8:00 P.M.

Extreme Fussiness/Colic-Temperament

Temperament characteristics of mood, intensity, adaptability and approach/withdrawal are related to one another, and infants who were described as negative in mood, intense, slowly adaptable and withdrawing were diagnosed as having difficult temperaments because they were difficult for parents to manage. These infants were also observed to be irregular in all bodily functions. When parents performed a temperament assessment at *two weeks* of age and a twenty-four-hour behaviour diary at *six weeks* of age, it was observed that more difficult temperaments at two weeks predicted more crying and fussing at six weeks. At *four weeks* of age, infants who were more difficult in general, more intense and less distractible (less consolable) in particular, cried more during their second month of life than other infants.

Another prospective study performed temperament assessments at the ages of *three* and *twelve months*. At *three months*, the extremely fussy/colicky infants were more intense, more persistent, less distractible and more negative in their mood. However, at *twelve months*, ratings on the temperament questionnaire showed no group differences between the extremely fussy/colicky infants and the control group, but the general impression of the mothers of the colicky group was that they were more difficult.

Infants who had extreme fussiness/colic, using Dr Wessel's criteria, are more likely to have a difficult temperament than non-colicky babies when the temperament assessment is performed at *four months* of age. Furthermore, this progression occurs even when extreme fussiness/colic is successfully treated with the drug dicyclomine hydrochloride. This drug may act centrally in the nervous system or relieve smooth muscle spasms of the gastrointestinal tract. Similar results were observed in another study: while behavioural management significantly reduced evening fussing and crying, there were no effects of successful treatment on later temperament ratings; the infants were still described as difficult. These results originally suggested to me that biological factors cause increased cry/fuss behaviour during the first three to four months of age and subsequently lead to difficult temperament assessments. I then thought that colic-induced parental distress or fatigue was a much less important factor. Now I have a slightly different view that I will share later.

Extreme fussiness/colic does not appear to be an expression of a permanently difficult temperament. In one study of extremely fussy/colicky infants, subsequent measurements of temperament at *five* and *ten months* did not show group differences between formerly extremely fussy/colicky and common fussy/crying infants.

Sleep Temperament

Continuous recordings of sleep patterns during the *second day* of life were linked with temperament assessments at *eight months*. It was observed that infants with the most extreme values on all sleep variables were more likely to have difficult temperaments.

Temperament assessments performed at a mean age of *3.6 months* showed an association between problems of sleep/wake organisation, difficult temperament, and extreme crying. *Mothers of crying infants scored high on depression, anxiety, exhaustion, anger, adverse childhood memories, and marital distress.* The authors concluded that factors related to parental care, while not causing persistent crying, did function to maintain or worsen the behaviour. The persistence of parental factors may explain why at *one year* there is reported to be *more difficulty in communication, more unresolved conflicts, more dissatisfaction and greater lack of empathy in families* with an extremely fussy/colicky infant, and after *four years*, formerly extremely fussy/colicky children have been reported to be more negative in mood on temperament assessments.

In my study of sixty five-month-old infants, the infants rated as difficult had average sleep times substantially less when compared to the infants rated as easy (12.3 versus 15.6 hours). Although nine infant-temperament characteristics were measured, only five are used to establish the temperament diagnosis of difficult. Four of these (mood, adaptability, rhythmicity, and approach/withdrawal) were highly associated with total sleep duration.

When my original study of sixty five-month-old infants was extended to include 105 infants, those with difficult temperaments slept 12.8 hours and those with easy temperaments slept 14.9 hours. This observation was subsequently confirmed in another ethnic group with different parenting practices. It thus appears that infants who have a difficult temperament have briefer total sleep durations when assessed at *four to five months* of age.

Support for a sleep-temperament association is also based on a study where objective measures of sleep/wake organisation, derived from time-lapse video recordings, were compared with parental perceptions of infant temperament at *six months* of age. Dr Keener stated that 'Infants considered [temperamentally] easy have longer sleep periods and spend less time out of the cot for caretaking interventions during the night.' However, the authors' analysis also led them to the conclusion that the night waking is also caused by environmental (parental) rather that biological factors. This increased time out of the cot for temperamentally more difficult children at six months is similar to the observation that increased night waking occurs in formerly extremely fussy/colicky infants at four, eight and twelve months.

Utilising a computerised movement detector, it was observed that for *twelve-month-old* children, those with the temperament trait of increased rhythmicity went to sleep earlier and had longer sleep durations, and by *eighteen months* of age there was again the observation that both subjective and objective improved sleep measures were associated with easier temperament assessments.

The exact same sixty infants that I examined at *four months* of age were restudied at *three years*. Again, temperamentally easy children had longer sleep durations compared to children with more difficult temperaments. However, there was no individual stability of temperament or sleep durations between the ages of four months and three years. Thus, temperament ratings and associated sleep patterns at age four months do not predict temperament or sleep patterns at three years.

Post-colic Sleep

I did another study of 141 infants between *four to eight months* of age from middle-class families and showed that the history of extreme fussiness/colic was associated with the parents' judgement that **night waking** was a current problem. The frequency of awakening was a problem in 76 per cent of infants, the duration of awakenings a problem in 8 per cent, and both frequency and duration a problem in 16 per cent. The more often a child woke up the longer were the durations of the night wakings. Other studies also reported more **night waking** at *eight* and *twelve months* and ages *fourteen to eighteen months* in post-colic children. Among those post-colic infants, the total sleep duration was less (13.5 versus 14.3 hours). These group differences decrease as children become older.

There are studies suggesting that both infant irritability and sleep deficits are moderately stable individual characteristics during the first year of life and beyond. One study showed that children with extreme fussiness/colic had more sleeping problems and the **families exhibited more distress** than a control group at age *three years*. The trend of decreasing group differences with age regarding sleep between colicky and non-colicky infants and the normal sleep lab recordings of colicky infants at nine weeks of age suggest that it is not biological factors that contribute to enduring sleep problems beyond nine weeks of age, it is **parenting practices**.

It may be difficult for parents of post-colicky infants after four months of age to eliminate frequent night wakings and lengthen sleep durations. Because of parental fatigue, parents may unintentionally become inconsistent and irregular in their responses to their infant.

It cannot be overemphasised that, as stated by Dr Parmelee, 'Parents are never truly prepared for the degree to which the babies' sleep/wake patterns will dominate and completely disrupt their daily activities.'

They may become overindulgent and oversolicitous regarding night wakings and not appreciate that they are inadvertently depriving their child of the opportunity to learn how to fall asleep unassisted. Some mothers have difficulty separating from their child especially at night, while other mothers have a tendency toward depression, which might be aggravated by the fatigue that results from struggling to cope with a colicky infant. In either case, simplistic suggestions to help the child sleep better often fail to motivate a change in parental behaviour. If a child fails to learn to fall sleep unassisted, the result is sleep fragmentation or sleep deprivation driven by intermittent positive parental reinforcement. This causes fatigue-driven fussiness long after the colic has resolved, which ultimately creates an overtired family.

Support for this view has come from research on infants at *five months* of age who were followed to *fifty-six months* of age. Dr Wolke showed that 'Long crying duration and having felt distressed about crying during the first *five months* were significant predictors of **night waking** problems at *twenty months*' but not at fifty-six months. In other words, the combined factors of long infant crying or fussing plus parental distress at five months of age make it more likely that a night-waking problem will develop. Even more powerful, later sleep problems are mostly related to the co-morbidity or linking of crying with sleep problems at *five months* rather than to crying problems alone. Sleep problems at *five months* remain the best predictor of sleep problems, especially night waking, at *twenty months*. Dr Wolke concluded that post-colic 'sleep problems are likely to be due to a **failure of the parents to establish and maintain regular sleep schedules** . . . This conclusion *does not* blame parents for sleep difficulties. Rather, it recognises why many parents adopt strategies to deal with **night waking** in the least conflictual manner by night feeding or co-sleeping. This may be especially true of parents who are dealing with a temperamentally more difficult infant.' The authors also concluded that post-colic sleeping problems are not due simply to increased crying per se, but appear to be the consequence of associated infant sleeping problems and altered caretaking patterns for dealing with **night waking** in infancy.

Dr Bates and associates recently directly evaluated the interaction between family stress, family management, disrupted child sleep patterns (variability in amounts of sleep, variability in bedtime and lateness of bedtime), and adjustment in preschool in children about five years old. Children with disrupted sleep did not adjust well in preschool. In their analysis, disrupted sleep directly caused the behaviour problems. They did not find any evidence that family stress or family management problems caused both disrupted sleep and behaviour problems. Dr Bates concluded that 'sleep irregularity accounted for variation in [behavioural] adjustment independently of variation in family stress and family management'. Dr Bates agrees with my hypothesis that sleep modulates temperament and told me that 'parenting responses to [sleep] issues would be involved in the continuity/discontinuity of temperament . . . If parents make the effort to manage their kids' sleep schedules consistently, I would think that over the years they are going to see less difficult and unmanageable behaviour'. Another recent study examined sixty-four children, aged eight to ten years, who had, as infants, 'persistent crying' defined as fussing or crying more than three hours on three days in the week. The authors concluded that they were at risk for hyperactivity problems and academic difficulties. In addition, at eight to ten years of age, the previous persistent criers took a longer time to fall asleep, suggesting to Dr Wolke that 'they were less effective in controlling their own behavioural state to fall asleep'.

Therefore, it appears that the increased crying/fussing behaviour in infancy is associated with less infant sleep, and the crying/fussing alone does not directly cause later sleep problems. Although the post-colicky child's family may be stressed, it appears that it is the failure to establish age appropriate sleep hygiene that specifically leads to later disrupted sleep and behavioural problems.

Summary

During the first four months, colicky infants, by definition, exhibit more cry/fuss behaviour. Data from parent diaries obtained at four and a half, six, seven and eight weeks of age show that extremely fussy/colicky infants sleep less than common fussy/crying infants (about 12–12.5 versus about 14–14.5 hours), but there is disagreement as to whether the decreased sleep occurs predominantly during the day or night hours. By nine weeks of age, sleep lab data does not show group differences regarding sleeping between extremely fussy/colicky and common fussy/crying infants. Group differences in sleeping duration between these two groups of infants, while present even at four months of age, disappear by six to eight months. This raises the suggestion that **parenting practices** might be especially important in affecting sleep patterns after nine weeks, especially regarding the development of a **night-waking** habit. Also, by six months of age, researchers are more apt to describe parents contributing to sleeping problems, especially **night waking**.

There appears to be agreement that infant crying alone does not predict the development of sleep problems. Rather the co-morbidity of crying plus parental distress at five months or crying plus sleep problems at five months predicts night waking at twenty months, but not at fifty-six months.

Temperament assessments at two and four weeks of age showed that infant difficultness predicted increased crying/fussing at about six weeks of age. Infants with extreme fussiness/colic are more likely to have a difficult temperament when assessed at four months of age, but not at twelve months. A difficult temperament is associated, at many ages, with problems in sleeping, such as shorter sleep durations and night waking, but this association is not predictive of later sleep problems. At four to five months of age, infants with a difficult temperament have total sleep durations of about thirteen hours versus about fifteen hours for infants with an easy temperament.

The association of difficult temperament and sleeping problems during and shortly after four months occurs despite successful treatment of colic. My revised view is that it is exactly those parents who have the willingness and resources to invest heavily in soothing during periods of fussing, who are able to prevent some of the fussing escalating into crying and to prevent some post-colic sleep problems. On the other hand, some parents are unable to manage severe infant fussing and become overwhelmed by crying. They feel they cannot influence their child's behaviour regarding crying and, later, sleeping.

It is important for parents to help post-colicky infants establish healthy sleep habits. Some of these children have difficulties falling asleep and staying asleep. At about four months they have not developed self-soothing skills, perhaps because parents had invested constant soothing to prevent fussiness developing into crying, or perhaps the inability to self-soothe is an integral component of colic. A successful intervention effort to help families cope with infant crying during colic will reduce parental distress. Continued age-appropriate sleep hygiene after colic ends is likely to prevent sleep problems persisting beyond four months. Unsuccessful intervention increases the likelihood that temperament issues, family stress, and sleeping problems will persist beyond four months.

Here is one vivid personal account of extreme fussiness/colic.

A Father Remembers Colic; or, Is the French Foreign Legion Accepting Applications?

Sleep? Hmmm . . . Oh, yes! I remember that! We used to do that frequently before Michelle was born.

Two years and another baby later, I still replay Michelle's birth in my mind at least daily. I joked in the delivery room that the newborn was 'ug-ly', but it was just a ruse to help me hold back the tears. A healthy, normal baby! The demons of the past nine months disappeared in a flash.

The first few days were spectacular. While my wife and baby recovered in the hospital from a long, tough, toxaemic labour, I played the role of red-eyed, tired-but-ecstatic new father to the hilt. I showed up at work the next day, ostensibly to guard against using up a holiday day, but actually to show off the Polaroid pictures I had carried home with me in the wee hours of that postpartum morning to avoid waiting an ungodly twenty-four hours for the 35-millimeter prints to be developed.

Everything was perfect. I was getting the house in shape, making the phone calls, bringing goodies to the hospital. Nursing was starting off fine for my wife, Sharon, and our new baby was peaceful and thriving.

The false security even lasted through the first few days Sharon and Michelle were home. Michelle would wake up about every three or four hours and, with a tiny, delicate cry, let us know that it was time to nurse again. We marvelled at the fact that no matter how soft the cry or what room it came from, we could always hear it. Isn't parenthood amazing? And as Michelle nursed, she would usually doze off again. When Sharon was finished, she'd put the baby back in her cot, and we would just stare down at her, enjoying the peaceful sight of our sleeping baby.

Just as Michelle crossed the boundary into her second week of life, the scene started to change. Same little cry. Same nursing routine. But then, when the nursing stopped, a new cry would start. This one was different. Louder. More agitated. More demanding. I rather enjoyed it at first, because it gave me a role – I could pick her up – and with a few minutes of rocking and patting, the crying would stop. It was my first fleeting sense of competence as a father.

But the crying grew worse and worse. Five minutes of rocking were replaced by hour-long midnight jaunts in the pushchair. On rainy nights I'd carry her around the kitchen-to-dining-room-to-living-room-to-kitchen circuit so many times that I actually started to vary my route for fear of embedding a path in the carpet. The left shoulder of every T-shirt I owned had spit stains on it. I switched to the rugby hold: holding Michelle facedown on her tummy with my fingers supporting her chin, I would swing from my hips, back and forth, back and forth, back and forth. At 3:00 A.M. I would strap on the sling and set off for another trek with my frantic daughter.

Each of these strategies worked for a short time. But Michelle had become a motion junkie. Absent motion, she would shriek and scream violently and tirelessly, literally for hours at a time. She would become hoarse, but even that failed to deter her.

Everyone we knew had a theory, even people we had only just met in the supermarket checkout line. All the advice was offered freely and generously, but never without the subliminal undercurrent that the real problem was our incompetence as parents. The baby was nursing too much. She wasn't getting enough food from nursing, so we should give her formula. Mix some cereal in with the formula. Wait four hours between feedings. Put her on a schedule. Relax, she senses your stress. And on and on and on. There was no end to the advice, all of it contradictory, much of it accusatory, and none of it helpful.

Michelle got worse and worse. And we got more and more tired, more and more frazzled, and more and more testy. Then we got the swing.

The swing was one of those wind-up numbers where you place the baby in the seat, turn the crank fifty times, and the seat swings back and forth with a mechanical click.

The swing was the true definition of a mixed blessing. While it was in action, clicking away, Michelle was quiet and often fell asleep. But within two minutes after the final click, Michelle would stir, stretch her arms, fill her lungs and scream.

One good cranking would last about twenty minutes. So we organised our lives into neat, twenty-minute intervals, always trying to catch the sound of lessening momentum so we could crank up the swing again before Michelle got cranked up. And it worked.

It worked so well that Michelle would accept no substitute. Unless she was hungry, there was no longer any time that we could hold our child without her screaming. All of our fears, all of the subliminal messages we had received, were coming true. We were rotten parents. A mechanical swing could calm our child, but we could not. We hated the swing, but we dared not, could not, put it away.

Dr Weissbluth gave us a copy of his book *Crybabies*. Sharon and I each devoured the book in one sitting. One section was particularly important and encouraging to us. It was a bell-shaped curve. Along the horizontal axis was the amount of what was laughingly called 'unexplained fussiness'. 'Unexplained fussiness' is medical jargon for unending, sharp, fierce shrieks that push parents to the edge of insanity.

The point is this: all newborn babies cry a lot. A portion of that crying is for no good reason, as far as we in the grown-up world can tell. If you normalise the daily variations in the amount of this crying, what you find is that it keeps going up for the first six weeks of life, then gradually falls off over the next six weeks. Then it's gone.

We weren't sure it was true, but we decided to delay our mutual suicide pact for twelve weeks to see if it was. As Michelle reached her eighth week of life, we started to notice a strange phenomenon: there were brief periods of time when she was awake and not crying! And those periods of calm were starting to increase! *We were believers.*

Of course, nothing kids do ever conforms entirely to what the books say. Getting Michelle settled down to sleep remained a long, drawn-out ritual well past her twelfth week. And getting her to sleep through the night was still an impossible dream. We were still tired (especially Sharon, who had gone back to work but still nursed her at night and expressed milk for Michelle to take during the day), but we were no longer frantic and frazzled. We had regained a sense of time, a sense of day and night. We no longer felt like miserable failures at the baby business.

We let it ride until Michelle reached five months. Then, after another series of consultations with our doctor, we decided to aggressively manage Michelle's sleep patterns so that both she and we could get some meaningful rest.

The theory was that Michelle was waking up at night at various times just as we all do. But instead of turning over and going back to sleep, she was demanding food and attention from us. She no longer needed the food, and the attention was robbing both her and us of a satisfying night's sleep.

The first rule was no more middle-of-the-night feedings. And because of that, we decided that Sharon should not go to the baby at all during the night, since the sight and smell of her would be too tempting for Michelle. When she cried, I would go in and rock, cuddle, sing or swing . . . whatever it took to get her back to sleep.

The next phase was no more talking. Now when I was summoned to her room for a soiree, I would just lean over her cot and pat her on the back until she was fast asleep. In fact, anything short of a full five minutes would lead to a revival meeting shortly thereafter.

A few days later we held our final strategic planning session with our paediatrician. He suggested that we make the room as dark as possible, put Michelle in her bed, and not open the door until morning. He recommended that Sharon spend the night with a friend, and promised us that this final step would not take more than three nights of prolonged screaming. Very encouraging.

Sharon decided to tough it out with me. When the designated time approached, we started the bedtime ritual. Then we put Michelle in her cot, turned, marched out of the room and shut the door. The crying started immediately. But it lasted only ten minutes. Ten minutes! That was it.

Neither of us slept well that night. We kept straining our ears to hear the cries. But there were none. When daylight came, we rushed into Michelle's room and, lo and behold, she was fine.

And that was it. Ten tough minutes, and the three of us were free from this five-month ordeal. As the days passed, we noticed some very positive side effects. Just like us, Michelle was becoming much more pleasant and fun now that she was well rested. She was thriving, and we were loving it. Life had resumed.

While this father's story may sound extreme, it is actually typical of the lengths parents will go to help their babies through their crying spells. I would like to emphasise that soothing a fussy or crying child is something both parents can do. Even if she is breast-feeding, it is not solely the mother's responsibility.

Fathers can, and in my opinion should, help with their children. If a father can be at home to help the mother for a time after she arrives home from the hospital and again for a period when the baby is about six weeks old, then the mother will be able to adjust to the changes in her baby. One father called this 'tag-team parenting' because whenever one parent became exhausted, the other one took over for car rides, walks or trips in the pushchair to let the other get some much-needed rest. Two exhausted parents don't make a good couple!

Although many remedies have been suggested for extreme fussiness/colic, including catnip or herbal tea, papaya juice, peppermint drops, heartbeat or womb recordings, hot-water bottles or trying new baby formulas, only three manoeuvres have been found to calm fussiness and crying. Additional treatments such as simethicone drops and chiropractic spinal manipulation have been proven to be completely ineffective. Gastroesophageal reflux disease is the newest popular diagnosis in fussy and crying babies, but research has shown it to be a coincidental finding and not the cause of irritability in babies. The three manoeuvres are:

1. ***Rhythmic motions:* rocking chairs, swings, cots with springs attached to the casters, cradles, prams, and pushchairs; walking, taking ceiling tours, using your baby for curling exercises to strengthen biceps, and**

taking car rides. Maybe all rhythmic rocking soothes babies by encouraging regular breathing, thus taking away the need for the baby to 'make' colic in order to breathe well. However, avoid water beds, which are dangerous because they may cause suffocation. Other dangerous colic 'treatments' include certain herbal remedies, which have caused poisoning; beanbag pillows, which have caused suffocation; and trampoline-like devices suspended in the cot, which have caused strangulation. Tryptophan was once used to help babies sleep well, but we now know that this is dangerous; similarly, melatonin should not be given to babies.

2. ***Sucking:*** **at breast, bottle, fist, wrist, thumb or pacifier.**
3. ***Swaddling:*** **wrapping the child in blankets; snuggling, cuddling and nestling. After the first few weeks, however, this manoeuvre is often less effective.**

You should avoid trying gimmick after gimmick; it will only make you feel more frustrated or helpless as the crying continues. You may also feel resentment or anger if your child, perhaps unlike your friend's child, doesn't seem to respond well to home remedies.

PRACTICAL POINT

Feelings of anger towards your crying child are frightening – and normal. You can love your baby and hate her crying spells. All parents sometimes have contradictory feelings about their baby.

Take breaks when your baby is crying. This will enable you to better nurture your child; it's a smart strategy for baby care, not a selfish idea for parent care.

You may feel, during the first few months, that you are not influencing your extremely fussy/colicky child's behaviour very much. And you are right, but consider this period to be a rehearsal. Your hugs, kisses and loving kindness are expressing the way you feel. Practise showering affection on your baby, even when he's crying. This loving attention is important for both of you.

However, unceasing attention showered on a fussing or crying baby, whether he is extremely fussy/colicky or just common fussy, during the first few months *can* have complications if you continue this strategy of intervention for the older, post-colic child at bedtime and nap times. Thus, after the extreme fussiness/colic passes, the older child is never left alone at sleep times and is deprived of the opportunity to develop self-soothing skills. These children never learn to fall asleep unassisted. The resultant sleep fragmentation or deprivation in the child, driven by intermittent positive parental reinforcement, leads to fatigue-driven fussiness long after the biological factors that caused the extreme fussiness/colic have been resolved.

Temperament at Four Months

When the excessive crying and fussiness of your baby's first few months have passed and the child seems more settled, what next? After about four months of age, most parents have learned to differentiate between their child's *need* for consolidated sleep and the child's *preference* for soothing, pleasurable company at night. Most parents can learn to appreciate that prolonged, uninterrupted sleep is a health habit they can influence; they can quickly learn to stop reinforcing night wakings and irregular nap schedules that rob kids of needed rest. A process of 'social weaning' from the pleasure of a parent's company at nap times and bedtimes is underway. As one young mother said, 'I see – I should now forget the company she [the baby] wants.'

But parents of post-colic children still have a few challenges to face. That's because children who have had extreme fussiness/colic appear more likely than other babies to develop a difficult temperament, shorter sleep durations and more frequent night wakings between four and eight months of age.

My research also has shown that parents of post-colic kids are more likely to view frequent (instead of prolonged) night wakings as a problem. Furthermore, boys are more likely than girls to be labelled by their parents as having a night-waking problem. Let's see how these patterns could have emerged.

Dr Alexander Thomas, a pioneer in child development, described temperament differences among babies. In a study based on both his own careful observations and parent interviews, Dr Thomas noted interrelations among four temperament characteristics: mood, intensity, adaptability and approach/withdrawal. Infants who were moody, intense, slow to adapt and withdrawing in Dr Thomas's study were also rated as irregular in all bodily functions. Thus they were diagnosed as having 'difficult' temperaments because they were difficult for parents to manage! We don't know why these particular traits cluster together, but we do know that infants with 'easy' temperaments had opposite characteristics. In Dr Thomas's study, four additional temperament characteristics were described: persistence, activity, distractibility and threshold. (Threshold means how sensitive or insensitive the child appears to be to noises or changes in lighting.) These four temperament characteristics were not part of either the easy or difficult temperament clusters.

The term 'temperament' means behavioural style or the manner in which the child interacts with the environment. It does not describe the motivation of an action. All parents naturally make their own assessment of their babies' temperaments. You may be surprised to know that there is a standardised system for evaluating infant temperament. It is not absolutely objective, and it has a number of limitations that I will point out later, but it has proved over the years to be very useful.

The researchers who developed this system did not have extreme fussiness/colic anywhere in their minds. There is not even a crying dimension in their system. No one connected temperament, as rated on this scale, with extreme fussiness/colic until much later. However, as you will see, the connection proved to be striking.

Infant Temperament Characteristics

Activity (General Motion, Energy)

Does your baby squirm, bounce or kick while lying awake in the cot? Does she move around when asleep? Does she kick or grab during nappy-changing? Some infants always appear to be active, others only in specific circumstances, such as bathing. Activity levels in infants have nothing to do with 'hyperactivity' in older children. I have examined a few babies who previously had been referred to a paediatric gastroenterologist because of extreme fussiness/colic. When he recognised that there were no gastrointestinal problems, he decided that the problem was 'hyperactivity'. This diagnosis was made on the false motion that wakeful, reactive or difficult infants are hyperactive. There is no proven association between high activity levels in infancy and hyperactivity when older.

Rhythmicity (Regularity of Bodily Functions)

Rhythmicity is a measure of how regular or predictable the infant appears. Is there a pattern in the time he is hungry, how much he eats at each feeding, how often bowel movements occur, when he gets sleepy, when he awakens, when he appears most active and when he gets fussy? As infants grow older, they tend to become more regular in their habits. Still, some babies are very predictable at age two months, while others seem to be irregular throughout the first year.

Approach/Withdrawal (First Reaction)

Approach/withdrawal is a temperament characteristic that defines the infant's initial reaction to something new. What does he do when meeting another child or a baby-sitter? Does he object to new procedures? Some infants reach out in new circumstances – accept, appear curious, approach – others object, reject, turn away, appear shy or withdraw.

Adaptability (Flexibility)

Adaptability is measured by observing such activities as whether the infant accepts nail cutting without protest, accepts bathing without resistance, accepts changes in feeding schedule, accepts strangers within fifteen minutes and accepts new foods. It is an attempt to measure the ease or difficulty with which a child can adjust to new circumstances or a change in routine.

Intensity

Intensity is the degree or amount of an infant's response, either pleasant or unpleasant. Think of it as the amount of emotional energy with which they express their likes and dislikes. Intense infants react loudly with much expression of likes and dislikes. During feeding they are vigorous in accepting or resisting food. They react strongly to abrupt exposure to bright lights; they greet a new toy with enthusiastic positive or negative expressions; they display much feeling during bathing, nappy-changing, or dressing; and they react strongly to strangers or familiar people. One mother described her extremely fussy/colicky baby's intense all-or-nothing reactions: 'Her mood changes quickly; she gives no warning – she can go from loud and happy to screaming.' Intensity is measured separately from mood. Infants who are not intense are described as 'mild'.

Mood

If intensity is the degree of response, mood is the direction. It is measured in the same situation described above. Negative mood is the presence of fussy/crying behaviour or the absence of smiles, laughs or coos. Positive mood is the absence of fussy/crying behaviour or the presence of smiles, laughs or coos. Most intense infants also tend to be more negative in mood, less adaptable, withdrawn. Most mild infants also tend to be more positive in mood, more adaptable and approaching.

Persistence

Persistence level, or attention span, is a measure of how long the infant engages in activity. Parents may value this trait under some circumstances but not under others. For instance, persistence is desirable when the child is trying to learn something new, like reaching for a rattle, but it is undesirable when the infant persists in throwing food on the floor. Unfortunately, some babies persist in their prolonged crying spells and their prolonged wakeful periods. One father described his persistently crying baby as follows: 'We have a copper-top, alkaline battery-powered baby and we're powered by ordinary carbon batteries. He outlasts us every time.'

Distractibility

Distractibility describes how easily the baby may be distracted by external events. Picking up the infant easily consoles a distractible infant's fatigue or hunger; soothing can stop fussing during a nappy change. New toys or unusual noises easily distract the infant. Distractibility and persistence are not related to each other, and neither trait is related to activity or threshold levels.

Threshold (Sensitivity)

Threshold levels measure how much stimulus is required to produce a response in the infant in specific circumstances, such as loud noises, bright lights and other situations previously discussed. While some infants are very reactive or responsive to external or environmental changes, other infants barely react.

Difficult Temperament

As previously mentioned, while observing many children and analysing many questionnaires, Dr A. Thomas and Dr S. Chess noticed that four, and only four, of these temperamental traits tended to cluster together. In particular, infants who were extreme or 'intense' in their reactions also tended to be slowly adaptable, negative in mood and withdrawn. This appeared to be a personality type.

According to their parents' descriptions and direct observation by the researchers, these infants seemed more difficult to manage than other infants. Consequently, a child whose temperament scores fall into this pattern is said to have a difficult temperament. One mother referred to her infant as a 'mother killer'. Infants with the opposite temperamental traits are said to have easy temperaments. These are sometimes called 'dream' babies. One father described his 'easy' infant as a 'low-maintenance baby'. The difficult temperament and the easy temperament are only descriptions of a behavioural style. Temperament research usually does not ask why a child behaves in a particular way. There is no scientific basis for labelling a child with a difficult temperament as a 'high needs' child. In fact, there is no scientific support for labelling a child a 'high needs' child under any circumstances.

Later, I will explain why so many so-called 'high-needs' children are really very overtired children/difficult temperament children.

Of the original group of infants Thomas and Chess studied, about 10 per cent fell into the difficult temperament category. These infants also tended to be irregular in biological function such as sleep schedules and night awakenings. They were more likely to have behavioural problems – particularly sleep disturbances – when they grew older. One of the most interesting differences between difficult and easy babies is the way they cry when they are past the extreme fussiness period – that is, when they are three or four months old. Published research found that mothers listening to the taped cries of infants rated difficult (not their own babies), described the crying as more irritable, grating and arousing than the crying of easy infants. They said that the first group sounded spoiled and were crying because of frustration rather than hunger or wet nappies. An audio analysis of cries helped explain why this should be. The crying of the difficult infants was found to have more silent pauses between crying noises than that of the easy babies. These silent pauses caused the listener to repeatedly think that the crying spell had ended. Also, at its most intense, the crying of difficult infants was actually pitched at a higher frequency. These two differences can make the crying seem much more frightening, piercing and annoying.

What causes the difficult temperaments? Do they learn to be this way? Is it genetically prewired or are they overtired?

Here's how child development specialist Laya Frischer described a post-colicky baby.

JANE AT AGE FOUR MONTHS

Jane is difficult and unpredictable, with less than average sleep and cuddling and more than average crying. Observations over five weeks have revealed an extremely sensitive infant. For a period of time, she could not even tolerate touches on her abdomen. Swaddling helps a little, and the rhythmic swing movement gives her some relief. If these things fail, the parents walk her around. Sometimes these efforts quiet her fussiness, but at other times it escalates to panic crying. Jane seems to have no capacity to console herself, and very little capacity to be consoled by usual methods of touch. The pacifier has been helpful, but not always successful. Jane does not have good state regulation. *She can be in a panic cry state when she seems to be asleep.*

Jane goes from sleep to distress in seconds. She becomes overtired and cannot sleep, which contributes to her irritability. She does not habituate easily to sensory stimulation of light and touch. Jane requires a very protective environment, which puts great stress on her parents, particularly her mother. Her cries are very hard to read; her parents feel she is unpredictable, and often uncommunicative.

Connecting Sleep, Extreme Fussiness/Colic, and Temperament

Different Approaches for Different Babies

As you read earlier, for every hundred babies, about 80 per cent will have common fussiness, and of these, 49 per cent (thirty-nine babies) will have easy temperaments, 46 per cent (thirty-seven babies) will have intermediate temperaments, and only 5 per cent (four babies) will have a difficult temperament. However, for that 20 per cent of babies who had extreme fussiness/colic, the outcome at four months is quite different. In this group, only 14 per cent (three babies) will have easy temperaments, 59 per cent (twelve babies) will have intermediate temperaments and 27 per cent (five babies) will have difficult temperaments. It is important to recognise that the largest group is the intermediate temperament group comprising of forty-nine babies, or 49 per cent of the total. Some of these babies will be closely but not quite resembling easy-temperament babies or difficult-temperament babies. So, for almost half of all babies, the advice regarding common fussiness leading to an easy temperament and extreme fussiness leading to a difficult temperament fits only approximately. So please read the entire section and take out of it only that which applies to your baby.

The risk of developing sleeping problems after four months of age probably looks something like this:

LOWEST RISK FOR SLEEP PROBLEMS AFTER FOUR MONTHS

39 per cent of common fussy babies who develop easy temperaments

3 per cent of extremely fussy/colicky babies who develop easy temperaments

37 per cent of common fussy babies who develop intermediate temperaments

12 per cent of extremely fussy/colicky babies who develop intermediate temperaments

4 per cent of common fussy babies who develop difficult temperaments

5 per cent of extremely fussy/colicky babies who develop difficult temperaments

HIGHEST RISK FOR SLEEP PROBLEMS AFTER FOUR MONTHS

Different temperaments and perhaps different paths to these temperaments will lead to different sleep strategies for each child. It appears to me that the difficult temperament at four months mostly represents an extremely overtired baby while the easy temperament represents an extremely rested baby. But keep in mind that biological factors within the baby, such as elevated serotonin levels or immature development of sleep/wake rhythms, may contribute to a baby's behaviour during the first four months. It is equally important to remember that there is enormous variability regarding the resources with which parents are able to soothe their babies. These are factors within the mother (for example, baby blues or postpartum depression), the husband (forcing a too-late bedtime, not helping to soothe the baby), the marriage (disagreements regarding family bed or breast-feeding), and the family (too many conflicting time pressures regarding other children, career events, not enough bedrooms, ability to hire housekeeping or baby care help, and so forth). So it is important to look at the big picture, your baby and your total soothing support structure, and resources that you have available. What will work for one family may not work for you. The goal is to develop a caring environment for the family, not a cure for extreme fussiness/colic.

'No Cry' versus 'Let Cry'

Some parents are strong believers in only one approach to soothing to sleep. They believe there should never be any crying and that by always holding their baby, frequently nursing their baby and sleeping with their baby, they can prevent extreme fussiness/colic from occurring and prevent sleep problems. They characterise their approach as 'gently to sleep', 'attached parenting', a gentle, warm, child-centred style that enhances a sense of security because the baby is taught that the mother is always there. They characterise other approaches as 'cry it out', 'detached parenting', a cold, rigid, parent-centred style that creates a sense of abandonment because the baby is taught that the mother is unresponsive. These parents say that when the baby stops crying and sleeps, he 'has given up' trying to communicate with his mother. This stark contrast in parenting styles is supposed to produce differences in babies and differences in the bonding between the child and her parents. However, there are some major problems with this way of thinking. First, there is no evidence that one style or another produces a specific outcome. Second, babies themselves contribute a lot to what will easily work or not work. Third, fathers, siblings and real-life family issues help shape your ability to soothe, comfort and put your baby to sleep. Fourth, there are methods in between always attending to night crying and never attending to night crying such as 'check and console' or 'controlled crying', whereby the child is allowed to cry for only short periods of time (see page 104).

'Attachment parenting' may or may not be your decision, but it may work well for 39 per cent of babies who had common fussiness and developed an easy temperament. For these babies, everything you read in popular books about soothing and sleeping will likely 'work'. This might even be true for the 40 per cent (3 per cent plus 37 per cent) of babies in the next two groups of babies at a low risk for developing sleep problems. So, perhaps the majority of families (39 per cent plus 37 per cent) will have a fairly smooth course to easy soothing and sleeping, and an additional 3 per cent will struggle to get to a place where sleeping becomes easy at four months of age. Perhaps, for the majority of parents, the path does not involve any crying. There is no reason to be judgemental and criticise other parents who are not so fortunate.

There is an unfortunate minority (9 per cent) of families who I believe become distressed or overwhelmed with the arrival of their baby because they lack sufficient resources to soothe the baby and/or the baby has extreme fussiness/colic so she develops into an overtired four-month-old with a difficult temperament. These parents may have started out with the cot and decided later to use the family bed for soothing and sleeping, and were still frustrated later because after four months the baby still did not sleep well. Flexibility and sensitivity to your own baby and your own family situation is key.

Common Fussiness: Low Risk for Sleep Problems After Four Months

Breast-feeding becomes much easier around four months of age or sooner for these babies because everyone is better rested and life is more predictable. At three to four months, your baby will start to show drowsy signs earlier in the evening. Instead of becoming sleepy at 8:00 to 10:00 P.M., she will become sleepy at 6:00 to 8:00 P.M. Respect her need to sleep and *begin the soothing process at night at the earlier hour*. If you are using a cot, simply put her to sleep earlier; but if you are using a family bed, you have to make some choices. The first is to go to bed much earlier yourself, but this is not usually practical. The second would be to lie down with her in your bed and create a safe nest or use a co-sleeper where she will sleep, and then leave her after she has fallen asleep. The danger in this is that she might roll off the bed and injure herself. The third is to transition her to a cot for the beginning of night sleep and until she awakens for her first night feeding, and then bring her to your bed for the remainder of the night. Because these are well-rested four-month-old babies, they are more adaptable and easy to transition to a cot. One strategy is to breast-feed at night, pass your baby to his father, who soothes him in his arms, and then puts the baby down in the cot. This breaks up the previous pattern of mother-breast-feeding-sleep in parents' bed. If your baby cries, soothe him without picking him up. But if this fails, pick him up and, after soothing, try again.

If you are bottle-feeding (formula or expressed breast milk) or breast-feeding and using a cot around four months of age, expect to feed your baby about four to six hours after her last evening bottle and again early in the morning around 4:00 to 5:00 A.M. until about nine months of age. Some bottle-fed babies are fed only once, around 2:00 or 3:00 A.M. If you are breast-feeding and using a family bed, you might feed your baby many times throughout the night.

If you are using a cot, there is more social stimulation as you pick up the baby, more time required to prepare the bottle, and more handling as you put the baby down to sleep again. Under these circumstances, feeding your baby more than twice at night after four months is likely to create a *night-waking habit*. If you are breast-feeding, the obvious question is whether the awakenings at night, other than the two times mentioned, are due to hunger. If your breast milk supply has not kept pace with your baby's needs or has decreased, then your baby will awaken more at night because of thirst and/or hunger. Are you thirsty throughout the day? If so, you are not drinking enough fluid. Are there some unusual stresses in your life such as an important trip that you have to take, are you worried about balancing child care and working, or worried about returning to work and continuing to breast-feed? Is your baby producing less urine? Has the volume of your expressed breast milk decreased? When offered a bottle of expressed breast milk or formula, does your baby now take a much larger feeding? Does he sleep better or longer after taking a bottle? If you think your child is hungry and you want to continue breast-feeding, then contact a lactation consultant through your paediatrician or maternity hospital.

If you are using a family bed, feeding often throughout the night is not likely to create a night-waking habit. This is because your baby is partially asleep or barely awake when fed. Therefore, the risk of sleep fragmentation for both mother and baby from too much social stimulation is low. With early bedtimes in place, the family bed does not create any sleep problems, and in fact, the family bed may have been part of the soothing solution during the first few months.

After the development of an earlier bedtime, the next sleep change is the evolution of a regular nap around 9:00 to 10:00 A.M. This nap may initially be about forty minutes, but it will lengthen to one or two hours. The rest of the day may be snatches of brief and irregular sleep periods. After the morning nap develops, when the baby is a little older, the next regular nap occurs around noon to 2:00 P.M. This nap will also lengthen to become about one to two hours. There may be a third mini-nap that is irregular and brief in the late afternoon.

These sleep rhythms are maturing for night sleep and day sleep. A common mistake is to approach the timing of naps and night sleep by strictly enforcing a 'by the clock' (BTC) routine. A temperamentally very regular baby might appear to be sleeping BTC, but watching your baby's behaviour for sleepy signs is more important than watching the clock.

Consider our original group of one hundred babies. At four months, of the forty-nine babies with an intermediate temperament, thirty-seven babies (about 76 per cent) had common fussiness when younger. Also, at four months, of the forty-two babies with an easy temperament, thirty-nine babies (about 93 per cent) had common fussiness when younger. So, out of the original eighty babies with common fussiness, the vast majority, seventy-six (thirty-seven plus thirty-nine), or **95 per cent**, is at a low risk for developing sleep problems because:

Parents are not likely to be stressed
Infant is likely to be well rested
Infant is likely to be able to self-soothe
At night, consolidated sleeping (long sleep duration) develops early
During the day, regular and long naps naturally develop early, without parental scheduling
If sleep problems exist, 'no cry' solutions usually work

Extreme Fussiness/Colic: High Risk for Sleep Problems After Four Months

Consider our original group of one hundred babies. Out of the original twenty babies with extreme fussiness/colic, a minority of only five, or **20 per cent**, is at risk for developing sleep problems. However, at four months, of the nine babies with a difficult temperament, five babies, or a majority of 56 per cent, had extreme fussiness/colic when younger. Another way to look at this is that only nine out of the original hundred babies, a tiny group, or **9 per cent**, develop a difficult temperament and subsequent sleep problems because:

Parents are likely to be stressed
Infant is likely to be overtired
Infant is likely to be only parent-soothed
At night, fragmented sleep (night waking) persists
During the day, irregular and brief naps persist
If sleep problems exist, 'let cry' solutions might be necessary

I believe it is in this small percentage of babies that you have the most severe and hard-to-solve sleep problems. There are two reasons for this. The first is that the biological factors that led to extreme fussiness/colic in the first place in five of the nine babies might persist and frustrate parents' best efforts to solve sleep problems. The second is that the social or family factors that led to parents' distress and difficulty in soothing for four of the nine babies who had common fussiness might persist and interfere with establishing healthy sleep habits. These social or family issues of course might also be a factor for those babies with extreme fussiness/colic, either caused by the extreme fussiness or independent of the extreme fussiness/colic.

Breast-feeding these babies may be difficult because everyone is tired. As the biological need for an earlier bedtime develops, the best strategy is to temporarily try to do whatever it takes to maximise sleep and minimise crying. The plan is to keep your child as well rested as possible in order to buy time for the development of more mature sleep/wake rhythms. Once these rhythms are developed, they may be used as an aid to help your child sleep better. For example, the breast-feeding mother might have to take the baby into her bed and nurse her to sleep at the earlier bedtime. However, real life events, such as returning to work or caring for other family members, might not permit the luxury of always sleeping with your baby whenever he appears to be sleepy.

You may have wanted to practise 'attachment parenting' and spend much of the first four months soothing your baby, but now, she is heavy when you carry her all day. More important, she is more alert and curious and able to resist and fight sleep for the pleasure of your company even when she needs to sleep. This 'natural' desire for social contact may interfere with the 'natural' development of healthy sleep habits. It is difficult to have clarity of thought and purpose when everyone is tired. As outlined in Chapter 1, it is not always clear what really is 'natural' or 'unnatural'.

It is 'natural' for all babies to fuss or cry, for all mothers to want to soothe their babies and to be distressed by their babies' fussiness or crying, that the more fussiness/crying for the baby means less sleep for the mother, that mother's distress increases with her own sleep loss, and that in some tribal cultures other people are available to help care for the baby. It is 'natural' to breast-feed, to change when soiled, to feed when hungry, to soothe when fussy, to sleep when tired, to sleep with your baby and to carry your baby everywhere in most, but not all, tribal cultures. In some tribal cultures, for example Yemen, mothers leave their baby totally alone all day while they work.

It is 'unnatural' to have urban stimulation (noises, voices, shopping trips, errands), day care (naps not occurring when sleepy, too late a bedtime at night), mother working outside the home (returning late causing a late bedtime), or social isolation (mother is alone and becomes exhausted with too many things to do). It is 'unnatural' to deliberately wake your baby and remove your breast before putting him down to sleep 'awake'. It is 'unnatural' to try to force-feed your baby at night to try to make him sleep better. Is all this brand new? Probably not. We know that during the Egyptian and Roman empires, wealthy women did not breast-feed their babies but instead hired wet nurses.

Can you change your lifestyle so that your child will receive the soothing to sleep at those times when she needs to sleep? Can you avoid too much social stimulation from interfering with sleep even if it means ignoring your child's crying only at those precise times when she needs to sleep? These are difficult questions that many families never have to confront. Many popular books on children's sleep give simple answers or easy solutions that often fail for this group of 9 per cent of infants.

Recent research on an initial group of 1,019 families supports my idea that at four months of age there are two subgroups of overtired children who appear to have a difficult temperament. Many mothers dropped out of the study, but the 560 mothers who stayed were more likely to be married, have completed more formal education, have higher household incomes, be nonsmokers, breast-feed and have 'higher levels of social support'. They noted that at three months of age there were thirty-five children who were crying enough to be called colicky. Of these, eighteen (51 per cent) had been this way at six weeks of age (typical colic) but seventeen (49 per cent) had not ('latent colic'). They felt that these represented two subgroups of colicky infants and went on to describe a third subgroup (14 per cent of colicky infants) that continued to cry substantially past three months of age. The authors considered this to represent a 'persistent mother-infant distress syndrome'. Comparing this study to my analysis, I would say that at four months of age there are about 9 per cent of overtired children with difficult temperaments representing two groups of whom five out of nine, 56 per cent, were formerly extremely fussy/colicky babies (similar to the 'typical colic') and four out of nine, 44 per cent, had common fussiness/crying (similar to the 'latent colic'). I believe that those families with limited resources for soothing their babies are at greater risk for the overtired/fussy/crying state to persist. However, I do object to the term 'mother-infant distress syndrome' because of the blame it directs to the mother. Obviously, fathers, grandparents, financial factors and so forth can stress a family independent of the mother's capabilities to nurture her child.

Post-colic: Preventing Sleep Problems After Four Months of Age

After extreme fussiness/colic winds down around four months of age or sooner, a child may be overtired, not sleeping well and difficult to manage. But not all difficult to manage four-month-olds had colic. I suspect there are two groups of children at four months of age, both of whom have difficult temperaments.

The first group with a difficult temperament comes from the large group (80 per cent) of infants with common fussiness/crying. Only about 4.5 per cent of these children, or four infants out of a hundred, fall into this category. I think they are less overtired than the second group. When parents put forth great effort to help them sleep better, there is relatively fast improvement. They are more adaptable and it is easier to change their sleep routines. 'No cry' sleep strategies are likely to work well.

The second group with a difficult temperament comes from a small group (20 per cent) of infants with extreme fussiness/colic. About 27 per cent of these children, or five infants out of a hundred, fall into this category. I think they are more overtired than the first group. When parents put forth great effort to help them to sleep better, there is relatively slow improvement. They are less adaptable and it is more difficult to change their sleep routines. 'No cry' sleep strategies are not likely to work and parents have to consider 'let cry' sleep strategies.

Here is a practical example of how different these babies are. Read the following advice on how to move your baby out of your bed. If you had decided that you wanted a family bed before your child was born, you might decide to continue the family bed for a long time, and when you move your baby out, the transition might be very easy if your baby had common fussiness/crying and now has an easy temperament. On the other hand, if your decision for a family bed was in reaction to extreme fussiness/colic and your child now has a difficult temperament, the transition might be very stressful for the entire family.

Transition from Family Bed to Cot

Q: *I am breast-feeding and my child sleeps with us, but I want to move him out of our bed. How do I do this?*

A: There is no one right way to do this, but however you do it, do it gradually and slowly over several weeks or a few months. Make the move when both parents agree that it is the right time. Always be mindful for your baby's safety. Initially, respond promptly when your baby calls for you. Later, you might delay your response. A baby might be placed in a cot secured to the side of your bed with the railing down. Later the railing is placed up and the cot is moved a few inches from your bed. Gradually, the cot is moved farther away until it is in baby's room. An older child might sleep on a mattress on the floor in your room, with or without the parent. Later, the mattress is moved to the child's room, with or without the parent. Sometimes you might just want your child to be in her cot or bed but in your room. If you are going to use a separate room and your child is older, announce the planned move in advance, make the room very attractive, or let her help decorate her room. Alternatively, move your baby into the room or bed where the siblings are sleeping. Some parents will begin the night all together in the parents' bed and then move the child to a cot after she has fallen asleep.

Q: *Do I have to wean my baby from breast-feeding before I move him out of our bed?*

A: I think the answer depends on your resources for soothing other than breast-feeding, especially the assistance of the father, plus your desire to continue or discontinue breast-feeding. I see no reason why weaning from breast-feeding has to precede or accompany your moving the baby.

The observation that brief and interrupted sleep often follows extreme fussiness/colic might suggest that some congenital, biological factors lead initially to extreme fussiness/colic, and that they are still present in the baby after the colicky period has passed. This is supported by the observation (mentioned earlier) that despite successful drug therapy that eliminated or reduced colicky crying, brief sleep periods were still the norm at four months of age. In addition, some, but not all, post-colic infants continue to behave as if they had heightened activity levels and excessive sensitivity to environmental stimuli.

Here is another example of sensitivity to environmental stimuli from my own experience. When my first son had colic, I had to keep the cot railing up and locked in place, because the clunk of the spring lock would always awaken him. This makes it awkward for me to place him in his cot, but fortunately I was limber from college gymnastics. For my wife, it was an impossible situation until we got a sturdy stool for her to stand on – but it still hurt our backs!

Interestingly, these two temperament characteristics (high activity and high sensitivity) are not part of the diagnostic criteria for babies who fall into the difficult temperament category. But some of these post-colic infants were exquisitely sensitive to irregularities in their nap or night sleep schedule. Disruptions of regular routines due to painful ear infections or holidays and trips subsequently caused extreme resistance to falling asleep and frequent night waking, lasting up to several days after the disruptive event. These prolonged recovery periods might reflect easily disorganised internal biological rhythms caused by enduring congenital imbalances in arousal/inhibition or wake/sleep control mechanisms. Alternatively, parents who put their baby to sleep slightly too late, or who often cause their children to skip naps after four months of age, keep their post-colic infant close to the edge of over-tiredness. What happens when some natural disruptive event occurs is that the child falls into the abyss of severe agitated wakefulness and irritability and the child is unable to easily get back into a regular sleep pattern.

Some post-colic kids have boundless energy. 'She crawls like lightning' was how one mother described her baby. These babies are constantly on the move. They would rather crawl up mum's chest to perch on her shoulder than sit quietly in her lap. But once having reached the shoulder, they immediately want to get down and check out that ball or some equally exciting object off in the corner. They appear easily bored; they also seem very stimulus-sensitive, especially to mechanical noises such as those of a vacuum cleaner, hair dryer or coffee grinder (which may have seemed to calm them down during colicky spells when they were younger). It's as if they have a heightened level of arousal, activity and curiosity. When overtired, they are always grumpy and socially demanding, needing mummy's presence and wanting to be held all the time. They also are quick to fuss when mum leaves the room for only a minute. But when they are well rested, it's a different story.

When they've had enough sleep, these same babies appear to have boundless curiosity, actively seeking opportunities to learn. Maybe these are very intelligent children who are so alert, curious and bright that they have difficulty controlling their impulses to explore or investigate the world. No data support the conclusion that post-colic kids in general are more intelligent, but there may be a small number who are so exceptionally bright that they gave birth to this myth. One study of infants published in 1964 connected increased crying (induced by snapping a rubber band on the sole of the foot at age four to ten days) to increased intelligence at three years of age. Whether this artificially induced crying and its link with intelligence can be generalised to colicky crying is an open question.

When you become your child's timekeeper and programme her sleep schedules, she will be able to sleep day and night on a regular schedule. For most parents, this is a relatively easy adjustment to make. But for post-colic infants, expect to put forth a greater effort to be regular and consistent. Your effort to keep the child well rested will be rewarded by a calmer, happier, more even-tempered child. One family that was finally able to permanently degrump their baby explained, 'The "other" baby is back!'

Here is a story of a child who probably had extreme

fussiness/colic, even though the parents wanted to call him sleep-deprived. There was no quick sleep solution, but improvement did come slowly. Patience is always rewarded if you are reasonably consistent.

When Jackson was four months old, he had never been on any kind of sleep schedule. He seemed to cry all the time and would only sleep about four hours at a time (if we were lucky!) My husband and I would spend hours on end, holding, rocking, bouncing, singing, playing, doing anything we could think to do to get him to stop crying. Our paediatrician said that he had colic and there was nothing we could do about it but to wait it out. Looking back on it all now, I am convinced that he didn't have colic at all, but was just plain sleep-deprived. At first we were hesitant to allow Jackson to cry without holding him. Given that we are both psychologists, we were scared that leaving him alone to cry would be emotionally scarring and would affect his attachment and self-esteem. But we were both sleep-deprived ourselves, stressed out and desperate to try anything. Dr Weissbluth's belief that not to allow him to learn to soothe himself to sleep was damaging in itself and was what allowed us to finally take the plunge. The first time I put him to sleep in his cot for a nap, I left the room and he screamed bloody murder. I sat at the top of the stairs and just cried and cried. I was convinced I was the worst mother in the world. After twenty minutes (which felt like an eternity), he finally fell asleep and slept for two hours. Unfortunately, later naps did not prove to be so easy. There were times in which he screamed for the whole hour (and I cried for the whole hour) and we would get him and try again later. Jackson was a bit resistant to the whole idea, and even though we were very consistent, he always put up a good fight. Even now, at nine months old, Jackson will still cry before most naps and bedtime. Sometimes it's thirty seconds, sometimes it's thirty minutes. He sleeps so much better and longer than he ever did. We calculated that before he was averaging ten hours of sleep per day, and after just a few weeks he was sleeping around seventeen hours a day. The best part of all was that he learned how to sleep through the night. Now, he goes to bed most nights between 6:00 and 7:00 P.M. and he wakes up

> usually between 6:00 and 7:00 A.M. He takes two naps per day, one around 9:00 A.M. and the other in the early afternoon. My husband and I finally got the sleep we needed and the stress level went down dramatically. We have our evenings together back, which we desperately needed. And Jackson's temperament is dramatically improved. I would still say he is a highly active baby, but would no longer say he is fussy. Before, I was certain we would never have another child because it was just too much on us emotionally. But now we are planning to conceive again within the next year.

Without your effort to maintain sleep schedules, a child will have a tendency to sleep irregularly and become unmanageably wild, screaming out of control with the slightest frustration, and spending most of the day engaged in crazy, demanding, impatient behaviours. The majority of post-colic infants do not fit this extreme picture, but they do require more parental control to establish healthy sleep schedules, compared to non-colicky infants. Thus it appears that after about four months of age, poor sleep habits are learned, not congenital.

PRACTICAL POINT

For all post-colic infants over four months of age, my clinical observations are that frequent night wakings may be eliminated and sleep durations lengthened if, and only if, parents establish and maintain regular sleep schedules for their child.

It appears that most post-colic sleep problems are not caused primarily by a biological disturbance of sleep/wake regulation; rather, the problem is parents' failure to establish regular sleep patterns when the colic dissipates at about four months of age. Both obvious and subtle reasons can be cited as to why parents have difficulty in enforcing sleep schedules when colic ends.

Three months of crying sometimes adversely and permanently

shapes parenting cycles. An inconsolable infant triggers in some parents a perception that their baby's behaviour is out of their control. They observe no obvious benefit to their extremely fussy/colicky child when they try to be regular according to clock times or to be consistent in bedtime routines. Naturally, they then assume that this handling will not help their post-colic child, either. Unfortunately, they do not observe the transition, at around four months, from colicky crying to fatigue-driven crying.

Alternatively, some parents may unintentionally and permanently become inconsistent and irregular in their responses to their infant simply because of their own fatigue. The constant, complex and prolonged efforts they use to soothe or calm their extremely fussy/colicky baby are continued. But these ultimately lead to an over-indulgent, over-solicitous approach to sleep scheduling when the colic has passed. Their nurturing at night, for example, becomes stimulating over-attentiveness. In responding to their child's every cry, the parents inadvertently deprive her of the opportunity to learn how to fall asleep unassisted. The child then fails to learn the important skill of self-soothing, which she will need her entire life.

In addition, my studies have shown that when daytime sleep is interrupted, the same consequences occur. The nap-deprived infant develops a short attention span. Remember, other studies have shown that the difficult child is irregular. It is exactly these two temperament traits, short attention span and irregularity, that have been shown to interfere with a child's ability to learn – beginning with learning how to fall asleep without his parents' help.

Effective behavioural therapy to establish healthy post-colic sleep patterns by teaching the child how to fall asleep and stay asleep may or may not be acceptable to you, depending on your ability to perceive and respond to the sleep needs of your infant. (A variety of ways to achieve healthy sleep will be discussed in detail in the chapters that follow.)

Other parents, usually mothers, have extreme difficulty separating from their child, especially at night, as will be discussed in Chapter 12. They may have some difficulty themselves being alone at night because their husband's work requires frequent or prolonged absences, or because nights have always been lonely times for them. They perceive every cry as a need for nurturing. These women are wonderful mothers, but they may be too good. The infant's every need is anticipated and met before it is experienced; in doing so, the mother unintentionally thwarts the development of her child's capacity to be alone. For example, she may block her infant's attempts to provide himself with a substitute (such as thumb sucking or use of a pacifier) for her physical presence.

These parents perpetuate brief and fragmented sleep patterns in their children. Their infants become, according to Dr Ogden, a child psychiatrist, 'addicted to the actual physical presence of the mother and [can]not sleep unless they are being held. These infants are unable to provide themselves an internal environment for sleep.' Although the *child* has disturbed sleep, here the focus of the problem and the key to its solution lies with the *parent.*

WARNING

Persistent sleeping problems in children have been linked to psychiatric symptoms in adolescents, hyperactivity in children, and depression in their mothers.

Extreme fussiness/colic certainly does not cause the parents to have difficulty separating from their child! But it is more than a sufficient stimulus to cause them to regress toward the least adaptive level of adjustment. The result is severe, enduring sleep disturbance in the child. In this setting, simplistic suggestions to help the child sleep better often fail to motivate a change in how the parents approach the problem. Thus, while it is the wakeful child who may be brought for professional help, it is often the parent who has the unappreciated problem.

Extreme fussiness/colic is the most obvious example of extreme crying, but please remember that any painfully overtired infant or child might cry. In some non-industrial societies, babies rarely cry, because they are always held close to the mother in a carrier. However, even in cultures where there is constant holding and unrestricted breast-feeding throughout the day and night, babies still cry and fuss. Here, too, the crying and fussing peak at about six weeks of age! Of course, these babies are less likely to have any congenital tendency toward fussiness exacerbated by overtiredness. These mothers do not drive cars, wear watches or keep many daily appointments to which they must drag their infants. Also, there is less environmental stimulation, so the baby might sleep well outdoors when the mother is planting rice or cooking. Our lifestyles are different, and may cause our children to be overtired more often.

IMPORTANT POINT

Because *all* babies fuss and cry, some a little and some a lot, it's best to think of colic as something a baby *does*, not something a baby *has*. It's a stage of life, not a medical problem.

Summary and Action Plan for Exhausted Parents

Sleep and Extreme Fussiness/Colic

All babies fuss and cry for no apparent reason during the first several weeks.

Babies who require more than a total of three hours a day of soothing to prevent crying, for more than three days in a week, for more than three weeks have extreme fussiness/colic. Fussing occurs more than crying. Fussiness is a pre-cry state that will often change into crying if parents are unable to soothe their baby; some fussing leads to crying despite parents' soothing efforts.

- **It starts around a few days of age**
- **It occurs in the evening**
- **It ends around three to four months of age**
- **They start to fuss/cry when awake and stop when asleep**

Twenty per cent of babies have extreme fussiness/colic.

During the first few months, these babies not only fuss and cry more, they also **sleep less**. Soothing these babies might lead to less crying, but not necessarily more sleeping. Review 'Drowsy Signs' on page 63.

Unfortunately, many extremely fussy/colicky infants do not show drowsy signs.

Review 'Soothing to Sleep' on page 63.

You cannot spoil your baby, so do whatever you can to maximise sleep and minimise fussing and crying.

Unfortunately, for extremely fussy/colicky babies, many simple soothing methods do not work. Constant holding, breast-feeding and sleeping with your baby may be required for soothing.

Review 'Resources for Soothing' on page 73.

Make plans to enlist extra help from family, neighbours, and relatives.

If sleeping with your baby is the only way to soothe him and get some sleep, then sleep with him, even if you did not want to do so, for four months.

It is far better to let your baby cry than it is to shake him, so if you are completely exhausted and in pain from sleep deprivation, take a break to recharge your battery . . . even if your baby is crying.

Maternal depression, anxiety, exhaustion and marital stress are likely to develop.

Extremely fussy/colicky infants are more likely to develop a night-waking habit after four months.

Extremely fussy/colicky infants are more likely to develop a difficult temperament after four months.

RISK FACTORS FOR ENDURING SLEEP PROBLEMS

1. **Extreme fussiness/crying plus maternal distress about fussing and crying at five months of age.**
2. **Extreme fussiness/crying plus sleep problems at five months of age.**

Extreme fussiness/crying alone is not a risk factor for enduring sleep problems.

Temperament at Four Months

How does your child interact with the environment? If he is intense, slowly adaptable, negative in mood, withdrawn and irregular, then he is difficult to manage. He has a difficult temperament. At four months of age, I think this represents an overtired child. Sleep modulates temperament, so helping your child sleep well will make him easier to manage.

Connecting Sleep, Extreme Fussiness/Colic and Temperament: Different Approaches for Different Babies

Plan for your baby's tendency to fuss/cry and your baby's temperament

For a hundred babies:

- At birth, 80 per cent of babies have common fussiness. Of these, 49 per cent (thirty-nine babies) will become *easy*,

46 per cent (thirty-seven babies) will become *intermediate* and 5 per cent (four babies) will become *difficult*.

- At birth, 20 per cent of babies have extreme fussiness/colic. Of these, only 14 per cent (three babies) will become *easy*, 59 per cent (twelve babies) will become *intermediate* and 27 per cent (five babies) will become *difficult*.

Match your parenting decisions to your baby's evolving temperament

- **Family Bed: All the time, part-time, never, with or without a co-sleeper.**

  For about 80 per cent of babies – those who have common fussiness – an early commitment to a family bed usually works well. Sleep problems later are unlikely.

  For about 20 per cent of babies – those with extreme fussiness – an early commitment to a family bed may be associated with sleep-deprived parents for several weeks, but the strong soothing power of bodily warmth, close physical contact, sounds of breathing, or hearing a parent's heartbeat when sucking at the breast, or the smell of breast milk may make the effort worth it. Sleep problems later might occur if the child is allowed to stay up too late when about four months old.

During the day, some parents with extremely fussy/colicky or common fussy/crying babies are overwhelmed because they may have limited resources for soothing. For babies whose parents initially did not want to have a family bed, but later made that decision because of its soothing power, sleep problems are more likely to occur. The sleep problems are more likely to occur not because of the family bed but because of limited resources for soothing to continue.

- **Breast-feed: All the time, part-time (expressed breast milk versus formula), never.**
  For about 80 per cent of babies – the common fussy/crying babies – mothers are better rested and feeding is mostly for nutrition. Breast-feeding is usually easy.

  For about 20 per cent of babies – those with extreme fussiness/colic – mothers are fatigued from being sleep-deprived. The stress from loss of sleep might inhibit lactation. Breast-feeding may be difficult because breast-feeding is used for nutrition and soothing. Nursing more frequently and for longer durations might cause more discomfort or pain if the skin of the breast becomes cracked or dry. The mother might worry that she doesn't have enough breast milk or that her diet is causing the breast milk to upset the baby because of the extreme fussiness/crying. Consider a single bottle of expressed breast milk given once per twenty-four hours by someone else.
- **Sleep Training:** Start early, drowsy cues, one- to two-hour window, consistent soothing style for naps, quiet and dark place to sleep, earlier bedtimes, synchronise soothing with drowsiness, by the clock. 'No-cry', 'maybe-cry', or 'let-cry' sleep solutions depend on your baby's tendency to fuss or cry, your baby's temperament and your resources for soothing.

Post-colic: Preventing Sleep Problems After Four Months of Age

- 49 per cent of babies have an intermediate temperament (thirty-seven had common fussiness; twelve had extreme fussiness/colic)
- 42 per cent of babies have an easy temperament (thirty-nine had common fussiness; three had extreme fussiness/colic)

Parents are not likely to be stressed
Infant is likely to be well rested
Infant is likely to be able to self-soothe
At night, consolidated sleep (long sleep duration) develops early
During the day, regular and long naps naturally develop early, without parental scheduling
If sleep problems exist, 'no cry' solutions usually work

- 9 per cent of babies have a difficult temperament (four had common fussiness; five had extreme fussiness/colic)

Those four babies who had common fussiness/crying might have been kept up too late, missed naps, or received too much attention at night. Or perhaps the families had limited resources for soothing and/or were overwhelmed by the demands of parenting. Reflect on how you handled sleeping during the first four months and how you might be able to get more help in caring for your baby.

Parents are likely to be stressed
Infant is likely to be overtired
Infant is likely to be only parent-soothed
At night, fragmented sleep (night waking) persists
During the day, irregular and brief naps persist
If sleep problems exist, 'let cry' solutions might be necessary

Different sleep styles work better for different temperaments.

What will work for one family may not work for you and your baby.

Concentrate on caring for your baby, not looking for a cure for extreme fussiness/colic.

1. Watch for an *earlier sleep time at night* developing and soothe your baby to sleep earlier.
    a. For the family bed, lie down in your bed and use a safe nest in your bed, a co-sleeper, or a cot only for sleep onset at the earlier bedtime.
    b. If you use a cot, *fathers can help* put their babies to sleep; at the first night feeding, return her to her cot or bring her to your bed for the remainder of the night.
2. If you use a cot, try to feed your baby no more than two times at night; otherwise, you might create a *night-waking habit*.
    a. For the family bed, breast-feed as often as you wish.
3. The *morning nap develops first, around 9:00 to 10:00 A.M.* Use this nap rhythm as an aid to help your baby fall asleep.
    a. Extremely fussy/colicky infants might have to go down for their first nap after only *one hour of wakefulness*.
4. The *afternoon nap develops second, around noon to 2:00 P.M.*
    a. Extreme fussy/colicky infants might still have to be put down to sleep after *one to two hours of wakefulness* following their morning nap.
    b. Switching from 'sleepy signs' to sleeping 'by the clock' (BTC) may occur in common fussy babies who are temperamentally very regular at three to four months of age.
5. For extreme fussy/colicy infants, the development of nap rhythms and long naps occurs when they are older.
    a. Try the 'Fade procedure' described on page 295 and 346 at four months.
    b. Try to 'focus on the morning nap', described on page 251 at four months.
    c. Plan to switch from 'sleepy signs' to 'BTC' only when much older.

Different Post-colic Groups

After extreme fussiness/colic winds down – around four months of age or sooner – your child may be overtired and not sleeping well and difficult to manage. But not all difficult-to-manage four-month-olds have colic. I suspect that there are two groups of children at four months of age, both of whom have difficult temperaments (see page 175).

The first group with a difficult temperament came from the large group (80 per cent) of infants with common fussiness/crying. Only about 4.5 per cent of these children, or four infants out of a hundred, fall into this category. I think they are less overtired than the second group. When parents put forth great effort to help them sleep better, there is relatively fast improvement. They are more adaptable and it is easier to change their sleep routines. 'No cry' sleep strategies are likely to work well (see page 103).

The second group with a difficult temperament came from a small group (20 per cent) of infants with extreme fussiness/colic. About 27 per cent of these children, or five infants out of a hundred, fall into this category. I think they are more overtired than the first group. When parents put forth great effort to help them sleep better, there is relatively slow improvement. They are less adaptable and it is more difficult to change their sleep routines. 'No cry' sleep strategies are not likely to work and parents have to consider 'let cry' sleep strategies.

PART II

How Parents Can Help Their Children Establish Healthy Sleep Habits

YOU CAN PREVENT SLEEP DISTURBANCES FROM INFANCY TO ADOLESCENCE

CHAPTER 5

Months One to Four

Every newborn baby is unique. And the closer we look, the more we can see differences. Some of these differences reflect inborn traits and are called genetic differences. Recent sleep research has focused on the gene that controls our biological clocks, and to mothers of fraternal twins, the finding that not all clocks run at exactly the same speed will not be surprising. But other congenital differences that are not inherited are due to whether the baby was born at thirty-seven or forty-two weeks of gestation, or whether the mother smoked or drank large amounts of alcohol during her pregnancy. A new area of research, based on animal studies, is how the mother's biological rhythms may help set or influence the rhythms of the foetus and the newborn baby. Based on the regularity or irregularity of the mother's sleep/wake patterns, activity/rest patterns or eating patterns, there may be a kind of prenatal programming affecting the baby's own rhythms.

All of these differences – in smiling, sucking, sleeping, physical activity, and so on – combine to make a baby an individual. This chapter will describe the individual sleeping patterns in babies and how these patterns change as babies grow.

THE ONE- TO TWO-HOUR WINDOW

Think and plan how you want to soothe your baby, but know that *when* you soothe your baby is more important.

- **Babies quickly become overtired after only one or two hours of wakefulness, and some cannot comfortably stay up for even one hour! During the day, note the time when your baby wakes up and try to help her nap by soothing within the next one or two hours before she becomes overtired. Try to keep the intervals of wakefulness brief.**
- **Babies less than six weeks old fall asleep at night very late and do not sleep very long during the day or night. Try to soothe your baby to sleep during the day before she becomes overtired. Always respond to your baby. Avoid the overtired state.**
- **Eighty per cent of babies more than six weeks old become more settled at night, sleep a little longer at night and begin to become drowsy for night sleep at an earlier hour. Try to soothe your baby to sleep at an earlier hour if she shows signs of drowsiness earlier. Do not let her cry.**
- **Twenty per cent of babies more than six weeks old do not appear to become more settled at night, do not appear to sleep longer at night and do not become drowsy at an earlier hour. Nevertheless, try to soothe your baby to sleep at an earlier hour even if she does not show signs of drowsiness earlier. Spend extra time soothing: prolonged swinging, long luxurious baths and never-ending car rides. Fathers should put forth extra effort to help out. Do not let her cry.**

Newborn: The First Week

While recovering from labour and delivery and perhaps the after-effects of anaesthesia, you may begin to experience new feelings of uncertainty, inadequacy or anxiety. After all, parenting skills probably was not one of your school or college courses. Unfortunately, hospital schedules can serve to underline these feelings. In hospitals without staff accommodation, an artificial schedule is imposed on baby care activities. This is determined by changes of nursing shifts, visiting hours and the need to measure vital signs, and not by your baby's needs.

PRACTICAL POINT

Your baby has no circadian rhythms or internal biological clocks yet, so you can't set your baby to clock time.

As soon as you arrive home, you need to disregard the clock and feed your baby whenever she seems hungry, change her when she wets and let her sleep when she needs to sleep. Full-term babies sleep a lot during the first several days. They also eat very little and often lose weight. This is all very natural and should not alarm you. If your baby sleeps a lot, don't confuse sweetness with weakness.

PRACTICAL POINTS

Unplug your phone when nursing.
Unplug your phone when napping.
Unplug your phone when your husband is with you.
Consider a relief bottle (one bottle a day of formula or expressed breast milk) if you are breast-feeding.

Presumably this calm, quiet period during the first days is somehow synchronised with the few days it takes for the mother's breast milk to come in. Babies sleep a lot, fifteen to eighteen hours a day, but usually in short stretches of two to four hours. These sleep periods do not follow a pattern related to day and night, so get your own rest whenever you are able.

Q: *I heard that I am supposed to put my baby to sleep when drowsy but awake. But every time I feed her, she quickly falls asleep. Am I then supposed to wake her up and then put her down to sleep?*
A: Newborns usually fall asleep during a feeding and it does not make sense to wake her. It goes against Mother Nature! Older babies will often be almost asleep when they finish sucking. When the breast or bottle is removed, older babies momentarily look around in a dazed fashion, just to check out that everything is okay, and then go into a deep, comfortable snooze with you in your bed or alone in their cot.

Why then have you heard that you should not let your child fall asleep during soothing or feeding? The theory is that your child is learning self-soothing skills, and that she would not learn these if you do not do this. Consider two scenarios. First, you keep the intervals of wakefulness brief, only one to two hours, and you watch for signs of drowsiness (see page 63). At the drowsy time, you soothe and/or feed your baby and she now may be more drowsy and entering the sleep zone, but she is not completely asleep at the end of the soothing and/or feeding. Now she is able to continue to self-soothe herself to deep slumber. This is easy because she was not overtired, and 80 per cent of babies (common fussiness/crying) can handle this well.

Second, you allow your child to stay up too long and he becomes overtired. He has passed through the drowsy zone and is entering the fatigue zone. Now, when you soothe and/or feed your baby, you discover that he will not be easily placed in his cot or stay asleep unless he is already in a deep sleep at the end of the soothing and/or feeding. Soothing himself to sleep is difficult because he was overtired, and 20 per cent of babies (extreme fussiness/colic) are often this way during the first few months anyway. The problem is not your failure to 'put him to sleep when drowsy but awake', rather, the problem is allowing your baby to become overtired or being unlucky and having an extremely fussy/colicky baby.

This translates into the observation that when parents are successful with the sleep strategy of 'put your baby to sleep when drowsy but awake', there are fewer sleep problems, and when parents do not (or cannot) do this, there are more sleep problems. The truth is, the success of this strategy is dependent on having a well-rested child to start with. If you innocently let your child get overtired or if you have an extremely fussy/colicky baby, this sleep strategy is not going to work well.

WARNING!

The first week of life is like a honeymoon. Newborns 'sleep like a baby'.

***For all babies:* It will become more and more difficult to soothe and settle the baby in the evening hours at six weeks of age, counting from the due date.**

***For 80 per cent of babies:* They settle down at night a few weeks later.**

***For 20 per cent of babies:* It will become more and more difficult to soothe and sleep the baby all the time starting at several days of age, counting from the due date. These babies settle down at night at three to four months of age.**

When your baby becomes more and more difficult to soothe and sleep, he appears to be more completely out of your control and your life will not be easy.

SLEEP TRAINING DOES NOT EQUAL CRY IT OUT

Sleep training involves several general principles to use the natural development of sleep/wake rhythms as an aid to help your child learn to sleep.

- **Respect your baby's need to sleep.**
- **Start early to plan for or anticipate for when your baby will need to sleep, similar to anticipating when your baby will need to feed.**
- **Maintain brief intervals of wakefulness, this is the one- to two-hour window.**
- **Learn to recognise drowsy cues (see page 63), though they may be absent in 20 per cent of extremely fussy/ colicky babies. Drowsy cues or sleepy signs signal that your baby is becoming sleepy; this is when you should begin your soothing efforts.**
- **When you put your baby down or lie down with him, he may be drowsy and awake or in a deep sleep. Either way works if you have good timing.**
- **Develop a bedtime routine.**
- **Matching the time when you soothe your baby to sleep to the time when he naturally needs to sleep is the key. For 80 per cent of common fussy babies, perfect timing produces no crying.**
- **During the first several weeks, many babies fall asleep while feeding or sucking to soothe even if not hungry. This is natural. It is not necessary to deliberately wake your baby before you put him down to sleep or lie down with him in your bed. Later, your older baby may or may not momentarily and partially awaken as you remove your breast or bottle before falling asleep. Do not force him to a wakeful state before attempting to settle him.**

Weeks Two to Four: More Fussiness

All babies are a little hard to 'read' during these first few weeks. Most activities such as feeding, changing nappies, and soothing to sleep occur at irregular times. Do not expect a scheduled baby, because the baby's needs for food, cuddling and sleeping occur erratically and unpredictably. When your baby needs to be fed, feed him; when he needs to have his nappy changed, change him; and when he needs to sleep, allow him to sleep.

What do I mean by 'allow him to sleep'? Try to provide a calm, quiet place for your baby if he sleeps better this way. Many babies are very portable at this age and seem to sleep well anywhere. You're lucky if your baby is like this, and you're even luckier if he is one of the few who have long night sleep periods. Most newborns don't sleep for long periods at night.

Studies have shown that for babies a few weeks old, the longest single sleep period may be only three to four hours, and it can occur at any time during the day or night. This is day/night confusion. Extremely fussy/colicky babies may not even have single sleep periods that are this long; premature babies may have longer sleep periods.

Parenting strategies such as changes in the amount of light or noise don't appear to greatly influence babies' sleep patterns now. In fact, specific styles or methods of burping, changing or feeding do not seem to really affect the baby. Try not to think of doing things *to* or *for* the baby. Instead, take time to enjoy doing things *with* your baby. Do the things that give you both pleasure: holding, cuddling, talking and listening, walking, bathing, and sleeping together. This active love is sufficient stimulation for now; you don't have to worry about buying the right toy to stimulate your baby.

A change will occur in all babies during these first few weeks, and you should prepare for it. When your baby is about to fall asleep or is just about to wake up, a sudden single jerk or massive twitch of his entire body may occur. As the drowsy baby drifts into a deeper sleep, the eyes sometimes appear to roll upwards. This is normal behaviour during sleep/wake transitions. Also, all babies become somewhat more alert, wakeful and aroused as the brain develops. You may notice restless movements, such as shuddering, quivering, tremulousness, shaking or jerking, twisting or turning, and hiccoughs. There may be moments when your sweet little baby appears impatient, distressed or agitated for no identifiable reason. This is normal newborn behaviour.

During these spells of unexplainable restlessness, the baby may swallow air and become windy. Often he appears to be in pain. Sometimes he cries and you can't figure out why. The crying baby may be hungry or just fussy. This is confusing to all parents.

All in all, now you may not have the baby you dreamed of having. She cries too much, sleeps too little and spits on you whenever you forget to cover your shoulder with a towel. Here are some concrete steps you can take to make it easier for everyone.

1. **Take naps during the day whenever your baby is sleeping**
2. **Unplug all phones in the house**
3. **Go out, without your baby, for breaks: a walk, a coffee date, a film**
4. **Plan or arrange for a few hours of private time to take care of yourself**
5. **Do whatever comes naturally to soothe your baby; don't worry about spoiling her or creating bad habits**
6. **Use swings, dummies or anything else that provides rhythmic, rocking motions or sucking**

If you find that your baby sleeps well everywhere and whenever she is tired, enjoy your freedom while you can. A time will come when you will be less able to visit friends, shop or go to exercise classes, because your baby will need a consistent sleep environment.

Q: *Why are breast-fed babies fed more often at night than formula-fed babies?*
A: It may be that the breast milk takes less time to digest so the breast-fed baby is hungrier sooner. It may be that the mother who has chosen to breast-feed is more sensitive or attuned to her baby and responds more frequently to the baby's sounds, both hungry sounds and sleep sounds. Maybe the breast-feeding mother is more committed to soothe or nurture her baby, using her breasts as a dummy even when her baby is just fussy and not hungry. Perhaps the breast-feeding mother responds more often because her breasts feel uncomfortably full. Or, the mother who is breast-feeding is unsure whether her baby has had enough because, unlike the formula-fed baby, she cannot see how much her baby has taken.

Q: *I've heard that my newborn should not sleep in the bassinet in my room or in my bed with me, that it will spoil him.*
A: Nonsense. For feeding or nursing, it makes it easier for both of you if your newborn is close. When your baby is older, say three or four months, both of you may sleep better if he is not in your room. Anyway, by then the number of night feedings is usually smaller.

Brief awakenings in young infants under four months of age are acceptable to most parents because these usually are thought to be caused by hunger. For the older child, especially if he had been sleeping overnight previously, night wakings are often thought of as a behavioural problem. The truth is that awakening at night or complete arousals are normally occurring events, as discussed in Chapter 2. Problems in the older child may arise when he has difficulty or is unable or unwilling to return to sleep unassisted. The more often these events occur, the longer each separate awakening lasts.

Q: *When will my child sleep through the night?*
A: Many infants between six weeks and four months will naturally go to sleep late around 9:00 to 11:00 P.M., and

sleep several hours without a need to be fed. Some call this 'sleeping through the night'. After four months, infants tend to go to sleep earlier, around 6:00 to 8:00 P.M., and some now need to be fed once or twice before they wake up to start the day. After nine months, these night feedings are not needed. Except for breast-fed babies in a family bed, more than two night feedings will begin to create a night waking habit.

Weeks Five to Six: Fussiness/Crying Peaks

At about six weeks of age, or six weeks after the expected date of delivery for premature babies, your baby will start to return your social smiles.

If you are lucky and have a calm baby who appears to have regular sleep periods, prepare yourself for changes resulting from your child's increased social maturation. The social smiles herald the onset of increased social awareness, and it may come to pass that your baby will now start to fight sleep in order to enjoy the pleasure of your company. This is natural!

> **PRACTICAL POINT**
>
> **Try to meet your baby's needs. If he's hungry, feed him. If he's tired, settle him.**

When your baby appears slightly fidgety, ask yourself two questions. First, when did you last feed her? Second, how long has she been up? Sometimes you need to settle her and not feed her.

Around the time your baby produces her first social smiles, at about six weeks of age, night sleep becomes more organised, and the longest single sleep period begins to occur with predictability and regularity in the evening hours. This sleep period is now about four to six hours long. (If your baby has extreme fussiness/colic, the longest sleep period might be less than this.) Your baby will also start to settle down more and more. She will become more interested in objects such as mobiles and toys, she'll have more interest in playing games and her repertoire of emotional expressions will dramatically increase.

Yet many parents find this time particularly frustrating, since many babies reach a peak of fussiness and wakefulness at about six weeks. Even extremely fussy/colicky babies may be at their worst at six weeks of age.

THE SIX-WEEK PEAK

All babies are most fussy, cry the most, and are most wakeful at six weeks of age.

One mother told me, 'He's a little excited about all the living going on.'

Here is a vivid description of the six-week peak.

Antonio's Sleep Story

Like many couples today, my husband, Arturo, and I got married in our late twenties/early thirties, and waited several years before deciding the time was right for starting a family. We felt that although our spontaneous, independent lifestyle would change, we were ready for the challenge of having a baby. Our friends with kids all told us that our lives would change, but it was impossible for us to imagine just how different our lives would be after our baby was born!

Antonio was born two weeks early and without difficulty. I remember thinking several hours after his birth that he was going to be a very easy boy, since my pregnancy and delivery were both routine and relatively easy. Three days after we brought him home, however, I realised that my expectations might have been a little off the mark. Looking back at the notes I took (I kept a spreadsheet with a sleeping/eating schedule and wrote many comments on it about Antonio's habits), Antonio started crying that day at about 8:00 P.M. and didn't stop until 5:30 A.M. After an extremely stressful night of walking Antonio up and down the hallway, rocking him and doing everything we could think of to soothe him, he finally fell asleep, exhausted, at about 6:00 A.M. It was a terrible feeling for parents who love their baby so much not to be able to soothe or comfort him! My husband and I felt like failures, and we called the doctor the minute the surgery opened that morning and pleaded for help. Luckily, we found out that part of his crying that night was due to hunger, as my breast milk hadn't come in yet. That was an easy problem to fix!

We remedied his hunger quickly, but he still seemed to cry a lot. Over the next three weeks we started to notice a pattern of crying that started at about 5:00 P.M. and usually lasted for about six hours. In addition to that, Antonio awakened every two hours to be fed (as most babies do) during the night and didn't take daytime naps! During these early weeks the only way Antonio would sleep, night or day, was if either my husband or I held him. Needless to say, both my husband and I were as desperately in need of sleep, as Antonio was! At the time, my husband said that he couldn't understand why our baby cried so much and slept so little when every other baby he knew didn't seem to have these issues. In fact, of all the new parents we met through my prenatal exercise classes (there were fifteen to twenty couples we knew who had babies at the same time), only one other baby seemed to have the same type of behaviour. In addition, couples with older babies and toddlers were no help whatsoever, as they all claimed to 'forget' whether or not their babies were fussy. I could not believe anyone could ever forget what we were going through. My husband thought we must be doing something wrong, and I was afraid he might be right, although I didn't admit it at the time.

When Antonio was about three weeks old, I took him to see Dr Weissbluth. We discussed his sleep patterns (or lack thereof), and he advised me that Antonio's evening fussiness would get worse until he was six weeks old, and then it would start to improve slowly and hopefully end at about twelve weeks. I was quite dismayed also to learn that since Antonio was born two weeks early, I had to count Antonio's age from his original due date, not his birth date. So instead of having only three more rough weeks, we would probably have at least five! That's an eternity when you're sleep-deprived! I really didn't know how we were going to make it through that rough period! At one point I remember counting out the weeks until week six, as I did at least every other day, telling my husband, 'We only have three and a half more weeks!' To which my husband replied, 'And what if he doesn't get better after that?!' I think the biggest worry we had was that Antonio's fussiness would *never* end. This being our first child, we weren't 100 per cent sure he would ever grow out of this! In the midst of this period, it seemed to us that this would be what our new lives would be like forever – endless nights of holding our crying baby followed by bleary days of holding him so he would sleep. We knew in our minds that he had to get better, but the big question was when.

Then, at about six weeks after Antonio's original due date, I couldn't believe it, but I actually started to notice that his evening fussiness was decreasing! It was almost six weeks to the day, and I was utterly amazed that Dr Weissbluth's timetable was so accurate. In addition, at the same time, his night-time sleep started becoming a little longer and he started falling asleep in his cot instead of having to sleep with me! The improvements were small, but at that point I was just ecstatic to have four solid hours of sleep at night! At about ten weeks I phoned the doctor and received encouraging advice. He suggested that I start putting Antonio to bed earlier at night, as this might help him feel less tired and make him fall asleep more easily. At the time, Antonio was going to bed between 10:00 and 11:00 P.M. So I moved his bedtime to around 8:00 P.M. for a few nights, and I could not believe how well this worked! I then started putting him in his cot even earlier, as I noticed that he actually became tired at around 6:30 P.M. Antonio is now almost five months old, and he has been sleeping from 6:30 P.M. through the night to about 7:00 A.M. He has been doing this since he was twelve weeks old. He does wake up occasionally at 4:00 or 5:00 A.M. if he's hungry, but for the most part he sleeps extremely well at night, and is even starting to take regular daytime naps! Arturo and I still can't believe that our 'colicky' baby is such a great sleeper now. If we had only known this back in week three, we would have been a little less stressed out! I hate to say it, but like most of my friends with older children, I'm forgetting the details of his fussy period, too! Antonio is such a joy to be with, I actually might want to have a second baby. Yikes!

Your baby may irritate and exhaust you. She may give up napping altogether and, to make matters worse, when awake may appear to be grumbling all day. You may feel battered at the end of each day; you may be at your wits' end. This, too, is natural. Being annoyed with your baby does not make you a 'bad' parent. Just understand why you're annoyed. Remember that your baby's immature nervous system lacks inhibitory control. The brain will develop inhibitory capabilities as it matures, but this takes time; things will settle down after six weeks of age.

Here is an account of one mother's first eight weeks.

'My First Bath in Eight Weeks'

Today my baby girl, Allyson, is eight weeks old. I celebrated by taking my first uninterrupted bath since her birth. Of course, she woke up just as I was towelling off, but I have learned to be grateful for small pleasures.

Allyson doesn't sleep much, and when she's awake she's usually either crying or feeding. It's been a little better the past week, but she still sleeps very little: six to eight hours at night and two to four hours during the day. And since I can't bear to hear her cry, that means she spends most of her time on my breast, where, mercifully, she can always be soothed. I feel as if I've merged with the brown corduroy chair where I nurse her.

Lately she's good for a couple of ten- to twenty-minute play periods (on the floor on her back, me leaning over her, or on the changing table while I change her nappy). I can't hold her and play with her; she's always squirming to get at my breast. So, anyway, she's on my breast ten to twelve hours a day.

Given Allyson's behaviour (constant crying or fussiness, and a constant desire to nurse or at least be near my breast), I naturally concluded that my baby was starving, that I did not have enough milk for her. If I did have enough, surely she would fall asleep and *stay* asleep. Obviously, I thought, she was waking after a few minutes or half an hour because she was hungry. A weighing at the doctor's, where I learned that she was in the seventy-fifth per centile for growth (at three weeks) did not reassure me.

When I talked with the doctor, he said it did seem my baby was colicky, and I took his book home to read. Finally, I found descriptions by other mothers of babies like mine! I was not alone. I came to understand how sleeping problems, like those of my baby, appear to be hunger, but really aren't. I also learned that there's nothing I can do for my baby that I'm not already doing, and so I might as well turn some of my energy around and start taking care of myself. Truly, I believe that in the case of a colicky baby, who in most cases cannot be treated for her condition, it is the *mother* who needs 'treatment' or help, and to this end I suggest:

1. **Get out of the house an hour or two a day, minimum**
2. **When out of the house, try to get some physical exercise to burn off the tension**
3. **Don't feel guilty about doing anything that makes you feel good**
4. **Socialise as much as possible outside the home**
5. **Keep a diary or log of your baby's sleeping/feeding habits**
6. **When the baby is asleep, get some sleep yourself, unless you're doing something for your own peace of mind**

And things are getting better. Last night Allyson woke up from a three-hour nap, fed calmly and wasn't fussy for several hours afterward. She didn't go back to sleep, but she didn't cry either. Later that evening she slipped back into her old ways, but I held her and played with her for over an hour; then she stayed calm in the swing for a while.

And I got my bath this morning.

If you are lucky enough to have an easy baby, at five to six weeks you may have already noticed her sleep patterns becoming slightly more regular. You can try to help your baby become even more regular by putting her down or lying down with her to sleep when she first appears tired, but, in any case, after no more than two hours of wakefulness. She may or may not drift into sleep easily. You do not need to let her cry at all, but some babies will fuss or cry in a mild fashion before falling asleep. If she cries for five, ten or twenty minutes, it will do her no harm, and she may drift off to sleep. If not, console her and try again at other times. Try to become sensitive to her need to sleep. The novelty of external noises, voices, lights and vibrations will disrupt her sleep more and more, so try to have her in her cot or your bed when she needs to sleep. Go slowly and be flexible.

Remember, sleep training means starting to respect your baby's need to sleep when he is a newborn by anticipating when he will need to sleep (within one to two hours of wakefulness), learning to recognise drowsy signs, and developing a bedtime routine. Then your baby will not become overtired.

Now you might want to try to help your baby sleep better at night. The ease with which you can accomplish this is related to whether your child is currently well rested or overtired. And this depends on whether he had common fussiness/crying or extreme fussiness/colic and whether you were able or unable to successfully soothe him during the first six weeks.

Alternatively, you might have no need or desire to try any of these three sleep training strategies. Your baby might be sleeping well at night, and there is no reason to rock the boat. Or, you are enjoying the family bed and do not wish to change or allow your baby to cry. This is fine for now, but after four months of age, you probably will want to consider some changes in sleep routines to accommodate your baby's need for an earlier bedtime. These changes do not necessarily mean that your baby will cry.

Always consider both your child's ability to self-soothe and your resources for prolonged daytime and night-time soothing. Do what works best for you and your baby.

FOUR SLEEP-TRAINING STRATEGIES: WHEN TO TRY

- **At six to eight weeks of age if you have to return to work and/or you are totally exhausted and unable to function. May work well for common fussiness/ crying babies, especially if they appear to have an easy temperament.**
- **At eight to sixteen weeks of age to help your baby sleep better at night for babies with common fussiness/ crying. Success may be quick and easy.**
- **After sixteen weeks of age to help your baby sleep better at night for babies who had extreme fussiness/ crying. Success may be slow and difficult.**

1. 'Let Cry', Ignoring, Extinction

Not responding to your child at night is most difficult for parents. It is also not always clear if your baby is or is not hungry. Between six to eight weeks and four months, babies might be hungry and need to be bottle-fed two or three times a night, but after four months, only once or twice, and after nine months, not at all. The idea is to respond if you think your child is hungry but not at other times. This determination may be harder for a mother who is breast-feeding because of uncertainty regarding her breast milk supply. Fathers should give a bottle of expressed breast milk or formula to help clarify whether the baby is hungry or not.

In addition, there is almost always a temporary increase in crying at night when parents do this. While appearing harsh, it is my impression that the total amount of crying with 'Extinction' is less than with 'Graduated Extinction' because success occurs faster. Research comparing these two methods showed that parents using 'Extinction' reported less stress in parenting. This supports my observation that parents are more willing to employ 'Extinction' again following changes of sleep routines such as holiday trips, special events such as birthdays, or illnesses. In contrast, because 'Graduated Extinction' often takes longer, parents are less willing to repeat the procedure when changes of sleep routines cause the child to become overtired. Another observation is that for older babies or children where there is less uncertainty regarding hunger at night, 'Extinction' is simpler to execute and parents can therefore be more consistent. In contrast, 'Graduated Extinction' requires a detailed plan of action to be modified gradually but consistently over several days or longer.

Here is one mother's account.

Ares

We brought Ares home from the hospital with only a ballpark notion of what it would it be like to care for a baby. As far as I knew, Ares would sleep when he needed to sleep. As the months progressed, I went to him whenever he cried and changed him and nursed him on demand. At night he woke often and slept in bed with me most of the time. Whenever Ares cried I would sort of panic. I seriously would have done anything to soothe him. All my adrenaline turned on and my heart raced. People would ask me if I had him on a sleeping or nursing schedule, and I didn't know what to say. He nursed on what seemed like a constant basis, and he hardly slept. I grabbed two-minute showers listening to him cry, feeling guilty the whole time. When I asked people about babies and their sleeping habits, they would say vague things like 'Babies sleep when they need to sleep, no less and no more' and 'Every baby is different, like a snowflake. Some just need less sleep than others.' I found this less than helpful. I kept waiting for Ares to 'sleep through the night', but it never happened. At night he was up seven or eight times. During the day he didn't sleep much, just little short naps. Sometimes, when I nursed him to sleep and put him down for a nap, he would wake up and cry as soon as I put him down. I started holding him while he slept.

I read that you should always take your baby everywhere and 'wear' your baby like the Native Americans did. I carried him around in a baby sling on walks and to do errands. By the time he was ten months old, his night-time routine was established. I would nurse him to sleep at 8:00 P.M., put him in his cot, and he would wake up at 10:00 P.M. and cry. I would change him and nurse him back to sleep, and carefully, oh so carefully, put him back in his cot, and repeat this process all night every two or so hours. Sometimes he would wake up when I put him back in bed and I would have to start all over again. As the night progressed, and he became more and more exhausted, he was more likely to wake up when I put him down and it took longer to soothe him back to sleep. By 6:00 A.M. he was up for the day, napping occasionally and only briefly. Sometimes I couldn't even put him down long enough to eat dinner. I held him while I ate. One night I went to him when he cried and nursing did not soothe him. He could not stop crying no matter what I did. I realised at that moment that he didn't need me so much as he needed to sleep. We were all exhausted.

We had heard about 'crying it out' before, and I thought it sounded cruel. But my husband wanted to do it, and it was clear that we had to change our methods, because although I was perfectly willing to deprive myself of sleep on his behalf, Ares was clearly suffering from sleep deprivation. Ares had all the symptoms of an overtired child. He was easily startled and cried uncontrollably at sudden or loud noises. He was unable to go to sleep on his own, and unable to stay asleep once he did. The book explained that in going to Ares every time he cried at night, I was stimulating him and keeping him awake, not soothing him and reassuring him as I had thought. All that stuff I had read about 'night-time parenting' and 'attachment parenting' was not only not helping, it was hurting Ares. We decided to try Dr Weissbluth's 'Extinction' method.

The first night I put Ares to bed at 8:00 P.M. as usual, but when ten o'clock came and he cried, I didn't go to him. It was one of the hardest things I have ever done, but I wanted to give it a try for his sake. He cried for forty-five minutes. I thought I would die. My nervous system went haywire. I cried, my whole body got hot, I was shaking and sweating and my heart pounded. *He's going to think I abandoned him,* I thought. *He will never trust me again.* But once he stopped crying he slept all night long. Ares had never slept for more than four hours in a row. I thought for sure he had died. But he woke up the next morning happy and rested and then fell back to sleep a couple of hours later on his play rug, another first. Ares had never in his life fallen asleep without nursing. From then on we were convinced that Dr Weissbluth knew what he was talking about. We worked to make sure Ares got the sleep he needed. At night we developed a sleep ritual of bathtime, reading to him and nursing him at 6:00 P.M., and putting him down sleepy but awake. He took two naps a day, following a slightly abbreviated sleep ritual, and slept for two hours in the morning and one hour in the early afternoon. For some reason he didn't cry at nap time, he just went quietly to sleep. At night, however, for several weeks he still cried for forty-five minutes when I put him down. This was extremely difficult, even painful. But once he fell asleep he stayed asleep for twelve hours, which was incredible to me, and he was so much happier during the day that we stuck with it. In the daytime, he was so much calmer; he even seemed sleepier for the first few weeks. He almost never cried any more, and his attention span was longer. Eventually, Ares went to sleep without crying, and he still sleeps every night all night long, for at least twelve hours a night.

2. Controlled Crying, Partial Ignoring, Graduated Extinction

This is a variation of 'Extinction'. One method is to leave your baby for about five minutes, then return and soothe him back to the sleepy state or put him down after soothing. If loud crying recurs, leave your baby for ten minutes and then repeat the soothing process. If loud crying again starts, leave your baby for fifteen minutes before repeating the soothing process. This sequence repeats with an additional five minutes of ignoring his crying until he falls asleep during one of the crying spells or does not cry after your soothing effort.

Another method is also to increase the time of ignoring before checking on your baby, but increase the time by about five minutes every two days. Research has shown this method to work well over a period of four to nine nights. Again, your success depends on your child's tendency to fuss or cry, how well rested or overtired he is and how consistent you are.

This method appears less harsh than 'Extinction' and works well for many children. It is my impression that for extremely fussy/colicky babies, by four months of age, parents are worn down from sleep deprivation and the child is way overtired. In this situation trying 'Graduated Extinction' often fails because the child's crying outlasts the parents' resolve to be consistent and 'Extinction' produces results sooner.

3. Check and Console

Responding to your child at night is least difficult for parents. You quietly enter whenever your baby cries to see that she is all right and gently soothe her in darkness but you try to not pick her up. Instead, you rub her tummy, stroke her hair or gently rock the cot. You do the least amount of rocking, singing and, if necessary, feeding to soothe her back to a calm, sleepy state. This method appeals to those who practise attachment parenting because they believe that it provides *emotional security*, that their cries will not go unanswered so they can learn to *trust* their mothers, and they will not *feel abandoned*. However, there is no evidence that babies are harmed when they are allowed to cry. Furthermore, this method could teach some babies to cry more frequently and longer in order to receive more soothing. In addition, it is very hard only partially to soothe a crying baby at night. On the other hand, if your baby is well rested and did not have extreme fussiness/colic, this method might work well.

4. Scheduled Awakenings

See page 298 in Chapter 6 for a discussion of this method.

REMEMBER

Different children require different approaches.

Here is an account from one mother who needed to get her child's sleep on a firmer schedule before she went back to work. Trying her methods with a more irregular, extremely fussy/colicky child probably wouldn't have worked at this early age. But an easy, regular, common fussy baby often responds quickly to sleep-training strategies at around six weeks.

In this story, the mother incorrectly equated sleep training with letting her baby cry.

'My Maternity Leave Would Soon Be Over'

When Ron and I had our first meeting with our paediatrician before David was born, we left his office comfortable with the care we felt our child would receive. Although we knew the doctor had a special interest in sleep disorders, we never dreamed we would be faced with a baby whose internal clock thought day was night and night was day.

Oh, it didn't happen right away. In fact, the first few weeks were spent nursing and changing nappies in between David's naps. Looking back at those first weeks, Dr Weissbluth must have really chuckled at some of the questions I asked him.

At the same time, I was beginning to relax and feel, yes, everything is going along normally, David became more alert; Ron and I knew it was a great step in his development. We looked forward to his periods of wakefulness as a time to interact with him. But a pattern began to develop: David didn't want to go to bed at night.

The doctor listened to what we were going through and assured us that, first of all, this was normal for some babies. David was really too young to go through sleep training at six weeks. So Ron and I resigned ourselves to some more of the same.

When David was two months old I began to panic. My maternity leave would soon be over. I could barely stand up most of the time, I was so tired. I also wanted to continue to nurse David whenever I was home. I knew we had to do something before I went back to work. So we called Dr Weissbluth and made an appointment to see him.

First, the doctor checked David's physical condition. He was in perfect health. Then we talked. Dr Weissbluth explained that we would have to make some changes in the way we handled David's sleep periods. David was to have a quiet, darkened room when sleeping. No more night-light, music, et cetera. Naps should last at least forty-five minutes to an hour. If David got up sooner, we were to leave him there until he got the rest he needed. Instead of letting David stay up late, we were to put him to bed between 7:00 and 9:00 P.M. No rides in cars, pushchairs or swings, where sleep occurred for a short time.

We decided to start that next Monday, since Sunday was Mother's Day. I nursed David at 9:00 P.M., and by 9:30 he was asleep in my arms. I tiptoed him into bed and crept back to the living room and turned on the intercom. It was quiet until 9:45, when I heard David sucking his fingers. I thought, Okay, he'll get back to sleep soon, but by 10:00 the crying began. David cried until 12:30 – two and a half hours. For every cry I heard I shared his frustration, anger and seeming pain. And I was angry – at David, the doctor, Ron and myself. Finally, David fell asleep, and he slept until 6:45 the next morning, when I woke him to nurse.

The morning wake-up was planned and agreed to with Dr Weissbluth. The idea was to get David to wake before I left for work so that I could nurse him. David seemed fine. I was exhausted.

Tuesday I let David wake himself up. That day he took naps ranging between two and three and a half hours, but his schedule was rather loose. At 8:30 that night, when he woke up, I fed, bathed and played with him until he had one last nursing and I put him to bed, although he was not asleep, at 10:50. This time he cried from 10:50 until 11:15. Only twenty-five minutes? Could it be this easy? I was very encouraged. Weeks of David's inability to get to sleep at night seemed to be at an end. Even Dr Weissbluth seemed surprised at David's progress. Once again he slept through the night.

Although we were still unsuccessful at getting David to bed early, the periods of crying himself to sleep were getting shorter. On day three he cried for twenty-one minutes and then didn't let out another peep until the next morning.

Just when Ron and I began to breathe a sigh of relief, David put us back in our places. On day four David cried for nearly an hour and a half. My spirits dropped. Was this just a temporary setback or had the last three days been a fluke? When I called the doctor the next morning, he told me to continue the training. David would have some off days, he explained.

We found that if we responded to him quickly, assuming he wanted to nurse, he became irritable and difficult to feed. Those were the nights the crying seemed to go on for ever.

We continued to check in with Dr Weissbluth, but less frequently. At the end of our third week of sleep training, David, Ron and I really had our acts together. Ron and I could tell when David was ready to call it a day, and we didn't push him to stay up any later than he wanted.

When Ron and I started sleep training, we kept a log of David's wakings and sleeps. We still do – not because he's still in training, but with my return to work and Ron's busy schedule, we are better able to understand David's moods and hunger patterns when the sitter lets us know what's gone on during the day.

Weeks Seven to Eight: Earlier Bedtimes and Longer Night Sleep Periods Develop

The major biological changes starting now are a tendency to go to sleep earlier at night and for longer periods of uninterrupted night sleep. Do not try to force an earlier bedtime on your child; rather, watch for drowsy signs developing earlier in the evening.

As we have seen, every baby behaves differently during these first few weeks. Your own baby most likely will fall somewhere in between the common fussy or 'easy' baby and the extremely fussy/colicky infant. And even if your baby has been 'easy', this may well be a period in which she 'forgets' what she has learned.

Common Fussy or 'Easy' Baby

'Easy' babies are placid and easy to manage, quiet angels most nights. They may have a fussy period in the evening, but it's not too long, intense or hard to deal with. They appear to sleep well anywhere and anytime during the day and quite regularly at night. In fact, the early development of regular, long night sleep periods – starting well before the age of six weeks – is a characteristic feature of 'easy' babies. These kids are very portable, and parents bask in their sunny dispositions.

But shortly . . . dark clouds may gather. The baby starts to have some new grumbling or grumpiness that does not occur only in the evening. In fact, the quiet evenings might now be punctured by new, 'painful' cries suggesting an illness. Or it might now take longer to put the baby to sleep. What has happened to your sound sleeper?

Irregularities of sleep schedules, nap deprivation and too late a bedtime are the chief culprits. Now is the time to become ever more sensitive to your child's need to sleep.

> **HINT**
>
> **Be careful, but . . .**
> **No set schedules.**
> **No rigid rules.**

After about six weeks of age, the best strategy still is to try to synchronise your caretaking activities with your baby's own rhythms. You should try to re-establish healthy sleep habits by removing the disruptive effects of external noises, lights or vibrations. Although it may be inconvenient for you, try to have your baby back in her cot after no more than two hours of wakefulness. Consider this two-hour interval to be a rough guide to help organise the day into naps and wakeful activities.

Q: *How long can I keep my baby up?*
A: No more than two hours.

Two hours of wakefulness is about the maximum that most babies can endure without becoming overtired. Sometimes a baby may need to go to sleep after being up for only one hour. Often this brief wakeful period of only one hour occurs early in the morning. Try to soothe him to sleep *before* he becomes overtired – *before* he becomes slightly grumpy, seems irritable, pulls his hair or bats at his ears. Expect this type of behaviour to develop within two hours of waking up if he is not put to sleep when he first shows signs of being tired. Look for drowsy signs (see page 63). Please do not mistake this two-hour guide to mean that he should be up for two hours and then down for two hours. Rather, two hours is the time interval during which you should expect to put him to sleep.

When you have been out for a walk or running an errand with your baby, watch the clock and try to have her asleep within two hours after she wakes up. If upon returning home during this time interval you notice that she is becoming overtired, say to yourself, 'I blew it this time; next time I'll return home sooner.' By paying attention to clock time, you will discover how much wakefulness your baby can comfortably tolerate.

Expect your overtired child to protest when she is put down to sleep. This is natural, because she prefers the pleasure of your soothing comfort to being in a dark, quiet, boring room.

Keep in mind the distinction between a protest cry and a sad cry. You are leaving your baby alone to let her learn to soothe herself to sleep; you are not abandoning her.

Q: *How long should I let him cry?*

A: Not at all if you want to lie down with him in your bed and soothe him to sleep, or start with five, ten or twenty minutes. Try to decide whether your child is tired, basing your judgement on (1) his behaviour; (2) the time of day and (3) the interval of wakefulness – how long he has been up.

When you have decided he is tired or overtired, put him down to sleep – even if he doesn't want to sleep. Sometimes he'll fall asleep and sometimes he won't. When he doesn't, pick him up and soothe and comfort him. You may try again after several minutes to allow him to go to sleep on his own, or you may decide not to try again for several days. But remember, if your baby cries hard for three minutes, quietly for three minutes and then sleeps for an hour, he would have lost that good hour-long nap if you had not left him alone for six minutes.

Remember that this baby was once a good sleeper, and is now fighting sleep for the pleasure of your company. At those times when he needs to sleep but wants to play, your playing with him is robbing him of sleep.

Keep a log or diary as you go through these trials to see if any trend or improvement occurs. Here's an account from Allyson's mother, who helped her baby make a dramatic – and permanent – improvement in her sleep habits at this time.

Allyson's Sleep Diary

Day 56: Allyson woke up from an afternoon nap, and I thought she was ill – she was so *calm*! No jerky movements or agitated behaviour, which I guess I'd assumed was just 'normal' for her. About this time, though, she still cried a lot when not feeding and she still had trouble falling asleep.

Day 59: Let her fuss one hour – and she went to sleep for three and a quarter hours (5:45 to 9:00 P.M.).

Day 60: Allyson fussed all morning and wouldn't sleep, but I kept her in her cot from 10:15 A.M. to noon, staying with her most of the time. Got her up to nurse at noon. That night she woke up at 2:30 A.M. – for the first time in several weeks. I nursed her until 3:00 and then put her down. She fussed off and on until 4:00, when she went to sleep.

Day 63: Breakthrough! She went to sleep for forty-five minutes in the morning and took a really long nap in the afternoon (12:45 to 5:00). But she woke in the middle of the night again (3:20 A.M.). She went back to sleep at 4:30 and slept until 8:30. She was happy in her cot – no screaming as I changed her nappy, which was new behaviour!

Careful records show that up to Day 59, the total sleep duration per twenty-four hours was about six to twelve hours. After Day 63, the total sleep duration was longer – twelve to seventeen hours. The four-day training really helped the child sleep longer.

Day 64: Two wonderful things happened. First, Allyson took a morning nap (10:45 A.M. to 1:30 P.M.), and when I put her down for the night, with her eyes wide open, she did not fuss at all. I quickly left the room and heard *no* crying. She slept from 8:35 P.M. to 5:05 A.M.

Days 87–96: Allyson is just about perfect. If she starts to fuss, I know she is hungry, wet or tired. If she's tired, I simply put her in her cot and *within two minutes* she is asleep. It's a miracle!

Sleep Log

The sleep log is a tool to help you see how your baby is sleeping – or not sleeping. A diary like Allyson's, which lists the events of the day, is difficult to scan visually; you want to see the forest, not the trees. Here's how to make a sleep log. Each twenty-four-hour day is shown as a separate bar on a graph with the horizontal axis as the day of the week and the vertical axis the time of day. So what you see is a series of bar graphs. Each bar is colour-coded for sleep times and wake times. Other times such as crying times, feedings, periods in cot awake, periods in cot asleep or periods asleep in parent's arms may be included. What happens is that you begin to pay closer attention to the timing of these events. You have some baseline data with which to compare an intervention such as an earlier bedtime. Spotting trends such as less crying or longer naps is often easy. When some success is observed, you are motivated to persist despite some crying or inconvenience for you.

For twins and triplets, instead of a single bar for each day on separate graphs for each child, put two or three bars, one for each child, next to each other for a given day on the same graph so you can see for any period of days whether one sibling's schedule can be slightly modified to help synchronise the entire group.

Extremely Fussy/Colicky Infants

In contrast to babies who are common fussy or 'easy', there are extremely fussy or colicky infants. Colicky babies are difficult to manage for three to five months because they are intense, wakeful, stimulus sensitive, irregular when they do sleep and sleep for brief periods. They have long periods of fussing and crying. And, unlike Allyson, often a portion of their crying is inconsolable. Because of their irregularity and alert/aroused state, it doesn't make sense to try to schedule their sleep at this time. They are hard to read. Most parents have difficulty telling whether they are hungry, fussy or plain overtired. So leaving them alone is confusing to everyone. The following hints and the information in Chapter 4 will help you get through the rugged first few months.

Helpful Hints for Parents of Colicky Kids

Pamper yourself; remember, this is smart for the baby, not selfish for you. If you feel better, you will be better able to nurture your baby.

Forget errands, chores, housework
Unplug the phone
Ignore your baby's sleeping sounds
Nap when baby sleeps
Hire help for housework or breaks when baby is most bothersome
Plan pleasurable, brief outings without baby (swimming, shopping, cinema)

Hints to Help Soothe Colicky and Non-colicky Babies

DEFINITELY HELP SOOTHE

Rhythmic rocking
Sucking (A dummy on a very short ribbon attached to a pillow cover or pyjama top; ribbon must be short so that it cannot go around the child's neck)
Swaddling

QUESTIONABLY HELP SOOTHE

Lambskin rug
Heartbeat sounds in teddy bear
Low-volume recording of vacuum cleaner or running water

Removal of stimulating toys from cot or bright night-light
Placing a soft blanket in baby's hand
Putting the child's head against a soft cot bumper

> **PRACTICAL POINT**
>
> **Don't save your smiles until colic ends.**

Crying should not be thought of as a test for you. Don't feel that you are creating a crying habit because of your prolonged, complex efforts. Your first test to help your baby sleep will come later, at three to four months of age, when the colic subsides.

You can't treat colic with smiles, but there will be less crying in a home where there is a lot of social smiling. Practice smiling; smile broadly; open your eyes wide, regard your child as you nod, and say 'Good boy' or 'Good girl'. Do all these especially when your baby calms down or smiles at you.

Months Three to Four: Extreme Fussiness/ Colic Ends. Morning Nap Develops at 9:00 to 10:00 A.M.

Let's consider the ways in which your child has changed. More smiles, coos, giggles, laughs and squeals light up your life. Your child is now a more social creature. She is sleeping better at night, but naps may still be brief and irregular.

Become sensitive to her need to sleep and try to distinguish this need from her desire to play with you. She would naturally prefer the pleasure of your company to being left alone in a dark, quiet bedroom. Therefore, she will fight off sleep to keep you around.

In addition to your presence, which provides pleasurable stimulation, your baby's curiosity about all the new and exciting parts of her expanding world will disrupt her sleep.

How interesting it must be for an infant to observe the clouds in the sky, listen to the trees moving in the wind, hear the noise of barking dogs or focus on the rhythms of adult chatter.

Become sensitive to the difference in quality between brief, interrupted sleep and prolonged, consolidated naps. Your child is becoming less portable. As her biological rhythms evolve for day sleep, your general goal is to *synchronise your caretaking activities with her biological needs*. This is no different from being sensitive to her need to be fed or changed.

When your baby needs to sleep, try to have her in an environment where she will sleep well. As she continues to grow, you will probably notice that she sleeps poorly outside of her cot.

I have examined many children who cry with such intensity and persistence that their mothers are sure they're ill. During their crying, they may swallow air and become very windy. If this happens, it is tempting to assume that their formula doesn't agree with them or that they have an intestinal disease – but only at night? These children are healthy but overtired. Not only do they cry hard and long when awake, they also cry loud and often during sleep/wake transitions.

PRACTICAL POINT

The crying baby may be hungry or just fussy. Or the crying baby may be *overtired*.

Most of these children are overtired from not napping well or from going to sleep too late. They are not napping well because they're getting too much outside stimulation, too much handling or too much irregular handling.

A sleep problem that is easy to deal with is the baby of about three months of age who had been sleeping well but now wakes up crying at night and during the day. The parents also may note heightened activity with wild screaming spells. These are regular, adaptable, mild infants who matured early but, at three months, began to decide they would rather play with their parents than be placed in a dark, quiet and boring room. Parents who have not had enough experience believe this new night waking represents hunger due to a 'growth spurt' or insufficient breast milk.

When these parents begin to focus on establishing a regular daytime nap schedule, when they put these babies in their cots when they need to sleep and when they avoid overstimulation, the frequent night waking stops. If the children had developed irritability or fussiness, this disappears, too.

REMEMBER

The more rested a child is, the more she accepts sleep and expects to sleep.

What is a good sleep strategy for your child at this age? As with the easy six- to eight-week-old, plan to put your three- or four-month-old child somewhere semi-quiet or quiet to nap after she's been awake for no more than about two hours.

Q: *When I put my child to sleep after no more than two hours of wakefulness, how long should he sleep?*

A: At this point, the naps may be either short or long without any particular pattern. This variability occurs because the part of the brain that establishes regular naps has not yet fully developed. Watch for signs of tiredness to help you decide whether a particular nap was long enough.

The two-hour limit on wakefulness is an approximation. Often there is a magic moment of tiredness when the baby will go to sleep easily. She is tired then, but not overtired. After you go past two hours, expect fatigue to set in. When the baby is up too long, she will tend to become over-stimulated, over-aroused, irritable or peevish. Please don't blame changes in weather – it's never too hot or too cold to sleep well.

Many parents misunderstand what over-stimulation means. A child becomes *over-stimulated* when the *duration of wakeful intervals is too long.* Over-stimulation does not mean that you are too intense in your playfulness.

PRACTICAL POINT

Do not think of over-stimulation as excessive intensity with which you play with your child, but rather too long a duration of baby's normal period of wakefulness. It's not too much of a good thing, it's just being up too long.

Become Your Child's Timekeeper: The Morning Nap Develops at 9:00 to 10:00 A.M.

Watch the clock during the day and expect the baby to need to sleep within two hours of wakefulness. Use whatever soothing method or wind-down routine works best to comfort and calm your baby. This may include a scheduled feeding, non-nutritive ('recreational') nursing, a session in a swing or a rocking chair, or a dummy.

After a while you may notice a partial routine or a rough pattern of when your child's day sleep is best. Based on your child's behaviour, the time of day and how long she has been awake, you may reasonably conclude that she *needs* to sleep at any given time. However, she may *want* to play with you instead. Please try to distinguish between your child's needs and her wants. Have the confidence to be sensitive to her need to sleep and lie down with her or leave her alone a little to let her sleep. How long should you leave her alone? Maybe five, ten or twenty minutes; there's no need for a rigid schedule. Simply test her once in a while to see whether she goes to sleep after five to twenty minutes of protest crying. If this approach fails, pick her up, soothe her, comfort her and then either try once more to get her to go to sleep, or play with her for a while and try again later.

This lack of rigid scheduling is appropriate for children a

few months old who are biologically immature. However, as the child gets older, extreme inconsistency will produce unhealthy sleep habits. Be flexible, but also become sensitive to your child's need to sleep.

When put down to sleep drowsy but awake, you are giving her the opportunity to develop *self-soothing skills*, to learn how to fall asleep unassisted. Some children learn this faster than others, so don't worry if your child seems always to cry up to your designated time. Perhaps she was too young; try the technique again another time.

Always going to your child when he needs to sleep robs him of sleep. Never letting your child cry might reflect confusion in your mind between the healthy notion of allowing him to be alone sometimes and your own fear that he will feel abandoned.

Here's an account from the mother of a three-month-old infant.

It Goes Against Human Nature

To leave a baby crying and not pick him up goes against human nature. However, after three days of teaching Katie to sleep and having to listen to her crying and being helpless, her hysteria was almost completely solved!

It started at just twelve weeks. Katie was so fatigued she would cry for hours, screaming completely out of control, scratching her head, pulling her ears. Holding her didn't help, so it wasn't hard not to pick her up – she screamed anyway.

Instituting a new day schedule was easy. As soon as she started getting irritable, I rushed her to her cot to sleep. She would watch her mobile, and then sleep for hours at a time. The first week, she was so tired that she only stayed up thirty to fifty minutes at a time and slept three to four hours in between. The key for me was to get her down before she got *really* upset.

The afternoon was when she was awake the longest, and then it was hard getting her to sleep at night. The first few nights under our new regime were the worst. Positive reinforcement from my doctor was important then. I had to hear several times that this 'cure' was the best thing to do.

The first night under our new strategy, my husband lay on the floor in her room (to make sure she didn't choke) while I sat crying in our living room. Finally after forty-five minutes Katie was *quiet*! Hurray! Each night she cried less and less, and I handled it better and better. After a week, her hysteria was gone! Sure, she cried a little sometimes, but now she was on a schedule. She napped two or three times a day, two to four hours at a time, and slept twelve to fifteen hours a night. Sleeping promotes more sleep, and makes it easier to fall asleep. It's a catch-22.

Writing down the sleep patterns helped, too. For one week I kept track of every time I put her down and every time I picked her up from her nap. At the end of the week I noticed a distinct pattern. She fell into it herself!

MAJOR POINTS

Letting your baby 'cry it out' is *not* the only way your baby will learn to sleep.

Babies and children learn to sleep when parents focus on timing, motionless sleep and consistency in soothing style.

As Katie's mother noticed, sleep begets sleep. This is a true statement. Even though it is not logical, it is biological!

Q: *My three-month-old used to take very long morning naps, but now at four months, they are shorter. What happened?*
A: Between three and four months, your child went to sleep later at night, he now goes to sleep earlier, wakes up better rested in the morning and no longer needs a very long morning nap.

Preventing and Solving Sleep Problems

Sleep periods develop as the brain matures. This means that there are times during the day and night when your baby's brain will become drowsy and less alert. These time 'windows', when the sleep process begins to overcome your baby, are the best times for him to be soothed to sleep, because it is easier to fall asleep at these times and because the restorative power of sleep is greatest when your baby's brain is in a drowsy state. Your child is able to sleep at other times, but going to sleep is more difficult and its restorative power is then much less. Unfortunately, your baby's brain may not be drowsy when you want him to sleep. You cannot control when he will become drowsy any more than you can control when he will become thirsty. As your infant's brain matures, these biologically determined periods of drowsiness will become more predictable and longer.

After your baby is born, there is a quiet and calm honeymoon during which he is very sleepy. This ends when he is a few days old, or a few days after his due date if he was born early. You may not have a honeymoon if your baby was born late! After a few days of life, the sleepy brain wakes up, and during the first six weeks of life infants display increasing amounts of fussiness, crying or agitated wakefulness, during which they swallow air and become windy. The duration of these periods peak and become more common in the evening hours at six weeks or six weeks after the due date. During these first six weeks, the longest single sleep period is not very long and can occur at any time; this is day/night confusion. At about six weeks of age, something dramatic occurs naturally. Your baby begins to produce social smiles, and the evening fussiness begins to decrease. One mother asked me if she could 'fast-forward to six weeks' and skip the hard part. Sorry.

REMEMBER

Long night sleep periods will develop first, so you will notice longer sleeping periods at night before you will notice longer naps.

The onset of social smiles followed by a decrease in fussiness reflects maturational changes within your baby's brain. In addition, the brain becomes more able to inhibit the stimulating effects of the sights, smells, sounds and other sensations around her. Your baby is more able to console herself – she is becoming more self-soothing. As a result of these biological changes, at six weeks of age your baby develops *night sleep organisation*. This means that her longest single sleep period now occurs at night. This is the end of day/night confusion. This longest night-sleep period may be only four to six hours long, but it regularly occurs at *night*. You cannot control the exact time when this long sleep period will occur, but at least you now know that you will get a little more rest at night.

Night sleep usually develops without problems at six weeks of age because:

1. **Darkness serves as a time cue**
2. **We slow down our activities and become quieter at night**
3. **We behave as if we expect the baby to sleep**

These three factors may be absent during the day, and so the major way to *prevent* sleep problems from developing is to focus your efforts on *helping your baby nap during the day*.

There are three factors that will help your baby sleep well during the day: timing, motionless sleep and consistency in soothing style. If you have experience because you have more than one child, start early; if you have a colicky baby, start later.

Timing

Keep the intervals of wakefulness short. Look at the clock when your baby wakes up in the morning or after a nap. After about one hour, begin a soothing process *before* your child appears grumpy, irritable, or drowsy. Usually the total duration of wakefulness plus the time of soothing should be *less than two hours*. This does not mean that you keep your baby awake for about two hours before trying to soothe him to sleep. The point is that young infants cannot comfortably tolerate long periods of wakefulness. In fact, some babies go to sleep after being awake for only *one* hour.

> **MAJOR POINT**
>
> **Perfect timing produces no crying.**

Think of surfing. You want to catch the wave of drowsiness as it is rising to enable your baby to have a long, smooth ride to deep slumber. If your timing is off and your wave crashes into an overtired state, then the ride is bumpy and brief. If your timing is off, you have accidentally allowed your child to become overtired, then there will be some crying, which you may ignore. Crying is the consequence of becoming overtired.

Think of how your baby behaves when she becomes overly hungry. She twists, turns and may dive-bomb at the breast for a few minutes before she settles down to suck well. Similarly, the overtired baby takes a few minutes to settle down to sleep. Crying is the consequence of becoming overtired. At this particular time your efforts to soothe – hugging, rocking, talking – may be stimulating and interfere with the natural surfacing of the sleep process. After all, your baby does not fall asleep immediately in the same way a light switch is turned off. Rather, the sleep process takes time. Remember, it is easier for her to fall asleep before she becomes grumpy, because when she becomes overtired – from nap deprivation or any other reason – her body produces stimulating hormones to fight the fatigue. This chemical stimulation interferes with sleeping well. This is why sleeping well during the day will improve night sleeping and why, conversely, *nap deprivation causes night waking*.

One mother told me that her child had been extremely fussy/colicky, but that at twelve weeks of age, he began to slip into a better sleeping routine at night and began taking longer naps during the day between twelve and sixteen weeks of age. She was breast-feeding and used the family bed; her child went to sleep at about 10:00 P.M. around twelve weeks of age. Her two-year-old son was not sleeping well at night either and he distracted her, and this allowed the baby to become overtired and now the naps were a mess. The baby was 'napping' between 5:00 and 6:00 P.M. By sixteen weeks of age, the baby was asleep for the night between 7:00 and 8:00 P.M. She recognised that the baby should be falling asleep for the night around 6:00 P.M., not napping then. Here was the solution that eventually corrected the overtired state.

Temporarily, her baby was put to sleep at a very early time, between 5:30 and 6:00 P.M. The plan was to help the child get more rested at night. The mother was to soothe her baby at night and then either lie down with him or put him in his cot. She wanted to use the cot because the hour was so early and she had a two-year-old to deal with. Because of his age, because he had been extremely fussy/colicky and because he had become accustomed to sleeping with his mother in her bed at the breast, we knew he would protest at our plan. We decided that we would ignore his protest crying at the onset of sleep and we would use the father to soothe him at night when he might cry but was not hungry. During the day, the mother would do whatever worked to maximise sleep and minimise crying to keep him as well rested as possible. The two-year-old made this part of the plan a little difficult. Within eight days, there was substantially less crying at night, and longer and fewer naps were occurring during the day. Now that he was better rested, he was able to stay up a little later at night. However, he still needed to go to sleep between 6:00 and 6:30 P.M.

EARLY BEDTIMES

A common complaint is 'We don't get to eat dinner as a family.' Or, 'How can we play outside as a family after dinner?' My answer is that what is most important is a well-rested family.

Motionless Sleep

How well do you nap in a car or on a plane compared to in your bed? I think babies have better-quality, more-restorative sleep when they are sleeping in a stationary cot, bed or bassinet. Vibrations or motion during sleep appear to force the brain to a lighter sleep state and reduce the restorative power of the nap. I explained to the mother of one child that her baby would not sleep well while she was shopping, walking in the park or doing something active with her friends. The mother discovered that this was true, that her baby napped best at home, but she also found it very difficult to spend more time at home during the day, as she and most of her friends were 'outdoor' people. On the positive side, her child no longer cried before going down for a nap.

You may wish to use a moving swing or a calm ride in the pushchair or car for a few minutes as part of the soothing process, but after your baby falls asleep, drive home, turn off the swing or stop walking with the pushchair. Although your baby may appear to be in an awkward position, don't disturb him if you notice that he always wakes as you try to move him to a cot. It doesn't hurt children to sleep in their swings or car seats. Your baby might also sleep well outdoors in a stationary pushchair, especially if it's a quiet neighbourhood. In general, however, as the brain matures, the child's increasing curiosity and social awareness make it more difficult to have good naps outside, so be careful.

Consistency in Soothing/Sleeping-Style Naps

Parents often assume that there is a right and wrong way to soothe a baby to sleep. This is not the case. Falling asleep is simply learned behaviour, a habit. Your child will learn best if you are consistent in how you soothe him to sleep for naps. Below are two popular ways to soothe a baby to sleep. Either will work as long as you are consistent.

> **IMPORTANT POINT**
>
> **One method is not better than another; both Method A and Method B can help your child sleep well. There is no reason to be judgemental about soothing styles or brand other parents as 'bad' simply because they do not agree with you. Different methods will seem more natural or more acceptable to different parents, and different methods work better for different children.**

Method A: At nap time your baby sometimes soothes himself to sleep unassisted. After soothing your baby for several minutes, you *always* put him down to sleep *whether or not he is asleep*. The soothing is a winding down, a transition from active to quiet, from alert to drowsy. Soothing may include breast- or bottle-feeding. Contrary to popular belief, your child will not develop night-sleeping problems if you include breast-feeding as part of the soothing process. Also, contrary to popular belief, it is not necessary that you always put him down fully awake. The key is that you consistently spend a relatively brief period of time soothing your baby to sleep for naps. Because he is not necessarily always asleep when you put him down, he eventually learns how to soothe himself to sleep without being held. Method A may be viewed positively (creating independence, learning self-soothing skills, acquiring the capacity to be alone) or negatively (creating insecurity, neglecting or abandoning your baby, selfishness in the mother).

Method B: Your baby always begins naps with your help. You *always* hold and soothe your baby *until she is in a deep sleep state, no matter how long it takes*. You may then lie down or sit down with your baby, nap with her or perhaps put her down only after she is in a very deep sleep state. Your child learns to associate the process of falling asleep with the feel of your breast, your breathing and heart rhythm, and your body's scent. Method B may be viewed positively (providing more security, is more natural) or negatively (creating dependence, spoiling). Contrary to popular belief, this association, in and of itself, does not automatically lead to a night-waking problem. A night-waking problem sometimes occurs when the mother indiscriminately responds to normal arousals, misinterprets them to reflect hunger and inadvertently fragments the child's sleep. Perhaps this situation occurs more often in those mothers who choose Method B for naps.

Be decisive; choose a soothing style and *be consistent*. Consistency helps your baby sleep better, because the process of falling asleep is a learned behaviour. Review the 'Resources for Soothing' on page 73. Grandparents and baby-sitters should handle your baby as you do. Sometimes grandparents are a major problem, interfering with the baby's sleep schedule. They want to come over to play with their grandchild when it is convenient for them. This is a difficult problem without a simple answer because, in addition to wanting your child to be well rested, you want to maintain family harmony. If the grandparents are the primary caregivers during the day, it may be difficult. Try to teach them how important sleep is for their grandchild.

Q: *When should I start to try to establish regular naps? When should I start to become consistent in how I soothe my baby before naps?*

A: Day-sleep organisation develops at twelve to sixteen weeks of age. A regularly occurring midmorning nap appears first, followed several weeks later by a regularly occurring early afternoon nap. The age when you start nap training depends on your experience and your baby's temperament.

Regardless of when you begin to start nap training, the sooner you develop a consistent approach, the easier it will be for the family. Please begin to be consistent around six weeks of age, when your child is clearly becoming more social and everyone is getting more rest at night. For babies born before their due date, these changes occur about six weeks after the due date, and that is when you start.

I encourage fathers to become as involved as possible – for example, at weekends – so that sometimes the mother breast-feeds the baby and then passes the baby to the father to be soothed to sleep. As I said, either soothing method works well, but my observation is that for well-rested babies whose parents have consistently used Method B and sometime later decide to switch to Method A, the transition is made with very little or no crying. However, the children of parents who use Method B *inconsistently* may never develop regular naps; they then become overtired, and when the parents switch to Method A, the overtired child cries a lot. For some parents, then, it is simply easier to be consistent using Method A.

If you have more than one child, it is very difficult to consistently use Method B, even with full-time help, as an older child's demands may make it impossible to devote so much time to getting the younger child into a deep sleep before putting him down. Therefore, it is more practical to use Method A. Because of your experience, you can begin helping your younger child sleep well as soon as you get home from the hospital. With two children, starting sleep training early for your newborn is especially important. Also, fathers need to help out more. As one basketball fan said, 'Now I have to shift from one-on-one to zone defence!'

Here is an account from a mother who started early with her second child using Method B.

Good Sleep Habits Start with Two. . .

As patients of Dr Weissbluth, we were ready to commit ourselves to promoting good sleep habits in our children. When our son, Hayden, was born, it was easier said than done being a new mother and not knowing what the different cries meant, we would pick Hayden up at the slightest whimper. We were quick believers when at four months we were a bit more seasoned and we decided not to rush in at the first cry. The cry lasted fifteen minutes and then it was smooth sailing; he gradually went to bed earlier and earlier until we reached a 6:00 P.M. bedtime with a 6:30 A.M. wake-up, and then naps at 9:00 A.M. and 1:00 P.M. This pattern still holds true minus the first nap and bedtime is at 6:30 P.M. at almost three years old. He is social, happy, sweet and most of all well rested.

With the birth of our second child, a girl, Lily, we were busy with Hayden, now a toddler, and were quite the experts on all the 'signs' babies give out. We had a rule: if she was not crying (even at a few days old), she was to be put in her bassinet. We still played with her and enjoyed her, but we were not walking around the house with her twenty-four hours a day. We also provided Lily with the same night-time routine we give Hayden, dim the lights, give a massage, bath, bottle, book and bed. This prompted Lily to develop a quicker sleep schedule, and we found by two and a half months she was sleeping through the late-night feedings. By three months she was going to bed at 5:00 to 5:30 P.M. and sleeping until 6:30 A.M. Also at three months we began putting her down for her morning nap two hours after she woke up, and that began her nap schedule. Now Lily, almost one, wakes up at 6:30 A.M., takes her first nap at 8:15 A.M., takes her second nap at 12:30 P.M. and is in the bathtub by 5:00 P.M. and asleep by 5:30 P.M.

We are vigilant about not letting either child nap in the car, pushchairs, or for that matter miss naps or have delayed naps. Once our children are in their cots for the night, we don't hear from them until the morning . . . no night waking or games! We greet them each morning with a smile on their faces.

We are committed to having well-rested children and will defend our decisions with anyone suggesting we don't get to be with our children at night or we are too strict with the daytime schedule. We find too often it is the parent who is putting the child on their schedule instead of vice versa.

Babies yearn for routines and respond unbelievably to them. Again, we feel that we have two of the happiest, sweetest children, and knowing that teaching them good sleep habits and, more importantly, the ability to fall asleep unassisted is the best gift you can ever give!

Your goal is to synchronise your caretaking with your baby's needs: feed her when she's hungry, change her when she's wet, play with her when she's awake and help her sleep when she's tired. Because of the irregularity with which these events occur, it is hard for first-time parents to 'read' their baby's needs, but experienced parents should trust their instincts and put the baby to sleep when she is tired.

If you have an extremely fussy/colicky baby, one who is more irritable, wakeful, harder to soothe and harder to read, you may find that only with Method B will these babies sleep or rest without crying. Later I'll give more specific advice on making a transition from Method B to Method A in the colicky baby.

COMMON NAP MISTAKES

Keeping the intervals of wakefulness too long
Using swings, cars or pushchairs during sleeping
Inconsistency in methods used to soothe your baby to sleep

Q: *Do I have to become a slave to my baby's nap schedule?*
A: Not at all. Simply respect his need to have good-quality naps. Try to distinguish between routine days and exceptional days. On routine days, try partially to organise your activities around the naps. On exceptional days, naps may be lost because of special events.

If you suffer the inconvenience of hanging around your house on routine days when you think your baby will need to nap, then between twelve and sixteen months (or somewhat later in colicky babies) you will notice that your child takes fewer and longer naps, longer periods of wakefulness will develop during the day, there will be no late afternoon fussiness and your baby will have longer periods of night sleep.

REMEMBER

Sleep quality depends on:

- **Timing of sleep periods**
- **Consolidation of sleep periods**
- **Duration of sleep periods**

Action Plan for Exhausted Parents

All babies become fussy a few days after they are born, or a few days after the expected date of delivery if they are born early. Parents do not cause the fussy behaviour. The exact cause is not known. About 20 per cent of babies will develop extreme fussiness/colic and, again, parents are not the cause. When babies fuss or cry, they do not sleep. When they do not sleep, mothers do not sleep. Mind-numbing fatigue from lack of sleep is your main enemy!

HOW TO SOOTHE AND HELP YOUR BABY LEARN TO SLEEP: BIRTH TO FOUR MONTHS OF AGE

Encourage sucking; do not worry if your baby falls asleep while sucking
Rhythmic rocking motions
Swaddling
Massage

Respect your baby's need to sleep: the one- to two-hour window. Think and plan how you will soothe your baby but *when* you soothe is more important.

- Babies quickly become overtired after only one or two hours of wakefulness. During the day, note the time when your baby wakes up and try to help him nap by soothing within the next one or two hours before he becomes overtired. Try to keep the intervals of wakefulness brief.
- Babies less than six weeks old fall asleep at night very late and do not sleep very long day or night. Try to soothe your baby to sleep during the day before he becomes overtired. Always respond to your baby. Avoid the overtired state.
- Eighty per cent of babies more than six weeks old become more settled at night, sleep a little longer at night and begin to become drowsy for night sleep at an earlier hour. Try to soothe your baby to sleep at an earlier hour if he shows signs of drowsiness earlier. Do not let him cry.
- Twenty per cent of babies more than six weeks old do not appear to become more settled at night, do not appear to sleep longer at night, and do not become drowsy at an earlier hour. Nevertheless, try to soothe your baby to sleep at an earlier hour even if he does not show signs of drowsiness earlier. Spend extra time soothing: prolonged swinging, long luxurious baths and never-ending car rides. Fathers should put in extra effort to help out. Do not let your baby cry.
- Use consistent soothing styles for naps.
- After a few weeks, sleep in a quiet and dark place.
- At six weeks of age, watch for an earlier bedtime in common fussy babies. Extremely fussy/colicky babies may show an earlier bedtime when older.
- At four months of age, your baby will have longer periods of wakefulness, but you should still synchronise the beginning of your soothing efforts with the beginning of your baby's drowsiness. For common fussy babies, this may appear to be highly predictable or 'by the clock'. Extremely

fussy babies may appear to have predictable and regular sleep times when much older.

- After four months of age, 'let cry', controlled crying, or check and console might be needed for a formerly extremely fussy/colicky baby. Rarely, this might be done for a younger baby.

Review

- Drowsy signs, page 63
- Soothing strategies, page 63
- Resources for soothing, page 73
- Bedtime routines, page 75
- 'Let cry' versus 'no cry', page 103

1. 'Let Cry' with no time limit *(Extinction)*
2. 'Let Cry' with time limit *(Graduated Extinction)*
   Delayed response for soothing
   Gradually increase the delay
   Increase the delay on the same night versus subsequent nights
   Soothe until drowsy versus soothe until deep sleep
3. 'Maybe Cry' *(Check and console, sleep away from parent)*
   Prompt response for soothing; never delay
   Repeat as often as needed
   Soothe until drowsy versus soothe until deep sleep
4. 'No Cry' *(Sleep with parent, family bed)*
   Prompt response for soothing
   Repeat as often as needed
   Soothe until deep sleep

WEEKS TWO TO FOUR

- Prepare for peak fussiness/crying to occur at six weeks of age. Try to get help then. If your baby is showing extreme fussiness/colic, read Chapter 4.
- Keep the intervals of wakefulness brief: one to two hours.

WEEKS FIVE TO SIX

- The worst is almost over for 80 per cent of babies.
- Keep the intervals of wakefulness brief: one to two hours.

WEEKS SEVEN TO EIGHT

- Look for drowsy signs earlier and move the bedtime earlier.

MONTHS THREE TO FOUR

- Watch for drowsy signs around 9:00 A.M.
- The morning nap develops around 9:00 to 10:00 A.M.

Motionless sleep is best.
Consistency in soothing style for naps.

A. Always lie down with your child or put him down only after several minutes of soothing.

B. Always soothe your child until he is in a deep sleep, no matter how long the soothing takes, before lying down with him or putting him down to sleep.

CHAPTER 6

Months Five to Twelve

Our goal is to establish sleep habits, so we don't want to get side-tracked by worrying too much about crying. When your two-year-old cries because he doesn't want his nappy changed or your one-year-old cries because he wants juice instead of milk, don't let the crying prevent you from doing what is best for him. Establishing healthy sleep habits does not mean that there will always be a lot of crying, but there may be some in protest. If you find this to be unacceptable when your child is four months old, then please reconsider this chapter when he is nine or ten months old.

Months Five to Eight: Early Afternoon Nap Develops at 12:00 to 2:00 P.M. Variable Late Afternoon Nap at 3:00 to 5:00 P.M.

As months three to four blend into months five to eight, behaviour does not change sharply. Nonetheless, a distinct shift occurs at about the age of four to five months. Increased sociability permits more playfulness and gamelike interactions between you and your infant. Your child may roll over, sit, imitate your voice with babbling or respond quickly to your quiet sounds. This increased social interaction certainly makes having a baby more fun.

Infants really do enjoy their parents' company; they thrive in response to your laughter and smiles. However, your baby is not like an empty vessel you can fill with love, warmth, hugs, kisses and soothing until it is full, thus leading to satisfaction, blissful contentment or undemanding repose. The more you entertain her, the more she will want to be amused. So it is natural and reasonable to expect your baby to protest when you stop playing with her. In fact, the more you play with your child, the more she will come to expect that this is the natural order of things. Nothing is wrong with this, except that there are times when you have to dress your baby or leave her to amuse herself for a while, and she will probably resist the partial restraint or curtailment of fun and games. When this happens, please remember that leaving your baby alone protesting for more fun with you while you get dressed is not the same thing as abandonment. Similarly, leaving your baby alone protesting for more fun when she needs to sleep is not neglect. You have become sensitive to your child's need to sleep, and she is now old enough to set her clock at a healthy sleep. Our goal is to synchronise caretaking activities with her need to be fed, to be kept warm, to be played with, and to sleep.

After four months of age, an infant's sleep becomes more adultlike. Infants younger than this enter sleep with a REM sleep period, but around this age they begin to enter sleep with a non-REM sleep period, like adults. Sleep cycling, from deep to light non-REM sleep with interruptions of REM sleep, also matures into adultlike patterns around four months of age.

As discussed previously, the five elements of healthy sleep are (1) sleep duration (night and day), (2) naps, (3) sleep consolidation, (4) sleep schedule and (5) sleep regularity. Now let's look at Figure 7 overleaf. This circle graph is a navigational aid for parents to help them understand sleep/wake rhythms. Although I designed this graph, I did not create it any more than a mapmaker creates the shape or location of an island. As your child gets older, the times when he will become sleepy are becoming more predictable. Another way of saying this is that the biological sleep/wake rhythms mature. This allows you to change your strategy for keeping your child well rested. Previously, the focus was on *brief intervals of wakefulness* to avoid the overtired state; now you can begin to use *clock time* as an aid to help your child sleep well. Some parents call this sleeping 'by the clock', or BTC. Stated simply, you are using your child's natural sleep rhythms to help him fall asleep. Let's start in the morning and go around the clock.

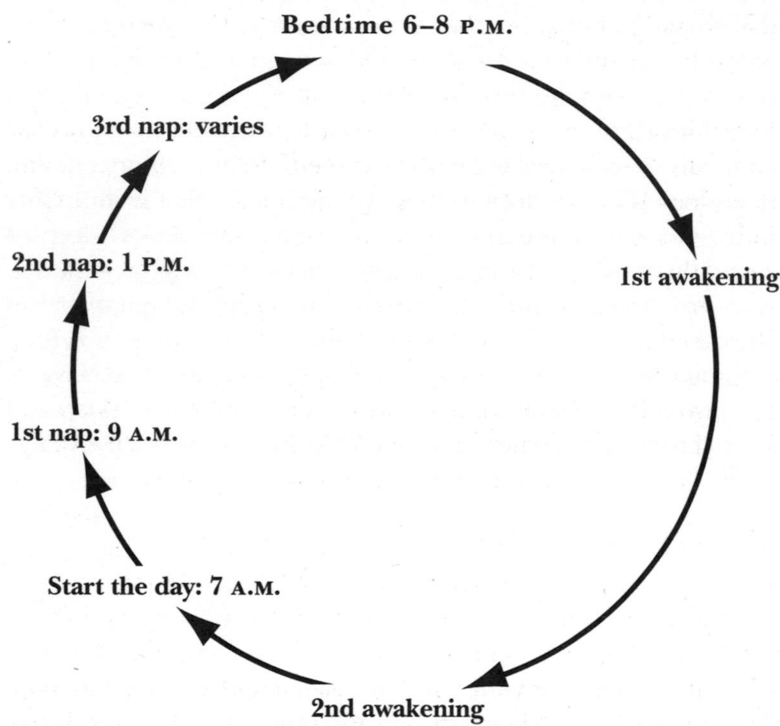

FIGURE 7: HEALTHY SLEEP SCHEDULE FOR INFANTS FOUR TO EIGHT MONTHS OLD

How to Teach Your Baby to Sleep or to Protect His Sleep Schedule

You are now about to learn how to help your child learn to sleep well and to protect a naturally developed, healthy sleep pattern.

The Wake-up Time

Some babies tend to wake up early, 5:00 or 6:00 A.M., and return to sleep after a brief feeding or nappy change. This is a true continuation of night sleep and not a nap. Other babies wake up later but start the day then. Most children will awaken to start the day about 7:00 A.M., but there is a wide range (between 6:00 and 8:00). In general, it is not a good idea to go to your child before 6:00 A.M., even if he is crying, because if you do, he will begin to force himself to wake up earlier and earlier in order to enjoy your company. The natural wake-up time seems to be an independent, neurological alarm clock in these young infants that is somewhat independent of the part of the brain that puts them to sleep or keeps them asleep. In fact, despite what is commonly believed, you *cannot* change the wake-up time by keeping your baby up later, feeding solids before bedtime or awakening your baby for a feeding before you go to sleep. The last seems insensitive, anyway. How would you feel if someone woke you from a deep sleep and started to feed you when you weren't hungry? The sleep strategy called 'Scheduled Awakenings' will be discussed later.

Morning Wakeful Time

Let's focus now on how brief intervals of wakefulness develop into 'windows' of clock time. These are periods during which you will watch your baby *and the clock* to determine the time when it is easiest for your child to take an age-appropriate nap. These windows of 'sleep propensity' open and close, and they represent times during which it is easiest to fall asleep and stay asleep. Morning wakeful time will last about two hours for four- to five-month-olds or about three hours for eight-month-olds. Some easy babies or babies born early may be able to stay up for only one hour at four months of age. Then, plan a wind-down or nap time ritual of up to thirty minutes. You decide what you want to do: bath, bottle, breast-feeding, lullaby, massage – but limit it, because hours of holding your baby produce only a light or twilight sleep state, which is poor-quality sleep. Begin this ritual about half an hour *before* the end of your baby's wakeful period, not after it's over. At the end of your predetermined nap time ritual, whether your baby is asleep or awake, lie down with her or put her in her cot. As one mother commented to me, 'I cannot tell you what a liberating experience it was to be able to put my baby down in her cot before she fell asleep in my arms.' She may now cry a little, a lot, or not at all.

The temperamentally easy child cries very little, and the routine is repeated for an early afternoon nap. The more difficult child, who may have also been a very fussy/colicky infant, might now cry a lot. The premature baby also may cry a lot, and the following approach might be delayed until four months after the expected date of delivery.

Nap 1: Midmorning

This nap develops first, usually between twelve and sixteen weeks of age or twelve to sixteen weeks after the due date for premature babies. It occurs about 9:00 A.M. and may last an hour or two. Sometimes you can stretch the child's morning wakeful period by a few minutes each day to get to this time, or you might wake him up at 7:00 A.M. in order for him to be able to take this nap. This violation of the rule 'Never wake a sleeping baby' is to help maintain an age-appropriate sleep schedule for the benefit of the baby. The rule mainly applies to waking babies for our social convenience, to their detriment. Try to anticipate your child's best nap time. If he takes this nap too early or too late, then it will be difficult for him to take the second nap on time.

We consider a sleep period to be a restorative nap if it is about an hour or longer. Forty to forty-five minutes is sometimes enough, but most babies in this age range sleep at least a solid hour. Certainly sleep periods shorter than thirty minutes should not count as naps.

If you are using Method A for naps (see page 235) or have a temperamentally easy baby, after putting your baby down for this nap, leave him completely alone to allow him to (1) learn to fall asleep unassisted and (2) return to sleep unassisted until he has slept about an hour in an uninterrupted fashion. Easy babies may cry very little or not at all; the temperamentally more difficult child may cry a lot. Remember, you are responding sensitively to his need to sleep by not providing too much attention. You are decisive in establishing a routine because you are upholding his right to sleep. Be calm and firm and consistent, because *consistency helps your baby learn rapidly*.

He will pick up on your calm/firm attitude and will learn quickly not to expect the pleasure of your company at nap time. You are not abandoning your child in his moment of need; you are giving him all the attention he needs when he is awake. Now he needs to be alone to sleep.

Q: *How long do I let my baby cry?*
A: No more than one hour.

Q: *What do I do if the nap is short? When I put my child down to sleep, she cries a long time, but for less than an hour, and then falls asleep, but she doesn't sleep very long. Do I let her cry again? Sometimes, she doesn't cry when I put her down for a nap, but she still doesn't sleep very long. Do I let her cry after the brief nap to see if she will sleep longer?*
A: If the nap is substantially less than thirty minutes, you might try to leave her alone for an additional thirty to sixty minutes, even if she cries, to see whether she will return to sleep unassisted. If the nap is substantially more than thirty minutes, it is less likely that she will return to sleep unassisted so you might want to leave her alone for an additional thirty minutes or go to her immediately and not let her cry any more. In general, the shorter the nap and the less restorative it appears, the longer you should leave her alone. Alternatively, you might want to try to lengthen the nap by rushing to your child at the first sound of awakening from a brief nap (less than an hour) and attempting to soothe your child back to sleep for a continuation of the nap. For some babies, this might be counterproductive and simply stimulate them to fight sleep more for the pleasure of the parent's company.

Q: *After one hour of crying, what do I do?*
A: Go to your baby and soothe her. Now you have two

choices. Your baby might be wakeful, and you might decide that this was so stressful for you or her that you want to go outside for a walk, relax and try again the next day to get a morning nap. Or your baby might be falling asleep in your arms after all this crying; if you feel that she will now be able to fall asleep, put her back down to see if she will nap. But do not let her cry for another full hour.

Q: *What's wrong if I quickly check my baby when she first cries and I give her a dummy or roll her back over? She always immediately stops crying and returns to sleep.*
A: Checking on your baby like this when she should be napping may not interfere with naps or night sleep in some infants between four and six months. But please be careful, because eventually all babies learn to turn these brief visits into prolonged playtimes. This learning process may develop slower if it is the father who does the checking and provides minimal intervention.

Q: *My child had extreme fussiness/colic and she is now about five months old. How do I get her on a 9:00 A.M. and 1:00 P.M. nap schedule?*
A: Make sure she is sleeping well at night.

Control the wake-up time; try to start the day around 6:00 to 7:00 A.M. by not going to her before 6:00 A.M. or waking her up at 7:00 A.M.

Try intense, but brief, stimulation outdoors. Expose her to wind, rustling leaves, moving clouds, street noises, voices, barking dogs, sand in the playground, motion in the jogger or soft sling on your chest, swings, 'swimming' pool splashing, and so forth.

Try to stretch her wakeful period to about 9:00 A.M. but be mindful not to allow her to become so frantically overtired that she will not be able to subsequently sleep well. She will get a little geared up and might get close to but not make it to 9:00 A.M.

Tone it down a little as you get close to 9:00 A.M.

Plan for a much longer and relaxing soothing-to-sleep routine before her morning nap because she will be a little overtired. Consider including a bath for relaxation, not for hygiene. Bathing might be stimulating but more often it is calm fun for babies.

Around 9:00 A.M., lie down to sleep with her or put her down to sleep. Review the sleep training strategies on page 211.

If she has a decent nap of close to one hour, repeat the same steps for her 1:00 P.M. nap.

If she does not nap in the morning, get out of the house and try to not let her sleep until about 11:00 A.M. Try the same soothing-to-sleep routine around 11:00 A.M. This means no car rides at 10:00 A.M.

Parents of post-colic babies or babies with a more difficult temperament (babies who are not self-soothing or who are irregular) might want to begin to practice Method A at this time. Many of these parents have been using Method B (your baby always begins naps with your help), as discussed in the previous chapter. Ideally, you have been very consistent with Method B up until now; the better rested your baby is when you make the transition from Method B to Method A, the easier it will be.

WARNING

It may be very difficult to establish regular naps at four to five months of age in some babies because their biological nap rhythms are maturing very slowly. Some babies don't evolve into a schedule of regular long naps until five or six months of age, especially if they had extreme fussiness/colic when younger or if their parents were inconsistent or irregular about naps during the first four months.

For the difficult-temperament or post-colic baby, establishing the morning nap may be the toughest parenting manoeuvre that you have attempted so far. By *focusing on the morning nap* we try to help a post-colic baby learn self-soothing skills. It's best to begin establishing an age-appropriate nap schedule with the morning nap because it is the first one to develop; it is the nap that should be the easiest to obtain, because your baby is most rested from the night sleep, and parents usually can be more consistent in the morning, when scheduling conflicts are less likely to develop, than in the afternoon.

After your child's day starts, look at the clock. *Within one hour of wakefulness,* clean, feed and soothe using Method A. This ultra-short period of wakefulness is designed to prevent the overtired state from developing.

Another reason why it is important to establish the morning nap by keeping the interval of wakefulness very short is that the morning nap might represent a continuation of night sleep. The morning nap contains more REM sleep than the afternoon nap, and large amounts of REM sleep are a characteristic feature of a baby's night sleep.

'He Did Best with His First Morning Nap'

The hours between 5:00 P.M. and 3:00 A.M. were the most difficult. When Eric was awake, he fussed or cried. The only way he would sleep was in our arms. My husband would cut up my food so I could eat with one hand while holding Eric with the other. I would nap from 8:00 to 10:00 P.M. to recharge for the next five hours. While I slept, my husband would alternately rock, walk and bounce Eric. The routine was nearly unbearable. Eventually we made a chart to show Eric's schedule to Dr W. We determined that we were holding Eric eighteen or nineteen hours a day. No wonder we were exhausted.

I'll never forget the night and early morning at about three months of age when Eric was so sleep-deprived he *could not* go to sleep. I tried everything – nursing, rocking, walking, bouncing, singing. Eventually he did fall asleep while I pushed him around the house in the pushchair listening to his favourite CD, only to wake up the second I tried to move him into his cot. The hours stretched on and Eric became more and more tired, overstimulated and agitated.

He began trying to pick the flowers off my pyjamas. Though he seemed to want to go to sleep, he appeared unable to get there. I felt I didn't have any choice but to put him in his cot – awake and crying. After about twenty minutes of crying, he fell asleep.

He did best with his first morning nap, crying only one or two minutes, if at all, before going to sleep. The evenings remained the most difficult. The longest crying episode was twenty-one minutes. My husband and I would sit in the den holding hands, listening to the baby monitor and engaging in self-doubt. Does he need us? Are we bad parents for letting him cry? We kept reminding ourselves that Eric was learning a valuable skill that would serve him (and us!) well for life. After about three days, we felt he had achieved success. He has been a terrific sleeper ever since. Now, at age eleven months, he sleeps from 7:00 P.M. to 7:00 A.M. and naps twice for an hour or two. Everyone who meets him says he is happy, joyful and alert.

If there is *bright morning light* during this hour, open up all your shades, because exposure to morning light might help establish sleep rhythms. If there is no bright natural light, make the room as bright as you can with room lights. Darken the room as you begin your soothing to sleep. After several minutes of soothing, which may include breast- or bottle-feeding, put your baby down. If there is crying, ignore the crying for between five and twenty minutes. You be the judge of how much crying you think is appropriate, but watch the clock, because three minutes of hard crying might feel to you like three hours. The reason we do not let difficult temperament or post-colic babies cry for an hour, as we can with easier babies, is that they have increased difficulty falling asleep unassisted. Their parents are usually extra stressed as well. I would, however, like to point out that some babies scream their brains out for two minutes, moan and whimper for three minutes and then go to sleep for a great nap! You might lose the chance for a long nap if you do not let your child blow off steam for a minute or two. As before, when you feel there has been enough crying, rescue your child and try it again the next day – or maybe put him back down if you think he will now go to sleep. For the remainder of the day, try to keep each interval of wakefulness to no more than two hours, do whatever works to maximise sleeping and minimise crying.

An alternative to putting children in their cot for naps is to sleep with them in your bed. This may work well for first-time mothers who do not have other children to care for. However, as your child becomes older, she becomes more aware of her environment while awake, drowsy and asleep. So you might have to position her cot next to your bed so she is not stimulated by your body movements, coughing or snoring.

As you read the following story, please try to notice features such as controlling the wake-up time, the ultra-short interval of wakefulness before the morning nap, making the bedtime earlier and transitioning from Method B to Method A.

'His Sleep Schedule Was Off Kilter'

Even when Patrick was only a few weeks old we noticed that he was becoming a night owl. He had what we called the 'late-night fussies' in which Patrick would fuss and cry until he fell asleep. This would begin between 7:30 and 9:00 P.M. and last until around midnight. He was going to sleep at night much too late and would not fall asleep unless one of us was holding him.

Our main concern was his grumpiness at night and his inability to fall asleep at a normal hour. Dr Weissbluth asked me to keep a record of Patrick's schedule for ten days. I created a bar graph for each twenty-four-hour period and colour-coded it to show when Patrick was awake, asleep or crying.

Dr Weissbluth's conclusion was that we needed to alter Patrick's sleep schedule. The goal was to get him to sleep earlier at night and to wake him up by 7:00 A.M. We began this by not letting him sleep past 7:00. If he awoke on his own between 6:00 and 7:00, great. If not, I had to get him up. I would then have one hour to change, feed and play with him. During this hour I was to keep him in bright sunlight or well-lit rooms to establish morning wake time. After he had been up for fifty minutes I was to begin 'quiet time' for ten minutes. This meant any soothing techniques I wanted to use to get him ready for his nap. I then had to put him in his cot awake and leave the room. If Patrick cried, my instructions were to leave him alone for five to twenty minutes to see if he would fall asleep on his own.

The first day I woke him at 7:00 on the dot. He was in a great mood as he ate, and we played in the light. At 7:50 I turned down the lights, read him a book in the rocking chair and walked him around the room singing lullabies. At 8:00 I put him in the cot and closed his bedroom door. He began to cry lightly as soon as I left. Knowing that it would be hard for me to listen to the crying and not go in to pick him up, I took my shower. This was the only way to force myself to stay out of his room. After exactly fourteen minutes he stopped crying and fell asleep for an hour! I couldn't believe how easy it was.

The next step was to put him down for a nap after he had been awake for two hours. We again did the same soothing techniques for ten minutes and I put Patrick in his cot awake. Unfortunately, things didn't go as well this time. Patrick cried for fifteen minutes and kept crying after I picked him up. His crying in my arms became louder, which was unusual, and eventually I was crying with him. I finally got him calmed down but had to wait until he fell asleep in my arms before I could put him back in his cot. I decided that we had to conquer the morning sleep before we could continue with the other naps.

I made my graphs of Patrick's sleeping habits and gave them to Dr Weissbluth. After reviewing them, he said that the progress was good, but now we needed to concentrate on getting him to sleep earlier at night. His ideal pattern should be to wake up at 7:00 A.M., with naps at 9:00 A.M., 1:00 P.M., and possibly 5:00 P.M., with bedtime around 7:30 P.M.

That night we began quiet time at 8:30. Although Patrick had been happily playing with us, he began to yawn. He eventually fell asleep in my arms without a fight and slept in his cot through the night. What a relief!

It was now time to start putting him down awake for his second nap. I began this by using the same soothing techniques for his second nap as I used for the first, only I did not have a time limit.

I would walk while singing quietly until Patrick began to close his eyes. I then put him in his cot awake but tired. Patrick would fuss for a few minutes and then fall asleep.

As the days went by and we felt comfortable with his ability to fall asleep for the first two naps, we tried the same technique on his occasional third nap and his evening bedtime. The end result is that we have a happy baby who takes great naps, falls asleep on his own at night and is an absolute joy. We still have some challenges. There are days when Patrick wants to take his nap after he has been up less than two hours and others when he wants to stay awake longer. If he fusses in his cot for more than fifteen minutes we pick him up and try again later. Bedtime at night is absolute. We put him in his cot for good around 7:30 P.M. Sometimes he fusses for a few minutes, but most nights we don't hear a peep until the next morning. It took a long time to get to this point and it was not easy, but it was definitely worth it.

Midday Wakeful Time

Expect your baby to be ready for another nap after two to three hours of wakefulness. In general, avoid long excursions, which might lead to mini-snoozes in the car or park. Although I've been emphasising sleep rhythms, remember that there are also wake rhythms – times when the body clock automatically switches to a wakeful mode, just as it switches to sleep mode at night and at nap times. Wakefulness turns on as sleep turns off.

If your child did not take a morning nap, do not allow him to take a snooze in the car or pushchair at a time when he should be awake. If your baby naps when he should be awake, it throws the remaining sleep/wake schedule off kilter.

The development of wakefulness is an active process; it is not just the turning off of sleep. During a wakeful mode, it is hard to fall asleep or stay asleep. If you do fall asleep during a wakeful mode, the ability of this sleep to restore alertness and a sense of well-being is less compared to the same amount of sleep occurring during a sleep mode.

For adults, there is a dramatic wakeful mode associated with a period of physical relaxation between about 6:00 and 9:00 P.M. Even if you are drowsy or sleep-deprived, it is hard to fall asleep during this time. This distinct zone of decreased sleepiness or increased arousal during the early evening hours has been called the 'forbidden zone' for sleep. This wakeful period has been recognised by television people, who have labelled it 'prime time'. This is the time when most adults do not and cannot sleep. Recent research also shows that there is a 'forbidden zone' for sleep in infants.

MAJOR POINT

It is as important not to let children sleep when they are in biological wake mode as it is to help them sleep when they are in biological sleep mode.

Usually if a nap doesn't occur, it is best to keep your baby awake and go to the next sleep period, whether it is another nap or night-time sleep. Probably this next sleep period will take place a little earlier because of the missed nap. Try to strike a balance between not letting your child become extremely overtired and preserving or protecting the age-appropriate sleep pattern.

Nap 2: Early Afternoon

The second nap usually occurs between noon and 2:00 P.M., most commonly around 1:00 P.M., but in any case it should usually begin before 3:00 P.M. The nap should last about an hour or two. Then go out afterwards and enjoy this longer period of wakefulness.

Please remember, this is an outline of a reasonable, healthy sleep pattern, not a set of rigid rules. In order to describe sleep patterns, we have to use clock time and the number of hours of sleep, but it is more important to watch your baby than to watch the clock. There is nothing absolute about napping at 1:00 P.M. or any other time in this sleep schedule. You'll have to make some adjustments to fit your own lifestyle and family arrangements. There will be special occasions when your child does not get the sleep he needs. He will recover from these exceptions faster if you have a regular pattern on most days. The problem with some families is that they never have a regular day, so the child is always somewhat overtired.

The most common problem with this second nap is that the interval of wakefulness following the first nap is too long. This causes your baby to become overtired, and he has difficulty either falling asleep or staying asleep. If you are using Method A, please leave your baby completely alone for one hour after soothing to see if he will fall asleep. If the duration of crying and sleeping associated with the early afternoon nap puts you way past 2:00 or 3:00 P.M., forget this nap and try to get your child to sleep in the late afternoon or early evening. If it is early, say around 4:00 P.M., limit this nap to about one and a half hours to protect a reasonably early bedtime. If it is later, say around 5:00 P.M., let your child sleep, because this 'nap' may simply continue into the night and it's important to maintain an early bedtime hour.

IMPORTANT POINT

This afternoon nap commonly continues until the third birthday, but after age three, it begins to drop out.

Nap 3: Late Afternoon: 16 Per Cent of Babies Have Three Naps

The third nap may or may not occur. If it does occur, the time when it starts may vary between 3:00 and 5:00 P.M. Also, the duration of this nap may vary, but it is usually very brief. This nap disappears by about nine months of age. A problem with allowing this third nap to continue much past this age is that the child is unable to fall asleep in the early evening, and bedtime battles may emerge around nine to twelve months of age because the bedtime is too late. In order to go to an earlier bedtime, eliminate the third nap. The earlier bedtime then abolishes the tiredness that had made the third nap necessary. Early bedtimes are especially difficult in families where both parents work outside the home, but, as will be discussed later, the entire family benefits.

Afternoon Wakeful Time

If there is no third nap, this is the time to go on longer excursions, errands or shopping trips. Exercise classes and outings to the park may be fun during this wakeful period. Many parents will give their baby solid foods in the late afternoon.

> **PRACTICAL POINT**
>
> **Never wake a sleeping baby except when you are trying to protect a sleep schedule.**

Nap Duration

Q: *How long should my child nap?*
A: Ask yourself this question: does your child appear tired?

If your baby is tired in the late afternoon or early in the evening, this *might* indicate insufficient naps. A possible solution is simply to put your child to bed earlier at night. Keeping a baby up too late produces fatigue and sleep deprivation, and will ultimately lead the child to resist falling asleep or to wake at night. This may be a problem, especially when a working parent or parents arrive home late, feeling guilty about being away from the family so long. As I mentioned above, after about six to nine months of age it is not a good idea to encourage a third, brief nap in the early evening just so the child can stay up later. This leads to an abnormal sleep schedule and the result is the equivalent of sleep deprivation.

Bedtime

Remember, you are establishing an orderly home routine and enforcing a bedtime hour. You are not forcing your child to sleep. When your child seems tired and needs to sleep, you will establish his bedtime routine, whether he likes it or not. The bedtime routine should be regular in terms of what you do: bathing, massage, story, lullaby, rocking or other soothing efforts. Approximately the same sequence each night helps signal to the child that it is the time for night sleep at approximately the same time. But don't be rigidly regular in terms of when you do it; there is enough normal irregularity in napping to produce some variability in bedtime. In much older children, extreme variability in bedtimes has been shown to be unhealthy.

PRACTICAL POINT

A parent who keeps a baby up past his natural time to sleep may be using this play time with the child to avoid time with the other parent if, say, they have argued.

Some parents make the mistake of always putting their baby down to sleep at exactly 7:00 P.M. For a few months this may work well, but when naps are irregular or the child stops taking the third nap, parents should learn to be more flexible in the timing of soothing to sleep at night, especially in the direction of an earlier bedtime!

Method A and Method B apply only to naps. At night, adopt whatever style seems comfortable to you. For example, at nap time, you may wish to put your baby down awake after soothing, and at night you may prefer to sleep with your baby. No problem. It appears that different parts of the brain are responsible for day and night sleep, so simply be consistent both in how you soothe to sleep for daytime naps and how you soothe to sleep at night, even if the two routines are different.

You are 'training' different parts of the brain at different times.

If it is your desire to put your baby down for the night after soothing and he is overtired, then there will be some crying. During the day, limiting the amount of crying to one hour in the hope of getting a nap at a time that will not mess up the rest of the schedule is reasonable, but at night, the crying that occurs as you put your child down should not be time-limited. Otherwise you train him to cry to your predetermined time limit. If you do not check on your baby, he will eventually fall asleep. He may cry more the second night, but each subsequent night he will cry less. This assumes that the bedtime is early, naps are in place, and night sleep is not fragmented.

This may be the first time you will ignore your child's protests, but it certainly will not be the last time. At some future point you will teach other health habits such as hand washing or tooth brushing. As he becomes mobile you will protect his physical safety by not allowing unreasonable risks involving playground equipment. Later still, you're not going to risk brain damage by letting him ride his bike without a helmet. In each of these cases, you won't let protest crying discourage you from implementing healthy practices and safety rules. Starting early and being consistent are the keys to establishing good habits.

Now is the time to let him learn to fall asleep at night by himself, to return to sleep at night by himself and to learn that being alone at night in slumber is not scary, dangerous or something to avoid. Keep everything calm and not too complicated as you go through a bedtime ritual. Fathers should be involved, especially if the child is breast-fed, because babies know dads cannot nurse them and so any protest crying is likely to be less intense or shorter.

Once your child is in bed, he is there to stay, no matter how long he cries, if you are using the Extinction method. Please do not return until your baby falls asleep. Little peaks or replacing dummies may be harmless when he is four months old, but they will eventually sabotage your efforts to help your child sleep well because intermittent positive reinforcement has enormous teaching power. Remember:

1. **When the duration of protest crying at night is open-ended, not limited, learning to fall asleep unassisted takes place.**
2. **When you put a time limit on how much protest crying at night you can tolerate or accept before going to the baby, you teach the baby to cry to that time limit.**

> **HELPFUL SUGGESTION**
>
> **When your child is crying and she is not hungry, say to yourself: 'My baby is crying because she loves me so much she wants my company, but she needs to sleep. I know the value of good sleep, and I love my baby so much that I am going to let her sleep.'**

Night Wakings for Feeding

Your baby may wake to be fed four to six hours after his last feeding. Some babies do not wake up then. Others are actually hungry at this time and you should promptly respond by feeding.

You may say, 'But when my baby was younger, he slept through the night.' Remember, in a child under four months, the bedtime was much later and the last feeding at night was much later. Now your baby is going to bed earlier, is fed earlier in the evening and may need a night feeding; this is normal. This night feeding, and a second night feeding, may be needed until the baby is about nine months of age.

As you may recall, partial awakenings or light sleep stages, called arousals, occur every one to two hours when your child is asleep. Sometimes your child will call out or cry during these arousals. If your child is not sleeping with you in your bed, going in to him at the time of these partial awakenings will eventually lead to a night-waking or night-feeding habit. This is because picking up, holding and feeding your baby will eventually cause him to force himself to a more alert state during these arousals for the pleasure of your company. He will learn to expect to be fed or played with at every arousal.

However, if you are sleeping with your baby and breastfeeding, you might promptly nurse at all of these arousals while you and the baby are still in a somewhat deeper sleep state, and then there is no real sleep fragmentation. No night-waking habit might develop.

Parents should not project their own emotions or misinterpret these naturally occurring arousals as signifying loneliness, fear of the dark or fear of abandonment.

If your baby wakes at night and behaves as if she is hungry, feed her. If your baby appears to want to play at night, stop going to her. At night, the question is 'Does my baby *need* me or *want* me?'

A second waking for feeding may occur around 4:00 or 5:00 A.M. Some children do not get up at this time, but those children who do awaken are wet, soiled or hungry, and a prompt response is appropriate. While you attend to your baby's needs, maintain silence and darkness so your child will return to sleep. A common mistake is to quietly play with your child, preventing the return to sleep. The return to sleep is important so your child will be able to comfortably stay up in the morning until the time of the first nap. Although many children do not need to be fed twice at night, others simply get up at 2:00 or 3:00 A.M. or not at all. A common mistake is to feed around midnight, 2:00 A.M., and again around 4:00 or 5:00 A.M. Please do not respond at the 2:00 A.M. time; the baby is not hungry then.

Summary: Your Baby at Five to Eight Months

In this age range, many babies accept naps without protest and fall asleep at night without difficulty. These easy babies may still awaken once or twice in the middle of the night. I consider this behaviour normal, natural, and not changeworthy – if it's for a brief feeding and not prolonged playtime.

Choose the one or two times when you'll go to feed your baby and change nappies, and don't go at any other time. Please review the earlier discussion on arousals (Chapter 2) if you are puzzled as to why babies sometimes get up or call out frequently throughout the night. If you have an intercom or baby monitor that allows you to hear all the quiet cries or sounds that occur during the arousals, turn it off. All you are accomplishing by listening to your child's awakenings is messing up your own sleep. A mother's sleeping brain is so sensitive to her baby's crying that any loud, urgent call will awaken her. You do not need an amplification system to ruin your sleep over every little quiet sound your baby makes!

Most mothers will partially synchronise feedings to sleep patterns so that the child is fed around the time he gets up in the morning, around the time of (before or after) the two naps, around bedtime and one or twice at night. In other words, bottle-feedings or breast-feedings now occur four to five times per twenty-four hours. Frequent sips, snacks or little feedings throughout the day are not necessary.

Gradually your child will begin to associate certain behaviours on your part, certain times of the day, his cot, and his sensation of tiredness with the process of falling asleep. This learning process, when started at about three or four months of age, usually takes only about three days in a fairly well-rested baby, or a little longer in an older or overtired baby.

Stranger wariness or stranger anxiety may be present in some babies by about six to nine months of age, and with this new behaviour, some mothers note some separation anxiety – that is, the child shows distress when the mother leaves. I do not think this type of separation anxiety directly makes it more difficult for a child to fall asleep unassisted. I have observed that babies with separation anxiety learn to sleep well as rapidly as any other babies when their mothers leave them alone at sleep times. The problem is that some mothers also suffer from the thought of separation and will not leave their children alone enough at sleep times to allow healthy sleep habits to develop. (This will be discussed further in Chapter 12.)

A major problem in implementing an age-appropriate sleep schedule is that it is *inconvenient*. Many parents resent the fact that their babies are now less portable. It is inconvenient to change their lifestyle to be at home twice a day so that the baby can nap. But when parents initially suffer through the process of establishing a good sleep schedule and their child is well rested, occasional irregularities and special occasions that disrupt sleep usually produce only minor and transient disturbed sleep. The recovery time is brief and the child responds to a prompt re-establishment of the routine.

> **REMEMBER**
>
> **Watch your baby more than your watch.**

Bluntly put, when parents are unwilling to alter their lifestyle so that regular naps are never well maintained or the bedtime is a little too late, then the child always pays a price. The child's mood and learning suffer, and recovery time following outings or illness takes much longer. These parents often try many 'helpful hints' to help their child sleep better. I'm not sure any or all of these hints can ever substitute for maintaining regular sleep schedules. Parents in my practice who have utilised regular sleep schedules have rarely, if ever, found these hints to be useful.

BUREAU OF 'HELPFUL' HINTS OF DUBIOUS VALUE TO SOOTHE BABY TO SLEEP

Lambskins
Heartbeat sounds
Womb sounds
Continuous background noises
Elevating head of cot
Maintaining motion sleep in swings
Changing formulas or eliminating iron supplement
Changing diet of nursing mother
Feeding solids only at bedtime

PRACTICAL POINT

You are harming your child when you allow unhealthy sleep patterns to evolve or persist – sleep deprivation is as unhealthy as feeding a nutritionally deficient diet.

Babies seem to respond quickly at this age to a somewhat scheduled, structured approach to sleep. If you can learn to detach yourself from your baby's protests and not respond reflexively by rushing in to her at the slightest whimper, she will learn to fall asleep by herself. As one mother said of her child, 'She now goes down like warm butter on toast!'

Month Nine: Late Afternoon Nap Disappears. No More Bottle-feeding at Night

Strong-willed, wilful, independent-minded, stubborn, headstrong, uncooperative. Sound familiar? These are the words parents often use to describe their toddlers. You may observe that your child is simply less cooperative. A psychologist might use the term *noncompliance* to describe this lack of cooperation, but the psychologist would also point out that these behaviours go hand in hand with the normal, healthy evolution of the child's autonomy or sense of independence. All infants can now express what they do and do not want with greater energy than previously. It is harder for you to distract your child. This increased ability to express intentional behaviour may be described as persistence, drive or determination. A child's expressing her own likes and dislikes may be called 'self-agency', which becomes stronger over time.

Usually, the experts tell us, the times when you should expect the most difficulties, or 'oppositional behaviours', are at dressing, during mealtimes, in public places and at bedtime.

Since this is the beginning of the 'stage' of autonomy (and noncompliance), some experts claim that it is natural for this independence/stubbornness to cause either resistance in going to sleep or night waking. I will explain later why I think this 'stage' theory is an incorrect interpretation.

Children in this age range also often develop behaviours described as social hesitation, shyness or fear of strangers. A child also might cry or appear distressed when his mother leaves him alone in one room while she goes to another room or when she leaves the child with a baby-sitter. Psychologists call this behaviour stranger wariness, stranger anxiety or separation anxiety. So if a child developed increased resistance in going to sleep at night at this stage, some experts might say that separation anxiety, or fear of being apart or away from the mother, was the cause. I think this is an incorrect interpretation also.

The major sleep change that occurs around nine months is the disappearance of the third nap. If the late-afternoon nap persists, it often causes the bedtime to become too late. Also, children who are bottle-fed after nine months of age are likely to develop a night-waking or night-feeding habit. If your baby goes right back to sleep after a feeding, then do not stop the feedings. But if he decides to play with you and does not easily and quickly return to sleep after the feeding, then stop going to him at night. Again, if you are breast-feeding in the family bed, no night-waking habit might develop.

Months Ten to Twelve: Morning Nap Starts to Disappear but Mostly Two Naps

A small percentage (17 per cent) of babies are now taking only one afternoon nap. Often the bedtime now has to be twenty or thirty minutes earlier because they tend to get more tired near the end of the day. Sometimes it is the afternoon nap that starts to disappear because the morning nap is too long. In this case, move the bedtime much earlier and/or wake your child after an hour or an hour and a half into the morning nap in order to protect the afternoon nap.

Nap Deprivation

When parents have invested the effort to create an age-appropriate sleep schedule and their child is well-rested, occasional disruptions due to illness, trips, parties or holiday visits cause only minor disruptions of sleep. Such a child requires only a brief recovery period before getting back on track. But when parents allow poor-quality sleep patterns to emerge and persist, then there is a gradual accumulation of significant sleep deficits. Now, even minor disturbances create long-lasting havoc.

In this age range, nap deprivation seems to be a major culprit in ruining healthy sleep patterns. It's only natural that you want to get out more and do more things with your child, who is now full of new social charms, is cheerful and crawling or maybe even walking . . . why not spend time together and enjoy the good weather at the park or beach?

Your child is likely to feel the same way. Self-agency might lead him to protest against naps because he would rather play than sleep. If you allow him to skip his nap, then he will become fatigued. The natural adaptive response to fatigue is to fight it with stimulating hormones, which allow him to maintain more wakefulness. However, this heightened state of alertness or arousal creates an inability to fall asleep easily or stay asleep for subsequent naps and night sleep. Not only does a vicious circle of sleep problems begin, but your child may also develop emotional ups and downs or a reduced attention span as a by-product.

As naps slip and slide, a trend of increasing fatigue clearly develops. First, the child becomes a little more grumpy, irritable or fussy, maybe only in the late afternoon or early evening. You might think it's normal for children this age to be easily frustrated or sometimes bored. Then he starts to get up at night for the first time ever, 'for no reason'. Later, maybe following a cold or a daylong visit with his grandparents, he starts fighting going to sleep at night, and you wonder why night sleep is a suddenly a problem.

When you re-establish healthy, regular nap routines, the night-sleep problem corrects itself (although non-compliant behaviours still exist and separation anxiety is unchanged). I have seen this over and over again. That's why I think nap deprivation and not a particular 'stage' is the culprit behind disturbed night sleep.

PRACTICAL POINT

Boredom may be masked tiredness. If your child's motor is idling and she's not going anywhere, maybe she's tired.

Normal Naps

You may think your baby needs only one nap now, but most babies in this age range still need two naps. One clue some parents have noticed is that their baby-sitter can have the child take two good naps, but they can only get her to take one, if that. The child is obviously more rested after the sitter leaves, and the parents wonder how the sitter does it. Well, children are very discriminating at this age. They know that the sitter, following parents' instructions, has a no-nonsense approach and will put them to sleep on a fairly regular schedule. But they figure that with mum or dad, enough protesting may gain them more playtime together. After all, sometimes it works. And so long as your child retains the expectation that you will come to her and take her out of her boring, quiet room, she will fight naps.

Here are three dramatic turning points in sleep maturation for young children:

1. **At six weeks of age, night sleep becomes organised.**
2. **At four months of age, day sleep is developing and night sleep is adultlike in terms of sleep cycles.**
3. **At nine months of age, the third nap is eliminated, naps are longer (especially for post-colic babies) and there is no need to be fed at night.**

These turning points are so highly predictable and independent of parenting practices that we know they reflect maturation of the brain. Anticipating these changes and allowing them to occur naturally will set the stage for preventing all common sleep disturbances.

Comforting Habits

Routines that comfort your baby include rocking, soft lullabies, stroking, patting and cuddling. Maintain these routines so your child learns to associate certain behaviours occurring at certain times in a familiar place with the behaviour called 'falling asleep'.

HELPFUL HINTS FOR COMFORTING

Soft, silky or furry-textured blankets, dolls or stuffed animals in cot
Dim night-light
Nursing to sleep

Nurse to Sleep?

There is nothing wrong with nursing your baby to sleep when there is no sleep problem. Most nursing mothers in my practice do this all the time. But if you have difficulty letting your child learn to fall asleep unassisted, your child *always* falls asleep at the breast and your child has disturbed sleep, then nursing to sleep might be part of the sleep problem. It may reflect the kind of separation problems discussed in Chapter 12.

Most mothers nurse their babies for soothing and comfort, and their babies either fall asleep at the breast or they don't. In either case, they are put in their cots when they *need* to sleep. I think that this intimacy between mother and infant is beautiful, and nursing to sleep, in itself, does not cause sleep problems.

Q: *Do I roll my older child over to his favourite sleeping position when he wakes up during the night? Do I help him get down when he stands up and shakes the cot railings?*

A: No. I doubt that you like playing these games with your child at night. Think, too, about what you teach him when you go to him at night to roll him over or help him down. If he rolls over only once at night or gets stuck in the railings of the cot, then help him go back to sleep.

Q: *Won't he hurt himself if he falls down in his cot? He can't get down by himself.*
A: No, he won't hurt himself. He may fall into an awkward heap . . . and sleep like a puppy.

Try to be reasonably regular by watching the intervals of wakefulness in babies four months of age or younger, and by watching your baby and the clock when he's over four months. However, try not to get locked into a fixed or traditional bedtime hour; vary the bedtime a little depending on duration of naps, when the second nap ended, and indoor versus outdoor activities. Often babies between nine and twelve months need to go to bed earlier because of increased physical activity in the afternoon and the absence of a third nap. Remember, too late a bedtime causes disturbed sleep just as nap deprivation does.

When you are somewhat organised regarding sleep schedules, sleep is accepted and expected. But don't feel you have to be this way for feeding or other infant care practices! When parents are creative, free-spirited and permissive regarding wholesome foods, feeding goes well. So respect the biological basis for regular sleep, but accept or reject the social customs for feeding as you see fit.

Preventing and Solving Sleep Problems: Months Five to Twelve

It cannot be emphasised enough: The major sleep problems in babies from five to twelve months old develop and persist because of the inability of parents to stop reinforcing bad sleep habits. Some parents don't see themselves as interfering with an important learning process in their child, namely, learning how to soothe themselves to sleep unassisted. The failure of children to fall asleep and stay asleep by themselves is the direct result of parents' failure to give their child the opportunity to learn these self-soothing skills. In other words, some parents can't leave their kids alone long enough for them to fall asleep by themselves. Don't under-estimate children's competence and ability to learn at these early months!

Helping Babies Sleep Also Helps Mothers

One recent study of 156 mothers of infants aged six to twelve months with severe sleep problems used controlled crying (Graduated Extinction) to help solve the problems. This intervention improved sleep problems in the children and reduced symptoms of depression in the mothers. Unfortunately, the benefits for the child and the mother lasted only about two months. Another study was comprised of 738 mothers of infants six to twelve months of whom 46 per cent reported their infant's sleep as a problem. They described a strong association between the maternal report of infant sleep problems and depression symptoms in the mother. After looking at all the variables that might have contributed to maternal depression and the observation that the better the child slept, the less likely the mother was depressed, they concluded that teaching how infants sleep should decrease or help prevent maternal depression. A third study consisted of 114 mothers enrolled when their infants were eight to ten months old; the mothers were again studied when their children were three to four years old. They concluded that infant sleep problems tend to persist or recur in the preschool years and are associated with more child behaviour problems and maternal depression. Analysis of their data led to the conclusion that the maternal depressive symptoms are a result, rather than the cause, of the children's sleep problems. It is uncommon for so many studies to be in agreement.

The Importance of Early Experiences: Theory versus Facts

> **WARNING!**
>
> **Sleep problems in children may cause maternal depression.**

What does it mean to be a 'good parent'? Parents feed and protect their young and provide comfort and guidance. When your baby cries, you go to him. On the surface, it certainly seems reasonable to say that the cry of your baby communicates messages: feed me, change me, pick me up, hold me, hug me or rock me. The question is, why is it that when a parent makes a complete response to these messages, some babies still cry? Alternatively, if crying is a form of necessary communication, why is it that many parents will deliver complete, loving and sensitive care even when their babies do not cry? Perhaps crying as a signal system is not perfect: some babies cry even when they don't need to cry because their needs are being cared for, and other babies don't cry but still receive the care they need. It may be an instinct: birds fly, babies cry. In infants, it is possible that crying is no longer tightly linked to infant survival but still occurs as a behavioural remnant of some distant past. An important fact is that the meaning of crying changes with age.

The baby may cry because he is hungry and needs food to survive. The toddler may cry because he wants a second helping of dessert after dinner. The child may cry when afraid. The teenager may cry when feeling hopeless. The adult may cry from happiness at a wedding. Not all crying signifies pain. Unfortunately, when parents talk about crying, the assumption is that crying equals pain. This leads to the sometimes hidden thought: 'If my baby cries, I am a bad parent.'

Thinking about how mothers relate to their babies during these early times and how they forge close relationships led to two popular concepts: infant bonding and attachment theory. Both focused almost exclusively on mothers and both claimed that future events would be strongly influenced by early experiences.

Infant bonding theories promoted the importance of early physical contact between baby and mother as a mechanism to a better adjustment later in life. The good news was that this concept caused the delivery of babies to become more comfortable even in a hotel-like environment. This was definitely an improvement for the family, compared to the cold, impersonal environment of a traditional delivery room. The bad news was that mothers who missed this experience because of complications around the delivery, and mothers who adopted older children, felt deprived and worried about their future relationship with their children. You see, infant bonding was thought to take place only during a critical period, very much like the imprinting of baby geese, who will follow any large, moving object they see at a specific time in their development. The fact is that there is no scientific evidence that a similar critical period exists for human babies, and there is no evidence that lack of 'bonding' at a specific time right at birth effects subsequent behaviour in either infant or mother.

Attachment theory not only considered the interaction between the mother and the child but claimed that if attachment doesn't develop well, the infant grows into an adult who has difficulty in peer relationships, romantic relationships or parenthood. The good news was that mothers were encouraged to be affectionate, tactile and warm without fear of spoiling their child. The bad news was that attention to children twenty-four hours a day was thought to be good.

The sad fact was that older theorists were unaware of the benefits of healthy sleep and how we are different in sleep and wake modes. Child psychologists, child psychiatrists and paediatricians did not know the benefits of healthy sleep until recently.

The improvement in educating child health care professionals has been slow; a recent survey in the USA of paediatric residency programmes showed that only 4.8 hours of instruction on sleep and sleep disorders took place during their three years of training. This explains why paediatricians in practice so often incorrectly advise parents that their child is likely to 'outgrow' the problem.

Popular distortions of attachment theory claimed that a twenty-four-hour parent – meaning one who attends to every cry day and night – would produce a more securely attached child than would a 'selfish' parent who ignores a cry at night so she can get some sleep. Accumulated scientific data do not support these claims. In fact, published research on children between seven and twenty-seven months of age has shown that when parents are instructed not to attend to their children's protest crying (the technique called 'extinction'), over time *measurements of infant security significantly improved and all the mothers become less anxious*. A similar study in sleep-disturbed infants also showed no evidence of detrimental effects on security. It's a simple but true statement that when the entire family gets more sleep, everyone feels better, even if the cries of one member of the family have to be ignored for a while to get there.

In discussing the myth of attachment theory, the famous child psychologist Michael Lewis emphasises how the development of social skills and peer relation skills are encouraged and protected both by family members other than the mother and by people outside the family. Further, this development depends more on current, ongoing relationships than on past experiences.

Extremely violent or catastrophic events aside, for ordinary families the power of past events has been extremely exaggerated and the singular influence ascribed to the mother is unjustified. Strong proponents of the importance of early events have created in the minds of many mothers a *false* conclusion: 'I am a bad mother if my child cries, because this may cause permanent emotional damage.'

Locus of Control

When your baby was younger, she slept when she needed to. She controlled your relationship with her, in the sense that you met her needs whether you wanted to or not. You didn't let her go hungry simply because you didn't feel like feeding her just then. You didn't let her stay wet because you didn't feel like changing her. Her needs determined your behaviour.

But from now on, a shift should occur so that *you* are in charge. For example, when your child is older, you may decide not to give her junk food simply because she asks for it. You will not risk her physical safety by letting her climb too high on a tree simply because she wants to. And you will not let her stay up to play when she needs to sleep. What, then, are we to do when the child does not cooperate, crying because she does not *want* to go to sleep even though she *needs* to sleep?

'Let Them Cry': A Division of Popular Opinions

There is disagreement among those who write for popular magazines about what happens when children cry after being left alone at night to sleep. In September 1984, *McCall's* said: 'Letting a baby "cry it out" will not teach him the basic trust of confidence he needs to feel secure in his new world.' While *Parents* magazine, in November 1983, said: 'It may give him the feeling that there's nobody out there who cares. The child may become a passive, ineffective person, or he may become angry or hostile.'

On the other hand, the editor in chief of *Parents* wrote in the October 1985 issue, after the birth of her third child: 'The trick was that after eight years of parenthood, my husband and I have discovered . . . [that] the first sound does not mean that the baby needs to be picked up immediately.'

Don't wait eight years to learn what experts discovered a long time ago!

'Let Them Cry': An Agreement of Expert Opinions

While the popular press may give all types of conflicting advice from a variety of sources, expert opinion is solidly together. In fact, all evidence accumulated by a wide array of child health specialists concludes that 'protest' crying at bedtime will not cause permanent emotional or psychological problems. In plain fact, the contrary is true. For example, Dr D. W. Winnicott, a British paediatrician and child psychiatrist, emphasises that the *capacity to be alone* is one of the most important signs of maturity in emotional development. In his view, parents can facilitate the development of the child's ability to soothe herself when left alone. Please don't confuse this with abandonment or, on the other hand, use this notion as an excuse for negligence.

Margaret S. Mahler, a prominent child psycho-analyst, has identified the beginning of the separation-individuation process whereby the infant begins to differentiate from the mother at four to five months of age. This is the age when children naturally begin to develop some independence.

Dr Alexander Thomas and Dr Stella Chess, two American child psychiatrists, followed over a hundred children from infancy through to young adulthood. One item they examined was the regularity of irregular sleep and how parents responded. They wrote: 'Removal of symptoms by a successful parent guidance procedure has had positive consequences for the child's functioning and has not resulted in the appearance of overt anxiety or new substitute symptoms . . . The basic emphasis [of the] treatment technique is a change in the parents' behaviour.'

So please don't fear when your child cries in protest at night, because he is being allowed to 'practise' falling asleep, that this crying will later cause emotional or psychological problems. By itself, it will not.

Let me be very clear about this. I am talking only about children over the age of four months and only during normal day and night sleep times. During these periods, emotional problems do *not* develop if parents ignore protest crying.

Drs Thomas and Chess were sensitive to irregular sleep patterns in the infants in their study. Many of those infants also had frequent and prolonged bouts of loud crying. When I asked Dr Thomas what advice he had given to the parents of those crying babies who did not sleep at night, he responded, 'Close the door and walk away.' Did this create or produce any problems? He said, 'No. None at all.'

Always going to your crying child at night interferes with this natural learning and growth. Such behaviour produces sleep fragmentation, destroys sleep continuity and creates insomnia in your child.

One study examined infant crying at one year of age. It compared children over six months of age whose parents indiscriminately responded to every cry, day or night, to those children whose parents were trained to respond promptly to every intense, stressed or demanding cry but to delay their response to quiet vocalisations or weak cries. The children in the first group, whose parents indiscriminately responded, cried much more than children in the second group. This suggests that crying for attention can be learned or taught by at least six months.

Mothers who in general do not feel loving or empathetic toward their children, who are insensitive or emotionally unavailable to them, and who have a lack of warmth or affection later come to the attention of professionals. Consequently, some psychologists or psychiatrists take the attitude that parents should be encouraged *never* to let their child cry, for fear of encouraging a cold parent-child relationship. As a general-practice paediatrician, however, I don't share this view, because I see that the vast majority of parents are loving and sensitive to their child's needs. These parents should not fear letting their child cry at night to learn to sleep.

Q: *How long do I let my baby cry?*
A: To establish regular naps, no more than one hour, but to establish consolidated sleep, there is no time limit at night if the child is not hungry or ill. If we place an arbitrary limit on the duration of crying at night, we train the child to cry to that predetermined time. When it is open-ended, the child learns to stop protesting and to fall asleep.

Q: *Why is it good for my child to cry? Why not delay sleep training until he is older and more reasonable?*
A: Crying is not the real issue. We are leaving the child alone to learn to sleep. We are leaving him alone to forget the expectation to be picked up. We *allow* him to cry; we are not *making* him cry in the sense that we are hurting him. When he is older and still not sleeping, it will be harder for him to learn how to sleep well. Plus, losing sleep is physically unhealthy, just as is too little iron or too few vitamins in his diet.

Q: *Isn't crying harmful?*
A: Not necessarily. In fact, studies have proven that *crying produces accelerated forgetting of a learned response*. So when a child cries, she may more quickly unlearn to expect to be picked up. When trying to stop an unhealthy habit, crying may have some benefit, because crying acts as an amnesic agent.

Let's look at several of the most common unhealthy sleep habits at this age, and the proven, effective strategy to deal with each one.

Abnormal Sleep Schedule

When the bedtime hour and sleep periods are not in synchrony with other biological rhythms, we don't get the full restorative benefit of sleep. Please refer to Figures 5 and 6 (see pages 43 and 44) for age-appropriate times when children fall asleep or awaken.

At any age, abnormal sleep schedules often lead to night wakings and night terrors in older children. The schedule often gets shifted to a too-late bedtime hour because mum or dad (or both), returning late from work, wants to play with the baby, or because parents deliberately keep their baby up late to encourage a later awakening in the morning.

The strategy for bringing sleep schedules back to normal is

based on developing an age-appropriate wake-up at 6:00 or 7:00 A.M.; a midmorning nap around 9:00 A.M.; an early afternoon nap, usually around 1:00 P.M., but always starting before 3:00 P.M.; an early bedtime, 6:00 to 8:00 P.M.; and unfragmented night sleep. This package of advice ensures good sleep quality, and it is quality, not always quantity, that really matters.

MAJOR POINT

The major fear that inhibits parents from establishing an earlier bedtime is that this will cause their child to get up earlier to start the day. In fact, the opposite will occur. An earlier bedtime will allow your child to sleep later, just as a too-late bedtime will eventually cause a too-early wake-up time. Remember, sleep begets sleep. This is not logical, but it *is* biological.

Q: *Why do you recommend 6:00 to 8:00 P.M. as an appropriate bedtime?*

A: Survey data from my earlier research showed that the vast majority of children between the ages of four and twelve months went to sleep between 7:00 and 9:00 P.M., and so I used to recommend those hours. However, as I have helped families correct sleep problems over the past thirty years, it has become clearer that children who go to bed earlier tend not to develop sleep problems in the first place. In addition, children in this age range who did have sleep problems almost always benefited from an earlier bedtime. I think we have simply grown accustomed to having overtired children in the evening hours, and because it is so common, we have assumed that fussiness or irritability near the end of the day was normal. Imagine what was a 'normal' bedtime before electric lights, radio, television, videos, commuting or dual-income families travelling from work to day care to home.

When your nine- to twelve-month-old child does not promptly go to sleep at his nap times, you should leave him alone for one hour, maximum. If a nap develops and you are trying to establish a healthy sleep schedule, you would want to limit that nap to about one or one and a half hours in order to have the next nap or bedtime occur on time. If your child is overtired and you allow a two- or three-hour nap to occur, then it will be difficult, if not impossible, to establish a good twenty-four-hour schedule.

PRACTICAL POINT

***You* are enforcing an age-appropriate nap and bedtime schedule. Your child initially may not cooperate by falling asleep immediately. Don't give up.**

Studies have shown that when sleep disturbances are associated with abnormal sleep schedules, control of the wake-up time may be sufficient to establish a healthy twenty-four-hour sleep rhythm. In other words, you set the clock in the morning!

Here's an account of one mother who left my office determined to set the clock that night and not wait until the morning.

'He Wakes Up Smiling'

Our son did not like to sleep. In fact, if it can be said that babies are born with an aversion to any particular thing, for Ryan, sleep was it.

From the day we brought Ryan home from the hospital, he had shown himself to be a night owl. Over and over, through the early hours (of the morning) we would pace and nurse until sleep would overcome us sometime near dawn. By the time he was four and a half months old, he was down to one nap a day. He didn't sleep through the night (and in my book, that's eight hours straight or better) until he was ten months old, and that lasted for only one night.

Not knowing any better, since Ryan was our first child, I thought this kind of behaviour was perfectly normal for a majority of babies. When other mums would talk about their children sleeping through the night at three months of age and napping twice a day for two hours or better at a crack, I thought that it was either so much idle boasting or their children had some sort of neurological disorder. But when our paediatrician told me at Ryan's eight-month check-up that it was not normal for a child his age to go to bed at 1:00 A.M. and sleep until 10:00 A.M., I started to realise we had a problem. The thought of my husband and me looking like a couple of zombies from years without sleep was not a pretty one.

We put Ryan to bed at 9:00 that evening and, as expected, he started to cry. We shut his door and went into the den, closing two more doors between the baby's room and the den in an attempt to muffle what were now becoming very loud screams. After a half hour had passed, the crying was more muffled but continued, so I headed for Ryan's room to 'reassure him'. 'Don't go in there now,' Tom suggested. 'He'll just get worked up again if he sees you. Do something else for a while.' I could see the logic and agreed to hold off. A half hour later, I eased the door open and again heard the crying. But now I could hear something else mixed in. Ryan was talking to himself. In a very hurt tone he was babbling and complaining between the sobs. My heart was breaking. 'My God,' I said to Tom. 'Now he's going to grow up hating us. I have to go to him.' For the second time that night, Tom talked me into leaving the baby alone.

The next fifteen minutes seemed like fifteen hours, but the next time I opened the door, there it was . . . *silence.* I could finally look in on Ryan without undoing all that we had just accomplished. So as not to awaken him with its squeaking, I turned the light on at its dimmest setting. In this low light and from across the room, I saw what appeared to be Ryan's blanket hanging over the side of his cot. As I moved closer to remove it, however, I discovered that it wasn't the quilt draped over the side – it was Ryan. Our son had fallen asleep standing up!

> The next night we again put him to bed at 9:00 and again he fell asleep standing up. But this time he only cried for one hour. The third night, he cried for twenty-five minutes and fell asleep lying down.
>
> These days, with few exceptions, he cries for only a few minutes before falling asleep. He also usually wakes up smiling, thus dispelling any fears I once might have had that he would grow up to hate us for letting him 'cry it out'.

One mother solved the problem of her child waking up and always standing up in the cot immediately after being put down almost asleep, by putting her drowsy child in the cot standing up. Now the child had only one way to go, down.

Nap Deprivation

Nap deprivation is a common occurrence between nine and twelve months of age. Children at this age are fearless, full of grace and self-confidence, and very explorative. Doing things with parents and siblings is simply a lot of fun. Unsure of when a child naturally shifts to needing only one nap, some parents try to get by with one nap before their child is ready. Afternoons full of activities help smooth over rocky moments of heightened emotionality or grumpiness. Anyway, mum or dad returns from work about then, so there is a loving play period early in the evening.

However, the fatigue from nap deprivation leads to increased levels of arousal and alertness, and this causes difficulties in falling asleep, staying asleep or both. These changes in the direction of disturbed sleep and behavioural changes during the day may be very gradual, so initially it may appear that a single nap is all right. The effects of persistent sleep deficits are cumulative, though, and eventually the fatigued child starts to behave differently.

I was consulted about two children, five and six months of age, who had severe bobbing, turning and jerking of the head and wincing or grimacing of the face. Both children had been hospitalised and evaluated for seizures or epilepsy, but all the test results were normal. Nap deprivation turned out to be the problem, and both children recovered completely when they were better rested, though the movements transiently returned to each child during a temporary period of overtiredness.

Here is one parent's account of how 'the programme' – that is, shortening the interval of wakefulness – helped her child sleep better.

'I Was Certain She Would Grow Out of This Bad Habit . . . Our Other Two Had'

On 19 November 1984, our third daughter, Rebecca, was born. Our other girls, Lauren, nine years old, and Karen, four years old, were busy with school activities, piano lessons and ballet. At that time I prided myself on how well I took our new baby around everywhere and how wonderfully she slept in and out of the car seat all day.

Our days were filled with errands and car pools, Rebecca nursing and napping on and off all day. What a cooperative baby, I used to think. But I was so exhausted by evening that I found the only way to survive was to sleep with the baby, waking up every hour or so to shift her so that she could nurse on the other side. I knew then that having her in bed with me wasn't such a terrific idea, but it was the only way for me to get any rest.

When Rebecca turned five months old, I placed her in her cot instead of going to sleep with her at my breast.

As I expected, every few hours she began to cry, expecting me to be by her side. I would quickly run into her room and rock and nurse her back to sleep . . . until the next time she woke up.

And so our next pattern began. She would wake up every few hours and I would faithfully run in and get her back to sleep. I was certain she would grow out of this bad habit . . . our other two had.

A few months passed. By now Rebecca was weaned to a bottle and I was sure things would change for the better. That didn't happen. In fact, things got worse. There were many nights when Rebecca would get up every hour on the hour. I tried letting her cry, fifteen minutes at a time, but it was much easier to just go in and give her a bottle.

When Rebecca was a year old, this pattern of frequent waking continued. It was difficult leaving her with a baby-sitter on the occasional evening we went out. I knew that within an hour or so of our leaving she would be up crying for me. I actually felt sick leaving her.

When Rebecca was almost thirteen months old we went to see Dr Weissbluth. Rebecca was charming for him. Could this delightful child really be causing all this trouble? I wondered.

Our appointment went well. After our story was poured out, Dr Weissbluth explained what steps we needed to take to change Rebecca's sleeping patterns. He cited studies, gave us graphs . . . this really was going to work! When we left his office I felt prepared for battle – armed with all the mental ammunition I needed to change Rebecca's nightly wakings. We started 'the programme' the next day.

In a week's time, the change in Rebecca was phenomenal! She was always a happy baby, but when she began to sleep better, she became even more relaxed, more affectionate and more fun to be with.

The change in her sleeping pattern has had an effect on everyone in the family. I don't yell and lose my patience with my older children quite as much, for I am better rested. Ironically, for the first few nights of our 'training programme' I continued to get up every two hours, waiting for her to cry. I now also have learned how to sleep through the night once again, and I feel so much better physically and emotionally.

Throughout some of Rebecca's crying periods, especially in the beginning, there were moments when I was sorry that we started this whole thing. I just wanted to soothe my poor, crying baby! Both my husband and I kept reminding ourselves that we were trying to teach Rebecca how to sleep and that we *had* to stay with it without sabotaging the plan. (Maybe knowing that we would be checking in with Dr Weissbluth every few days helped us to stick with it.)

This has been one of the most rewarding and positive experiences that we have shared as parents. We are so proud of Rebecca and also pat ourselves on the backs for a job well done.

Shhh! Rebecca's sleeping!

The treatment strategy involves (a) shortening the interval of wakefulness before the first nap and re-establishing the early afternoon nap by focusing on the midday interval and making sure this wakeful period is not too long, (b) making sure the afternoon nap does not start too late in the afternoon, in order to protect a reasonable evening bedtime, and (c) consistency in the nap time ritual.

If the afternoon nap is needed but that is when the child fights sleep the most, consider shortening the midday interval of wakefulness. Start the afternoon nap earlier. Perhaps you were allowing him to stay up too long and he became overtired and overaroused.

It's not uncommon for a child to sleep well at night but not nap well, especially in the afternoon. At night it is dark, everyone is more tired and parents want to be regular with bedtimes because they themselves want to go to sleep. During the day, it is light, everyone is more alert and parents are more irregular because they want to run errands or enjoy recreational activities.

So during a retraining period, it's easiest to establish good night sleep and easier to establish regular morning naps than afternoon naps. Don't expect improvement to occur equally at all times. Still, it's best to implement a twenty-four-hour sleep retraining programme, because if you focus only on one feature, such as bedtime, and ignore naps, you will be less likely to succeed.

In general, I recommend a twenty-four-hour sleep package to help restore healthy sleep habits. Here is an example of an exception. The single mother has limited resources for soothing and is completely exhausted. The child does not sleep well day or night. The mother wants to continue breast-feeding but now wants to transition the baby from her bed to a cot. The first step might only be a temporarily ultra-early bedtime in the mother's bed to help the child get more sleep. Everything else stays the same. The advice is to do whatever is necessary to maximise sleep and minimise crying during the day. After the child is a little better rested, the second step might be to make the transition to the cot. This might involve crying, but because both child and mother are better rested, the crying may be very little and the mother is more able to cope. The third step is to work on naps. This will now be easier because everyone is better rested. If, instead, this mother had an enormous soothing support system to help her, she might try to do everything at the same time. Her child might become better rested faster and the greater stress in making all these changes abruptly would be shared by people other than the mother.

Some families have found it difficult to establish naps because their bedrooms are too bright or noisy during the day. One family I know was fortunate enough to have a large walk-in cupboard, which they furnished like a little bedroom and which was used only for naps. Other families have problems because they live in a one-bedroom flat and it is difficult for anyone to sleep well when a child shares a bedroom with the parents. Such parents sometimes relocate to the living room and turn the bedroom over to the child so that the entire family can stay well rested. If you do not want to have a family bed, expect it to become difficult for your child to sleep well in your room. Plan ahead, before the family becomes overtired.

PRACTICAL POINT

As long as your child retains the expectation that she can convince you to play during nap time, she won't nap well. If she thinks she can outlast you, she won't give up her protesting.

Brief Sleep Durations

If your child is on an apparently normal sleep schedule and napping well, you might presume she is getting enough sleep. Overall, she doesn't look tired. But what if around ten, eleven or twelve months she starts waking at night? What's happening? Many times, physical and mental activity increases around nine months. The child is now moving around more, exploring more, becoming more active and independent.

If the customary bedtime hour had been around 8:00 or 9:00 P.M. before the onset of night waking, the problem will often disappear when bedtime is shifted to an earlier hour. Most families find that if they gradually shift the bedtime earlier in twenty-minute increments, they reach a time when night wakings melt away. Usually this change is easy for the baby; sometimes it is hard for the parent who returns home late from work to accept. But small changes in sleep patterns often make big differences in sleep quality. Even a change as small as twenty minutes' more sleep at the front end of the night can cause a big change in your child's behaviour during the day.

Early Awakenings

Most children five to twelve months of age should go to bed between 6:00 and 8:00 P.M. and wake up between 6:00 and 7:00 A.M. Some also get up once around the midnight hour for a brief feeding. This pattern is very common, but many parents don't like the idea of starting the day so early! In this age range, though, it seems that the wake-up part of our brain is like a neurological alarm clock.

For well-rested children, this neurological alarm clock is fairly regular, and I don't think we can ignore crying around 6:00 A.M. simply because we don't want to get up so early. Because they are well rested, having slept overnight, it seems unreasonable to expect children to go back to sleep without any kind of response. Instead, I would suggest a prompt, brief, soothing response so that perhaps both child and parent can return to sleep. If responding before 6:00 A.M. turns out to be more stimulating than soothing, then I would suggest not going in until 6:00 A.M. The reason is that children who get too much attention too early in the morning fight sleep to get up earlier and earlier for the pleasure of their parents' company. Increasingly, it makes it difficult to stay up to catch the first midmorning nap around 9:00 A.M., so the whole day gets thrown off balance. Sometimes overtired children develop new patterns, such as waking up at 4:00 A.M. and not returning to sleep after a prompt, soothing parental response. These kids are *really* up and want to play, yet they are often not well rested. When the parents put these children to bed earlier, they get more sleep at the front end and they sleep later in the morning because they are more rested and are thus able to sleep better. Even though this is counter-intuitive, it is true.

This means that when your child has disturbed sleep and an abnormally *late* wake-up time, you might decide to control his schedule by waking him up earlier so that the naps and bedtime hour all occur earlier. If your child has disturbed sleep and an abnormally *early* wake-up time, shorten the intervals of wakefulness before naps and make the bedtime hour earlier. When your child is well rested and has no disturbed sleep, an early wake-up hour may be inconvenient but not necessarily changeable.

METHODS THAT USUALLY FAIL TO PREVENT EARLY AWAKENINGS

Keeping your child up later at bedtime
Waking him for a feeding when you go to sleep
Giving solid foods late at night

If your child is near his first birthday, you might consider some of the items discussed in the section on older children.

Different Sleep Patterns: No Problem – Temporarily

Sleep patterns are as varied as children themselves, family sizes and parental lifestyles. One five-month-old always awoke briefly at 6:00 A.M. and then promptly returned to sleep until 10:00 A.M. A long midday nap occurred from noon to 3:00 P.M. and a brief nap from 5:00 to 5:45 P.M. Between 7:30 and 8:00 P.M. the child went to sleep for the night, until about 6:00 the following morning. This child was well rested, and the midday nap coincided with his older brother's single nap. For the time being, this pattern met both children's sleep needs. By six or seven months, this child developed the more common pattern of a midmorning nap and an early afternoon nap.

However, other children begin to accumulate a sleep deficit that grows, often slowly, over time. Eventually, daytime mood or behaviour problems develop, as do sleep disturbances at night.

PRACTICAL POINT

A temporary disturbance or mild variation in sleep schedules, nap patterns, amount of sleep or early awakenings may not be changeworthy. But if chronic or severe problems cause your child to become tired, then try to help your baby become more rested. Watch your child's behaviour, not some inflexible schedule.

Night Wakings

In this age range, night wakings are typically the complete arousals from sleep associated with disturbed sleep in post-colic babies (see Chapter 4), partial airway obstruction during sleep (see Chapter 10), general disorganisation of sleep with chronic fatigue (see Chapter 2) or parent reinforcement of such wakings.

Two separate groups of infants between four and eight months of age seem especially prone to night waking.

The first and larger group – about 20 per cent of infants – includes those infants who had colic when they were younger. These infants not only awaken more often, their total sleep time is less. Although boys and girls in this group awaken the same number of times, parents are more likely to state that it is their sons who have a night-waking problem. In fact, boys are handled in a more irregular way than girls when they awaken at night. This was shown in studies using videotapes in dim light in the children's own bedrooms at home. Even when the colic has been successfully treated with a drug during the first few months, by four months of age the children still were reported frequently awakening at night.

My conclusion is that some biological disturbances in infants can cause an over-aroused, too wakeful, hyper-alert, irregular state full of crying, especially in the late afternoon or early evening. This is commonly called 'colic'. In the past, the crying part of colic has been thought to be the major problem. But while this evening crying diminished at about three to four months, the wakeful, not sleeping, state may continue and thus be more serious and harmful in the long run.

This is because the parents have the correct impression that regular and consistent parenting does not much affect the colic, and, unfortunately, they give up the effort permanently. They do not know that after four months of age, regular and consistent attention to bedtimes and nap times really does help the older infant sleep better. The parents' failure to develop and maintain healthy sleep patterns in these older post-colic babies then leads to prolonged fussiness driven by chronic fatigue. (This is discussed in more detail in Chapter 4.)

The second group of frequent night wakers in the four- to eight-month-old age group includes the 10 per cent of infants who snore or breathe through their mouths during sleep. This difficulty in breathing during sleep might be due to allergies (see page 382). These infants awaken as frequently as do those with post-colic night waking, but their parents do not label this night waking as a problem. Probably the parents had not worried about night waking because the infants had not suffered from colic. Those infants who snored also had shorter sleep durations than other infants. As in many sleep disturbances, when one element of healthy sleep is disrupted, other elements are disturbed. (I will discuss why snoring is more than an acoustical annoyance in Chapter 10.)

A third frequent cause of night waking in this age group is sometimes associated with abnormal sleep schedules. Going to bed too late and getting up too late seems to set the stage for frequent night waking. Sleeping out of phase with biological rhythms produces an overtired and hyper-aroused child. One child I cared for took two to two and a half hours of soothing, rocking or holding before she would go to sleep, and then would usually awaken three to four times each night, sometimes as often as ten times. This prolonged period to put a child to sleep is called 'increased latency'. It's also called a waste of parents' time because the off/on twilight sleep for the child during the rocking, walking and hugging represents lost good-quality sleep.

> **PRACTICAL POINT**
>
> **Fatigue causes increased arousal. Therefore, the more tired your child, the harder it is for him to fall asleep, stay asleep, or both.**

One consequence of increased arousal is that disturbed sleep produces more wakeful, irritable and active behaviours in children. Also, these children often have increased physical activity when asleep. Although all babies can have gross movements involving the entire body or localised movements or twitches involving only one limb, these are brief motions lasting only a second or less. But chronically fatigued babies who are overly aroused move around more in a restless, squirmy, crawly fashion when sleeping. It seems that their motor is always running at a higher speed, awake or asleep. I will explain how you can reduce your child's idle speed by making sure he gets the sleep he needs.

What is disturbed sleep?

Abnormal sleep schedules (going to bed too late, sleeping too late in the morning, napping at the wrong times)
Brief sleep durations (not enough sleep overall)
Sleep fragmentation (waking up too often)
Nap deprivation (no naps or brief naps)
Prolonged latency to sleep (taking a long time to fall asleep)

Too active sleep (lots of tossing and turning)
Difficulty breathing during sleep

Night waking is not caused by:

Too much sugar in diet
Hypoglycaemia at night
Zinc deficiencies
Gastro-oesophageal reflux

Teething, contrary to popular belief, does not cause night waking. If you ask parents what happens when teething occurs, the answer is: everything! All illnesses, fevers and ear infections that happen to occur around the time a tooth erupts are blamed on teething. Throughout medical history, doctors used the diagnosis 'teething problems' as a smokescreen to hide their ignorance. In fact, at the turn of the twentieth century, 5 per cent of deaths in children in England were attributed to teething.

A proper study of problems caused by eruption of teeth was performed in Finland. Based on daily visits and the testing of 233 children between the ages of four and thirty months, it concluded that teething does not cause fevers, elevated white blood cell counts or inflammation. And most important, teething did not cause night waking.

Night waking between the ages of six and eighteen months is more likely due to nap deprivation, overstimulation or abnormal sleep schedules – not teething.

PRACTICAL POINT

Putting your baby to bed, allowing the child to hold a bottle of milk or juice, or resting the bottle on a pillow, will cause 'baby-bottle cavities'. Protect your child's teeth. Hold your baby in your arms when you give a bottle.

Growing pains also do not cause night waking. One study examined 2,178 children between six and nineteen years of age and found that 16 per cent complained of severe pain localised deep in the arms or legs. Usually the pain was deep in the thighs, behind the knees, or in the calves. The pain usually occurred late in the afternoon or in the evenings.

But when the growth rates of these affected children were compared to children without pain, there was no difference. In other words, growing pains do not occur during periods of rapid growth! Blaming night waking on growing pains is a handy excuse. But the rubbing, massaging, hot-water bottles or other forms of parent soothing at night are really serving the emotional needs of the parent or child and not reducing organic pain.

Night waking may be caused by:

Fever
Painful ear infections
Atopic dermatitis, eczema

PRACTICAL POINT

Do not attempt to correct unhealthy sleep habits unless you see a clear period ahead when you will be in control. Don't rely on most relatives or baby-sitters to do as good a job as you can to correct unhealthy sleep habits. Also, if your child's sleep improves during a retraining period but suddenly he becomes worse, appears ill or seems to be in pain, let your paediatrician examine him for the possibility of an ear or throat infection.

Let's consider the child who naps well, has a reasonably normal sleep schedule, does not appear overly tired, but simply gets up too often and/or stays up too long in the middle of the night. We want to help this child learn how to soothe herself to sleep unassisted when she wakes up. This skill also will help her fall asleep at bedtime, so the two strategies outlined here can be used when a child fights going to bed, too. The first technique, called 'fading', is a more gradual approach, while the second, called 'extinction', is an abrupt, cold-turkey solution. Let's look at how each works, and their pluses and minuses.

Fading

A gradual approach to reduce the number of night wakings until the baby can return to sleep independently is called 'fading'. Over a period of time you gradually reduce your efforts at night, so that your child takes over for himself and falls asleep or returns to sleep by himself. This is like teaching an older child how to ride a bike. You first provide balance and support and then gradually withdraw as the child gains confidence and skill. Here is an example of a fade sequence to eliminate night wakings.

Respond promptly, spend as much time as needed
Father gives bottle or mother doesn't nurse
Change from milk to juice
Dilute juice to only water
No bottle
No picking up
No singing, talking, verbal communication
Minimal contact, patting or hand-holding
No eye contact; sober, unresponsive face
No physical contact; sit next to child
Move chair away from cot towards door, slowly over several days
Reduce time with child
Delay response

This has been called the 'chair method' when done with an older child in a bed because you are basically slowly moving the chair further from your child until you are just outside the door.

The apparent advantage of gradually weaning the child from prolonged, complex contact is its seeming gentleness. A disadvantage is that it takes several days or weeks, during which many brief crying spells may occur. The major reasons why this approach usually only partially succeeds, or fails completely, are (a) unpredictable, real-life events interfere with parents' best plans and schedules, (b) parents do not appreciate the enormous power of intermittent positive reinforcement to maintain a behaviour ('I'll just nurse him this one time'), and (c) parents' resolve weakens from their own fatigue and sometimes from impatience. Here is an account of one mother's attempt to use a gradual approach.

Exhaustion Wins Out Over Patience

Lauren was eight months old when I finally sought help from the doctor; her sleep schedule could only be described as unbearable.

When we brought her home from the hospital after her birth, she would have a very long, wakeful period in the evenings from about 8:00 P.M. to 1:00 A.M. We can't say that she was colicky, as she was really quite pleasant most of the time. Only about once a week did she have an extended crying spell during which she would be inconsolable.

At around seven months or so, we decided to try nursing Lauren and putting her back in her own bed consistently. That's when the trouble really began! Lauren would wake up every few hours, and it would take one and a half to two hours to get her back to sleep. By now she had learned how to stand up, and I think that made it even more difficult for her to settle down.

The other thing Lauren did was to fall asleep easily at about 9:00 P.M. and wake up a half hour later, inconsolable. Eventually (after nursing, rocking, and so on), she would perk up and become very pleasant and often stay up and play happily for anywhere from two to four hours. At the same time, naps were totally irregular and unpredictable. She would usually sleep twenty minutes, but sometimes it was two hours.

When I saw the doctor, I explained that I was one of those people who didn't think I could let my baby cry herself to sleep.

The doctor recommended a plan of action that involved a gradual withdrawal process that would stretch out over seven to ten days. The response to Lauren's waking was supposed to be consistently prompt, but there was to be less handling of the baby at each step of the plan.

I put Lauren in her cot, kissed her good night, walked out and closed the door. She screamed for forty-five minutes and finally went to sleep. They were the longest forty-five minutes of my life – longer than labour! But it worked!

A few nights after our first success, we decided to leave her alone when she woke up at 9:30. Well, that crying session lasted for about thirty-five minutes. The next night Lauren went to bed about 9:00 P.M. and got up at 7:30 A.M.! I kept thinking that it must be horribly frightening for a baby, who is unable to communicate except through crying, to be left alone in a room to cry. What helped to convince me, however (in addition to utter and complete exhaustion), was the realisation that as long as I stayed in Lauren's room she screamed anyway. Walking, rocking, singing – none of these quietened her anymore. The only thing that calmed her was endless, nonstop nursing! I finally came to the conclusion that as long as Lauren was going to be miserable crying anyway, she might as well be learning something positive from it – learning to go to sleep. Even now, if I stay in her room after I put her in bed, she stands up and cries, but as soon as I kiss her good night, walk out and close the door, she lies down and goes to sleep.

Extinction (Going 'Cold Turkey')

When parents, however well intentioned, stop reinforcing a child's night waking, the habit can be eliminated quickly. In fact, psychologists have shown that the more continuous or regular you are in reinforcing the night waking during the first few months, the more likely it will rapidly be reduced simply by stopping the reinforcing behaviour. The advantages of ending the habit of going to your baby at night are that the instructions are simple and easily remembered, and the whole process usually takes only a few days. But the seeming disadvantage is that a few nights of very prolonged crying are unbearable for many parents. This procedure strikes many people as too harsh, too abrupt, or cruel. Those are personal value judgements, but bear in mind that this procedure is effective. It works.

The sleep strategy that I have emphasised is called 'extinction', and the alternatives are 'graduated extinction' and 'check and console' (discussed on pages 214–215). An additional sleep strategy that might be tried at this age is 'scheduled awakenings'. Parents note the approximate times when their child wakes up at night and then they awaken him before those times. The child is changed, if needed, and soothed back to sleep. Research has shown that extinction works much faster than scheduled awakenings but scheduled awakenings does work.

Here is an account of one mother who decided to stop going to her child cold turkey in order to eliminate her child's night wakings.

'One of the Hardest Things I've Ever Had to Do'

At six months of age, Stephen was strong, happy and healthy in every respect but one – he didn't sleep well. He did all his daytime napping in the car, the pushchair or our arms. If we put him in his cot, he awoke immediately and cried until we picked him up. His night-time pattern was different but equally exhausting. He went to sleep in his cot promptly at 8:00 P.M., but usually awoke within the first hour for a brief comforting, and two or three times between 11:00 P.M. and 5:00 A.M. for a feeding.

This routine was taking its toll. I was almost as tired as when Stephen was a newborn and I had no emotional reserve for handling everyday problems. I was sharp with the rest of the family and got angry if my husband was even ten minutes late getting home from work. We needed to make a change.

The doctor gave us explicit instructions for instituting morning and afternoon naps and unbroken night-time sleeping. At the end of the appointment, I was full of resolve. We had the weekend ahead of us, when my husband would be around for support, so we decided to start that night.

We put the baby to bed at 8:00 P.M., and he awoke for the first time around 9:30. We didn't go in to him, and he cried for twenty minutes before going back to sleep. He awoke again around 2:00 and 4:00 A.M. and cried about twenty minutes each time. When he cried at 6:00 A.M., I rushed into his room, anxious to hold him and be sure he was the same healthy, happy baby I had put down the night before.

Over the next few days it was amazing to see how quickly he fell into the schedule we had set up for him. He cried ten to fifteen minutes several times, but never again for an hour. Now he naps regularly and sleeps all night, occasionally crying for one or two minutes during the night as he puts himself back to sleep.

Letting my baby cry was one of the hardest things I've ever had to do. Now that the experience is behind us, however, I have no doubt at all that it was right. It gave me more confidence in my abilities to handle tough issues as a parent.

PRACTICAL POINT

Small, soothing efforts such as kissing the forehead, rearranging the blankets, comforting and patting appear trivial to parents, but they interfere enormously with learning to fall asleep unassisted.

A father told me that 'it was painful for him and his wife to admit that what they had been doing was wrong and not good for their child'. What were they doing? At several months of age, they were going in about every two hours, every time the child cried a little. He said that it would have been much easier to blame or get angry with someone like me who said that too much attention at night was not good for their baby, and accuse me of giving bad advice, than it was to recognise that they were the ones responsible for her continued night wakings and irritability during the day. Another mother said that the reason some mothers and fathers have such strong emotional rejection of my advice is quite simple: parental guilt. Since they spend so little time with their child because they are both working, they feel bad and try to spend more time after work in the evening playing with their child. They cannot consider that the bedtime is too late for the child's health, so they conclude that my advice regarding early bedtimes must be incorrect.

HELPFUL HINT

Use thick layers of zinc oxide paste in the nappy region so that no rash will develop when you do not go to your baby at night to change nappies. Ordinary baby oil will make removal of the paste easier in the morning.

Here are some typical questions and answers for this age group.

Q: *I've heard that if I nurse my baby to sleep, I'll create a night-waking problem.*
A: The issue is not whether nursing to sleep is good or not, but rather whether nursing too frequently or night-time nursing is part of a night-waking problem. Please include nursing, if you wish, in nap time or bedtime rituals, but after you finish nursing, whether the child's asleep or awake, put her down, kiss her cheek, say good night, walk away, turn the lights off and close the door.

Q: *I heard that because she learns to associate my breast with falling asleep, she will be unable to return to sleep later in the night if my breast is not present.*
A: Nonsense! Almost all the mothers in my practice nurse their babies to sleep, and at night, when they are hungry, either the mother nurses or the father bottle-feeds the baby.

I believe it is perfectly natural to nurse a baby to sleep, and by itself this act does not cause sleep disturbances. Older children can be very discriminating; they can learn to expect dessert after dinner, if that is the family custom, but not after breakfast. I think babies can also become very discriminating; they can learn to expect to be fed when they are hungry but not to be fed when they are not hungry.

Q: *Once I let my child cry a long time and she vomited. Won't I be trading one problem for another?*
A: Consider other sleep strategies that involve less crying. However, if the vomiting always occurs, I think you will want always to go in to clean her promptly and then leave her again. If the vomiting is irregular and occasional, you should try waiting until after you think she is deeply asleep before checking, and then quickly clean her if needed.

Q: *Won't my baby simply outgrow this habit?*
A: Believe it or not, eighteen-year-old college students who don't sleep well had difficulties sleeping as infants, according to their mothers, as reported in one study. It seems that if the child doesn't have the early opportunity to practise falling asleep by herself, she'll never learn to fall asleep easily.

Q: *Even if she won't outgrow this habit, what's really wrong with my still going to her at night?*
A: Consider your feelings. Good studies at Yale University in the USA show that all mothers eventually become anxious, develop angry feelings towards their child, and feel guilty about maintaining poor sleep habits. These feelings may persist for years. True, you will also feel guilty letting your baby cry in protest, but this will last only several days. Here's one mother's account.

'I Felt Cruel, Insensitive, and Guilty'

The moment my daughter, Amanda, arrived home from the hospital, she came down with a very bad case of colic. I took her to see the paediatrician several times, only to be told there was nothing wrong and to relax. I also received several suggestions about nursing and a pat on the back. All of these suggestions irritated me, and I felt as though I was being perceived as an anxious, first-time mother.

After twelve weeks of crying and screaming, Amanda was evaluated by two child development specialists. I decided we should work with one until my daughter's crying and screaming settled down. We also saw a psychiatrist, who recommended medication and also suggested that we continue to be followed by the development specialists. In the meantime, our lives had become a nightmare. Amanda cried most of the day and always screamed in the evening. To our horror, this behaviour had worked itself into the night hours, too.

By five months, we were referred to Dr Weissbluth for what we hoped was a sleep disorder. I say 'hoped', because we were at the point of seeing a paediatric neurologist and having an EEG done. I was very frightened for my daughter, and my husband and I were exhausted. I was eager for the consultation. My daughter had definitely been cursed with colic. Could this now be wired exhaustion from a sleep disorder caused by the treatment for colic – rocking, swinging, motion all the time? It was.

Amanda was old enough now to try 'crying it out'. It was the most difficult thing I've had to do as a new mother.

The first night Amanda screamed, choked and sobbed for thirty-two minutes. I remember feeling sick to my stomach.

The first two days weren't too terrible. However, the third and fourth were almost intolerable. Amanda would cry through her entire nap time. Then I would get her up to keep Dr Weissbluth's time frame going. Her temperament after these episodes is known only to mothers who have been through the same ordeal! When she would scream for *over an hour* during nap time and in the evening, I felt cruel, insensitive and guilty.

Three things kept me going: my husband's support; Dr

Weissbluth's concern, encouragement and compassion; and the fact that I knew it had to be done – Amanda had to learn to sleep.

It took Amanda about a week to catch on to the idea. The bags under her eyes faded, her sporadic screaming attacks stopped and her personality was that of a predictable baby – a sweet-heart when rested and a bear when she's past a nap time or her bedtime.

I would offer these suggestions to other mothers and fathers who have to take this measure in order to teach their babies to sleep:

You, as parents, have to understand and believe intellectually that it is the right thing to do. Otherwise feelings of guilt will overpower you, and you will give in. You must have the support of your spouse, as it will be too much of a strain to bear alone.

You are doing what is best for your baby. It seems cruel and unacceptable as a loving new mother to let your baby cry. But it is a fact of parenting – many, many things will bring tears and protests in the years to come.

Enlist the support of a sympathetic friend as much as you feel the need to. I found close telephone contact a tremendous help. Some parents may not need this close interaction, but many of us do.

In your role as parents, teaching your child to sleep may be the very first difficult task you have to undertake. Those parents who do should feel a special sense of accomplishment, for it *is* a very difficult task! Those of us who have been through a baby with a sleep disorder know what misery is. But so does the baby, who is miserable and exhausted all the time. Once patterns and the practice of sleep are established, everyone benefits and finally life can be somewhat predictable again.

It will get better!

A few more typical questions and answers:

Q: *I don't believe in this kind of unnatural programming.*
A: Consider the 'unnatural' effects of chronic sleep fragmentation on your child.

Q: *I don't think I can do just nothing when my baby cries for me at night.*
A: Letting your baby cry is not doing nothing. You are actively encouraging the development of independence, providing opportunities for her to learn how to sleep alone, and showing respect for her ability to change her behaviour.

If, after reading the preceding sections, you want to try allowing your child to learn to soothe herself to sleep but still feel you wouldn't be able to listen to her cry, consider the following:

WHY CAN'T I LET MY BABY CRY?

1. *Unpleasant childhood memories.* These may surface and remind you of feelings of loneliness or being unwanted.
2. *Working mother's guilt.* You may feel guilty about being away from your child so much.
3. *We've already tried and it didn't work.* Maybe the child was too young then; maybe you taught her, by your behaviour, that if she cried for more than a certain amount of time, you would go to her; maybe you unknowingly provided partial reinforcement by going to her at some times but not at others.
4. *I enjoy my baby's company too much at night.* This may be because you're not a good sleeper yourself.
5. *If I don't nurse my baby at night, she might lose weight.* This is not true.
6. *We're under a lot of stress.* In *My Child Won't Sleep*, Jo Douglas and Naomi Richman write:

If you are feeling stressed, your child may respond by not sleeping so well. If the stress is related to difficulties between you as parents, you may think that your young child will not notice, but the chances are that he will. His way of waking at night and coming into your bed can be a way of preventing

you from talking to each other and sorting out your problems, and his presence can act as a useful contraceptive.

Although this quote applies to older children, it's possible that maintaining the baby's night waking or having the baby sleep with you when he or she is younger also serves the purpose of avoiding marital problems.

7. ***I feel that I am a bad parent if my baby cries.*** **You are not a bad parent if you are helping your baby learn healthy sleep habits.**
8. ***I am afraid that letting my baby cry will cause her permanent emotional harm.*** **There is no evidence that protest crying while your child is learning how to sleep better will cause any kind of emotional problems later in life.**

PRACTICAL POINT

When your overtired child first starts to sleep better during a retraining period, he may appear, in the beginning, to be more tired than before! You are unmasking the underlying fatigue that had previously been present but was hidden by the turned-on, hyper-alert state.

Summary

Infants' sleep patterns begin to resemble those of adults at around four months of age. It may help to think of sleep as having two related components. The first is *sleep/wake organisation*, which means how long the sleep period lasts and when the sleep periods are occurring. The second is *sleep quality*, which here means whether the sleep is consolidated or fragmented and the duration of the different sleep stages.

Let's Walk Around the Clock

Here is the package of advice to prevent or correct sleep problems for children four to twelve months.

1. **Control the wake-up time**
2. **Short interval of wakefulness (ultra-short for post-colic kids) before first nap**
3. **Consistent soothe-to-sleep method (A or B) for midmorning nap, around 9:00 A.M.**
4. **Limited nap duration to protect next nap**
5. **No snoozing during period of wakefulness if midmorning nap is not taken**
6. **Consistent soothe-to-sleep method (A or B) for early afternoon nap, around 1:00 P.M.**
7. **Limited nap duration to protect bedtime**
8. **Variable third nap; you be the judge (but no third nap after nine months of age)**
9. **Early bedtime (time varies based on how your child appears, the quality of naps, and past performance) with regular soothing routine**
10. **No more than two feedings at night up to nine months of age (exception: unrestricted if breast-feeding in family bed)**

Action Plan for Exhausted Parents

Months Five to Eight: 16 per cent have three naps, 84 per cent have two naps

- If your child is post-colic or has a difficult temperament put him to sleep, after soothing, within only one hour of wakefulness for the morning nap.
- During the one hour of wakefulness, if possible, expose your child to bright natural light.
- If he cries, leave him alone for at least ten to twenty minutes. If the child has an easy temperament, prepare to leave him alone for one hour.
- Try to establish naps around 9:00 A.M., 1:00 P.M.; and if needed, a late-afternoon nap. Try to avoid naps at other times.

Month Nine: 5 per cent have three naps, 91 per cent have two naps, 4 per cent have one nap

- Eliminate late-afternoon nap to protect early bedtime.

Months Ten to Twelve: 1 per cent have 3 naps, 82 per cent have two naps, 17 per cent have one nap

- Morning nap starts to disappear.
- When morning nap starts to disappear, move bedtime twenty to thirty minutes earlier.
- If afternoon nap starts to disappear because morning nap is too long, move bedtime much earlier to shorten the morning nap. Protect and preserve the afternoon nap.
- If there is resistance for the afternoon nap, start the nap earlier.
- Consider your resources for soothing (see page 73).
- If resources are limited, go slowly and tackle one problem at a time – for example, bedtime battles.
- If resources are unlimited, go quickly and fix the twenty-four-hour schedule at once: bedtime battles, night waking and fighting naps.
- If your baby cries hard and vomits, consider changing sleep strategies to one that involves less crying.

CHAPTER 7

Months Thirteen to Thirty-six

When your child starts to walk, babble and show more personality, you will naturally begin to treat him less as an infant and more like a person. Please try to avoid the trap of endlessly explaining, negotiating or threatening when it comes to sleep times. Save your breath; let your behaviour do the talking.

Months Thirteen to Fifteen: One or Two Naps

At twelve months of age, 82 per cent of children have two naps and 17 per cent take only a single afternoon nap. But by fifteen months of age, 43 per cent of children are taking two naps and 56 per cent take a single afternoon nap. This is a dramatic change occurring over a short time period.

This transition, however, may not be smooth. You might have a few rough months when one nap is not enough but two are impossible. Here are some ideas for making the transition easier.

Move the bedtime earlier. The morning nap is always the first nap to disappear naturally. We do not know why. If the bedtime is moved up a little, most parents will notice that the morning nap becomes briefer or turns into a quiet playtime without sleep. Most of these children do not appear to become very tired.

Other children take longer and longer morning naps and then appear to actively resist or be unable to take the second afternoon nap. Because this second nap was short anyway, many parents forget it. The result is a child who is tired late in the afternoon or early evening and who quickly becomes overtired by bedtime. One solution is an earlier bedtime because your child will wake up rested and take a briefer morning nap. In addition, you might want to shorten the nap by waking your child after about one or one and a half hours so she will be more tired around the midday nap time. Also, try to get out of the house immediately following the morning nap to provide intense stimulation but tone it down as you get to the middle of the day. Provide extra long and relaxing soothing to sleep for the midday nap. Maybe consider moving the midday nap to a slightly later hour so your child is a bit more tired. Sometimes your child continues to take a morning nap but none of the above causes her to take a midday nap, so here's another plan. At the time of the morning nap, delay its onset by ten or twenty minutes. This might require more intense and prolonged soothing to sleep. Slowly, over many days or weeks, continue to delay the morning nap until it is occurring near the middle of the day. During this transition, the bedtime might have to be temporarily ultra-early because your child gets tired every afternoon. Some of these children appear to hate their bedroom in the afternoon and scream as you approach it. One mother solved this by doing all the pre-nap soothing in the living room and then quickly went into his room.

The earlier bedtime means that a working parent coming home late does not see the child then. If that is the case, that parent can get up extra early to have a longer morning playtime with the child before going off to work. Another solution is to declare some days as two-nap days and other days as one-nap days, depending on when the baby awakens, how long the morning nap lasts, scheduled group activities or the time you want your baby to go to sleep at night. Flow with your child and arrange naps and bedtimes to coincide with his need to sleep as best you can. Be sensitive to the growing need for earlier bedtimes.

Here is one mother's account of how an early bedtime helped her child.

> Sophie has always been inconsistent when it comes to napping. Some days she would sleep for half an hour, others she wouldn't sleep at all. And if I was lucky, she would take an occasional hour nap. I decided it was time to get help before the situation became worse.
>
> Sophie was thirteen months old when I met with Dr Weissbluth. She was sleeping for thirty minutes in the morning; her afternoon naps were unpredictable. At night, getting her to sleep was even more frustrating. Sophie had always been a great night-time sleeper. Then, all of a sudden, she was waking up several times throughout the night. Not only was her mental state unbearable, but physically she did not look well. As for me, I was becoming mummy the monster. There were days when I thought I was going to lose it. I blamed myself for her sleeping disorder, even though I was doing everything right – putting her to bed early, keeping a consistent nap time and putting her down in her cot for her naps instead of allowing her to sleep on the go.
>
> After looking over Sophie's sleep log, Dr Weissbluth gave me several options: try an earlier bedtime (5:00 P.M.), lots of stimulation when awake and soothing her longer at night. The goal was to allow her to catch up on her sleep.
>
> My husband and I put the plan to work. He supported the decision of an earlier bedtime, even though his time with her was already limited. Unfortunately, Sophie's sleeping did not improve. She continued to take one nap for thirty or forty-five minutes and then skip her afternoon nap. She and I were both exhausted and my frustration level was sky high at this point.
>
> During our follow-up conversation, Dr Weissbluth asked if I would consider dropping her morning nap. He recommended the continuation of an earlier bedtime (5:00 P.M.), which, surprisingly, she welcomed. Although I was hesitant to drop her morning nap, I was determined to get my happy child back.
>
> So, I put plan B to work. For the first several days, Sophie could

barely keep her eyes open past 10:30 A.M. I was able to keep her up until 11:00 A.M. and then 11:30 A.M. for the next several days. She continued to take thirty-minute naps. I called Dr Weissbluth and he reminded me that she was still trying to catch up on sleep, that it would take several days for her to feel rested. After day four, she was staying awake until 12:30 and sleeping for an hour. And she was sleeping through the night – no more night-time waking. By the end of the week, she was starting her nap at 12:30 and waking up at 2:00 P.M. And Sophie and mummy were happy.

Sophie continues to have thirty-minute naps every once in a while, and she looks forward to her nap time. She no longer cries; instead, she falls asleep quickly. As for me, I am feeling more confident. Sophie is not the only one who is sleeping better. I am spending more time enjoying her and less time being tired and frustrated.

Obviously, any combination of parents' scheduling for their convenience and the baby's need to sleep can determine nap patterns. If you are a napper yourself, you may protect your child's nap schedule differently from the parent who does not customarily take naps.

Q: *How long should my child nap?*
A: Does your child appear well rested? You be the judge. All of us have good days and bad days, but if you notice a progression toward more fussiness, brattiness or tantrums, your child may need longer naps.

Months Sixteen to Twenty-one: Morning Nap Disappears

The morning nap is on its way out. At eighteen months, 77 per cent of children take a single afternoon nap; by twenty-one months, 88 per cent sleep only in the afternoon. Sometimes the child is taking only the morning nap and the plan discussed above does not work because the general recommendation of an early bedtime backfires. You try an early bedtime and all you get is an earlier wake-up time, which makes your child more tired in the morning and makes him need the morning nap all the more. Under these circumstances, you might temporarily put your child to bed a little later at night with the hope that he will sleep in later. If you put him to bed much too late, he will have difficulty falling asleep and staying asleep, so this will require some patience and trial and error. Still, wake him, if he is asleep, at 7:00 A.M. and then proceed with one of the plans previously described to get an afternoon nap.

Q: *What do I do if my child is healthy but cries at night, and the crying stops as soon as I pick him up?*
A: Ask yourself if there is anything you can do to regularise the total sleep pattern, such as timing naps better or making the bedtime earlier. Was there anything that recently disrupted his schedule to cause him to become overtired? Does he snore or mouth-breathe during sleep, or might he be starting to become ill? Look at the big picture, not just the night crying. In general, you will not want to attend to the night crying because you want to encourage consolidated sleep. If you go to your child, you will cause fragmented sleep, which is poor-quality sleep. If your head says that not going to your child is the right thing to do, but your heart won't let you do it, try some of these suggestions.

One parent tied a ribbon around her ankle and her husband's ankle so that she did not shift into autopilot mode at night and go to her child when he cried. Another mother waited for her husband to go away on business for a few days so she could ignore the crying without having her husband undercut the plan. Sleep temporarily further away from your child; use earplugs, earphones, pillows over your head; take a shower. Do what is best for your child, but don't torture yourself.

Months Twenty-two to Thirty-six: Only a Single Afternoon Nap

Naps

At twenty-four months of age, only 5 per cent of children have two naps and 95 per cent are taking a single afternoon nap. By thirty-six months of age, no children are taking two naps, 91 per cent are taking a single nap in the afternoon and 9 per cent are not napping at all. A common problem occurs when the nap disappears but the child appears very tired during the day and really seems to need to nap. The closer the child is to his second birthday, the more likely you should try to re-establish the nap, because most probably it is biologically needed. But if he is almost three, you might not be as successful in re-establishing the nap because he might have outgrown the need for it.

Here are two plans to try to re-establish a nap. First, consider the situation where the bedtime is already quite early or you observe that when you moved the bedtime earlier it only caused your child to get up earlier in the morning. Slowly try to move the bedtime later by about twenty to thirty minutes each night with the hope that your child will sleep in later, wake up better rested and be more able to take an afternoon nap. Second, if the bedtime is quite late, slowly move the bedtime earlier by about twenty to thirty minutes each night with the hope that your child will wake up better rested. In either case, try intensive stimulation in the morning, followed by a wind-down, then a prolonged pre-nap soothing routine, and try to nap him when he's tired but not too overtired. Consider lying down with your child in your bed temporarily, mother or father, to re-establish the nap routine. After five to seven days, re-evaluate and make adjustments of bedtimes and nap times.

Between twenty-two and thirty-six months, most children still need to nap. The average amount of daytime sleep at thirty-six months is about two hours. But there is much individual variation; the range is from one to three and a half hours. If your child is at either extreme of this range, ask yourself if he appears well rested at all times.

The majority (80 per cent) of children between the ages of two and three years have a nap length in a narrower band between one and a half to two and a half hours. Most children nap for about two hours. The model nap duration is two hours between the ages of two and six years. The stability of the two-hour nap over different ages is another argument for a strong biological influence over sleep, but it does not necessarily mean that your child needs a two-hour nap. Some children need less and some need more daytime sleep.

Q: *When do I transition my child from a cot to a bed?*
A: As he approaches his third birthday, let the child ask for a big bed. If you move him too soon, he will not stay in his bed because he is curious and wants to see what's going on elsewhere in the house.

Fears

Nightmares, monsters, fear of separation, fear of darkness, fear of death, fear of abandonment . . . don't fears cause disturbed sleep at this age? Many experts tell us that night fears are common among children between two and four years old. Thunderstorms, barking dogs, loud trucks and many other events over which we have no control can frighten children. If your child has been a good sleeper up to now, you should expect any disturbed sleep triggered by these events to be short-lived.

Some child care experts believe severe sleep disturbances are caused by night fears. Usually, though, children with serious sleep problems did not sleep well at younger ages, and their current difficulty is simply misinterpreted as caused by an age-appropriate concern or 'stage'.

Reassurance, frequent curtain calls, open doors, night-lights, or a longer bedtime routine will help your child get over his fears. My recommendation is to spend extra time soothing your child to sleep or go to him once for reassurance, but use a kitchen timer to control the duration of the extra time. The timer is set to the number of minutes you want to spend with your child and is then placed under a pillow or cushion to muffle the noise. Tell your child that when the buzzer or bell sounds, you will kiss him and leave. The child learns to associate the sound of the time with your departure and learns that this signals the end of your hugging, massage or lullabies. This is called 'stimulus control', which is discussed further in Chapter 9. Just as when the final curtain call ends, you know the play is really over, or just as you know to slow down as the green light turns to yellow, your child learns to associate the sound with the end of your soothing effort. Because crying will not bring you back, the crying ends.

If your child has never been a good sleeper and now also appears during the day to be extremely frightened, withdrawn in new surroundings, shy or fearful, then it is very difficult for parents to give less attention at night, even if the goal is to enhance consolidated sleep. If this is the case with your toddler, a child psychologist can give you good advice on where to draw the line between supporting the child and encouraging him to learn to overcome his fears.

Routines and Schedules

At about two to three years of age, although most children in my research survey go to sleep between 7:00 and 9:00 P.M. and awaken between 6:30 and 8:00 A.M., I think that an earlier bedtime is better. A single nap between one and three hours occurs in over 90 per cent of children. Try to be *reasonably* regular about nap time and bedtime, and be consistent in your bedtime rituals. There are no absolute, rigid or firm rules, because every day is somewhat different. *Reasonable* regularity and consistency implies *reasonable* flexibility. Be aware that your lifestyle helps or hinders your child's sleep patterns, and remember that there will be changes due to growth and rearrangements in relationships within the family.

How about scheduled, organised activities that take place when your child needs to take her afternoon nap? If she is unable to take her afternoon nap two or three times each week and you are able to get an extra-early bedtime on those days, then there may be no problem, as long as the child is sleeping well in general. For the child who is not sleeping well, for whatever reason, losing a few naps can be quite problematic. Also keep in mind that children are likely to pick up minor illnesses from each other in group settings, and not feeling well may disrupt your child's sleep and push her into an overtired state. In general, be cautious. Have fun with your child, but occasionally have what my wife called a 'declared holiday'. Missing a swim class, gym class or any other preschool event now and then because your child is tired and needs to nap, or leaving soon after you arrive because the other children look sick will not jeopardise your child's college plans!

A Regular Bed and the Arrival of a New Baby

One rearrangement is moving your child to a 'big kid's' bed. There is no special age when you should make this change. As long as the cot is large enough, you should not feel that your child must be placed in a normal bed by a certain age. Many parents make the switch around the second or third birthday. Let your child ask for a big bed. One mother described how she felt that she had made the move too soon and the big bed must have seemed 'oceanic' compared to the cot, because her son always slept curled up in one corner of the bed – that is, when he slept. He slept better when returned to his cot. Before she made the move back to the cot, his mother wondered whether this would cause a 'regression' in her child. It did not. But it did result in a better-rested family.

If the move to a bed is needed because of a new baby brother or sister, consider making the move when the newborn is about four months old. By then, the newborn has regular sleeping habits. Before the baby reaches this age, there is a constant shifting of household routines due to the infant's naturally irregular sleep pattern. This may cause confusion or insecurity in the older child because he does not know when mum or dad will be available, or why he has to wait when he wants to go outside and has been used to doing just that. When the newborn is four months old and her sleep pattern is stable, events in the house are much more predictable. The older child now becomes adjusted to the new family arrangements. The baby goes to the cot and the older child graduates with pride to the big bed for big kids. He does not feel displaced. Before the newborn is actually moved from the bassinet to the cot, feel free to leave the cot up and empty for a while with the understanding that if the older child gets out of bed once, then it's back to the cot.

Moving to a big bed too early, before the birth of the new baby, often invites a problem: The commotion and excitement surrounding the arrival of a new baby creates confusion or insecurity in the older child, who may call out or cry at night. The more difficult situation is when the older child starts to get up every night to visit his parents.

If the move to a regular bed prompts frequent nocturnal visits, curtain calls, calls for help going to the bathroom or calls for a drink of water, think before you act. A habit may slowly develop in which your child learns to expect you to spend more time with her, putting her to sleep or returning her to sleep. Imagine what would occur if a baby-sitter gave your two-year-old sweets every day instead of a real lunch. Once you discovered this, you would immediately stop the sweets for meals. Your child might protest and cry, but would you give in and let her have the sweets? No. If you are spending too much time at night with your child when she should be sleeping, consider that you are giving 'social sweets' – not needed and not healthy for the child. Be firm in your resolve to ignore the expected protest from your child when you change your behaviour.

Preventing and Solving Sleep Problems

In one study of children between one and two years of age, about 20 per cent woke up five or more times a week, while in a study of three-year-old children, 26 per cent woke up at least three times a week. Unfortunately, you simply cannot assume that difficulty returning to sleep unassisted will magically go away. Returning to sleep unassisted is a learned skill; you should expect problems to persist in your child until she learns how to soothe herself back to sleep without your help.

Also, in the study of one- and two-year-old children, those who woke up frequently were much more likely to have an injury such as a broken bone or a cut requiring medical attention than those who slept through – while only 17 per cent of good sleepers had injuries, 40 per cent of the night wakers were injured! (Chapter 11 will discuss further the connection between injuries and disturbed sleep.)

The majority of children between the ages of one and five have a bedtime routine less than thirty minutes long, go to sleep with the lights off and fall asleep in about thirty minutes after lights out. Night waking occurs in the older children in this group once a week; only a few awaken more than once a night. If your child's pattern between the ages of one and five is substantially different, consider the possibility that your child is among the 20 per cent of children in this group with disturbed sleep. If so, then you might also later notice the excessive daytime sleepiness that has been observed in about 5 to 10 per cent of children between the ages of five and fourteen years.

Your child's developing personality and awareness of himself as an individual means that his second and third years will be a time of testing, non-cooperation, resistance and striving for independence. Your child has stronger self-agency. Sleep problems in twelve- to thirty-six-month-olds are related to this normally evolving stubbornness or wilfulness in children, who now want to do their own thing. For example, they may want to get out of their bed or cot at night, not take naps, get up too early to play and, of course, resist falling asleep and wake up at night. This last problem might have started during the first year and may now continue during the second year as an ingrained habit. Let's look at each of these major problems in turn.

PRACTICAL POINT

Don't confuse these issues:

- **Needs versus wants**
- **A sad cry versus a protest cry**
- **Being abandoned versus being alone**

Getting Out of the Cot or Bed: The Jack-in-the-Box Syndrome

It's quite natural for two- and three-year-olds to climb out of the cot or bed to check out the interesting things they think their parents are up to. Or maybe they just want to watch the late, late movie or have a bite to eat. Of course, what they like to do most is to come and see their parents and/or get into their bed. This not only disrupts their parents' sleep, but it also harms the child. Here's how.

When a child has a naturally occurring partial arousal during sleep, instead of soothing himself back to sleep, he learns to force himself completely awake to get out of his bed or cot. The result is sleep fragmentation – for him, and for his parents, too. Here's a five-step treatment plan to put your Jack back in his box at night.

Step 1: Keep a chart, log, or diary to record key sleep events: time asleep, time awake, number of times out of bed and duration of protest calling, fussing or crying. This will make you a better observer of both your child's behaviour and your own. The chart or log enables you to determine whether the strategy is working, and helps remind you to be regular according to clock times and to be consistent in your responses.

Step 2: Ask yourself whether your child behaves as if he is tired in the late afternoon or early evening. If the answer is yes, then consider the possibility that naps are insufficient or that the bedtime hour is too late. Deal with these problems at the same time you are working on his getting out of the cot or bed. If needed, keep data in your sleep chart regarding naps, such as the time he falls asleep, how long he sleeps during the day, how long he cries in protest before napping and the interval between the end of his nap and when he goes to sleep for the night.

Also, consider whether your child is snoring or mouth-breathing more and more at night. Please read the section on snoring in Chapter 10 if this is now a problem.

Step 3: Announce to your child that there is a new rule in the house: down is down – no getting out of bed until morning. Tell him that you love him very much but that you need your sleep, and he needs to put himself back to sleep by himself; getting out of bed is not allowed. Tell him that when he gets out of bed, you are going to put him back to bed and you are not going to talk to him or look at his face while you are doing so. Let's call this *'silent return to sleep'*. Silence when you take your baby back to bed is important, because if you are sweet or stern while trying to explain why everyone needs sleep, the verbal attention will reinforce your child's desire to get out of bed to get more attention. Attending to a problem will cause the problem to occur more often. Many parents do not understand that negative attention – yelling or getting angry – is still attention, and it will encourage your child to continue the behaviour.

Depending on your child's age, he may or may not understand what you are saying. But he will certainly sense that tonight something different is going to occur.

PRACTICAL POINT

Be *silent* and unemotional; appear disinterested or mechanical. No more night entertainment.

Step 4: Place yourself where you can easily hear him get out of his cot or bed. Place a bell on a rope on his door to signal when he leaves his room or enters your room, or use an intercom if you must be out of earshot. The signal makes him aware of what he's doing and it helps you to be consistent.

Every time you determine that he is out of his cot or bed, or discover him in your bed, gently place him back in his bed. *Maintain silence.* Plan not to sleep the first night, as he may try many, many times to get back to his old style. Parents might want to alternate nights so that at least someone gets some sleep. Do not take turns on the same night, because the child might think one parent would behave differently. Children learn quickly that there's no benefit in getting out of bed, so they stay in bed and sleep through the night.

Step 5: Every morning, shower the child with praise or affection for cooperating with the new rule. Perhaps offer a favourite food that was previously withheld or go on a special outing. Try small rewards for partial cooperation and larger rewards for more complete cooperation.

In addition to praising or rewarding your child when he cooperates, you might consider changing some of the routines when he *doesn't* cooperate. For example, past fifteen to eighteen months, you might close the door in a progressive fashion every time he gets out of bed. You can put three or four white tape marks on the floor, and for the first three or four times he gets out of bed, the door is closed a little more until it is barely open or completely closed. If he stays in the bed, the door is left open to the first tape mark. A similar progressive strategy could be used with brighter or dimmer night-lights.

Expect this plan to dramatically reduce or eliminate the getting-out-of-bed routine within a few days, usually three or four. All you had to do was remove the previous night-time social interaction (whether pleasant or unpleasant) as a reinforcer to the habit of getting out of his cot.

In short, every time your child gets out of bed, he encounters a silent, unemotional parent who gently picks him up and returns him to bed.

Here are some typical questions and answers about this strategy.

Q: *Won't my child hurt himself when he climbs or falls out of his cot?*
A: This is a common worry and often used as an excuse to go to your child or buy a 'big kid's' bed. But the truth is that serious injuries rarely occur when the child bumps on the floor as he lets himself down.

Q: *Can the plan fail?*
A: Yes, when both parents aren't committed, so that one partner passively or actively sabotages the programme. One father in my practice loved to sneak a bottle of formula to his baby once or twice a night. This caused the baby to suffer excessive wetness and a severe, persistent and painful nappy rash. Only in the course of trying to eradicate the rash did the father's behaviour come to light. Failures also sometimes occur when the child is still chronically fatigued from too late a bedtime hour or nap deprivation.

Q: *What if he stays in his cot but cries?*
A: Letting your child cry when he protests against going to sleep or staying in his cot is not the same as making your child cry as if you were hurting him. Leave him alone (extinction) or try controlled crying (graduated extinction).

One family instituted this five-step programme when their daughter was twenty-six months old – after twenty-six months of poor sleeping. She had always had difficulty in falling asleep and difficulty in staying asleep. Nicole always wanted to, and did, get out of her bed and go into her parents' bed. After the birth of Daniel, her brother, her parents decided this had to stop.

Their record showed the following results:

Night 1: **Between 8:13 and 9:45 P.M. – 69 return trips to bed. Slept until 8:30 A.M. with one brief awakening at 2:15 A.M.**

Night 2: **Between 8:20 and 10:30 P.M. – 145 return trips to bed. Slept until 7:20 A.M. with one brief awakening at 2:15 A.M.**

Night 3: **After 9:14 P.M. (bedtime) – 0 return trips to bed! Slept until 7:40 A.M., awakening once at 3:20 A.M.**

PRACTICAL POINT

Do not underestimate the enormous power of partial reinforcement to ruin your efforts to overcome baby's habit of getting out of the cot. If you are not *silent* and you discuss getting out of bed when it is occurring, your social behaviour reinforces getting out of the cot.

That's it!

An important point is that almost all of Nicole's getting out of bed occurred within the first hour or two of the night. Many children follow this pattern, so don't expect that you will necessarily lose a complete night of sleep during this training period.

After the third night of Nicole's programme, the curtain calls at bedtime ceased. Furthermore, at naps her mother would now leave after fifteen or twenty minutes of reading, whereas before she stayed in the room until Nicole fell asleep. The parents described Nicole as easier in many ways: less resistant in dressing, less argumentative, more charming and better able to be by herself.

Crib Tents and Locking the Door

Some families know that they are unable or unwilling to do the silent-return-to-sleep routine when their child climbs out of the cot. For a minority of children, moving them to a bed solves the problem; they want to sleep in a bed and they will stay put to enjoy it. In others, moving to a bed simply means it is now easier to go and visit mum and dad.

A crib tent will prevent your child from getting out of the cot, and it allows you to remove yourself from his protest crying without fear that an injury might occur. Sometimes duct tape is needed to cover the zipper because your child otherwise can work out how to escape. Don't worry about some theoretical sense of failure if the child has to return to the cot with a crib tent. Some parents feel that the crib tent 'locks their child in the cot like an animal caged in the zoo' and they would prefer to lock the door instead. Most families find the crib tent more acceptable and effective, but let's talk about locking the door.

To me, this is absolutely the last thing a desperate family might want to try, and because it sounds so extreme I want to share with you my observation in some detail. The reality is that not all marriages are made in heaven, not all jobs allow parents to spend much time with their children, not everyone can begin sleep training early and prevent sleep problems and, to be perfectly honest, it is difficult and inconvenient to be consistent in handling sleep routines. Circumstances beyond your control, such as twins in a one-bedroom flat, sick relatives who need your attention, or medical problems such as frequent ear infections conspire to rob children of healthy sleep. So what are we to do when all else fails and the entire family is stressed from sleep loss?

Locking the child's bedroom door to prevent social interaction at night, which interferes with sleep, is discussed further in the next chapter for older children, about three years old or more. But for younger children, around age two, some parents find that if they lock their bedroom door, while protecting the child's safety with gates if needed, everything begins to turn around. First, however, you'll need earplugs in order to ignore the banging, crying, or yelling. Second, place the child back in his cot or bed after he falls asleep. Third, praise him well when he eventually stays asleep in his own room.

Sleep Rules

A crib tent may be most appropriate for a child close to one year of age, and locking the parents' door might be needed for a two-year-old. However, as the child gets closer to the age of three, consider *sleep rules*. Sleep rules should be implemented for both nap time and night-time in order to be consistent. The family makes an elaborate, decorative, theatrical poster, which they put on the wall in the child's bedroom. Use stars and stickers; the more colourful and dramatic it is, the more motivational it will be. The poster looks like this:

SLEEP RULES

At bedtime we . . .

1. **Stay in bed.**
2. **Close our eyes.**
3. **Stay very quiet.**
4. **Go to sleep.**

Insert your child's first name before the title so that 'John' will listen carefully when a parent recites 'John's sleep rules' every time he is put to sleep. You simply say, 'John, remember your sleep rules. One, stay in bed; two, close your eyes; three, stay very quiet; and four, go to sleep.'

Rewards and privileges are an important component of this plan.

One family placed next to the poster a calendar called a 'bedtime star chart'. The mother read the rules at bedtime. If the child followed the rules, she got to put a star on the chart the next morning, which meant that she could choose a treat later that day. No star, no treat. She caught on very quickly to the relationship between following the rules and getting treats.

In general, even if there is no problem around naps, for the sake of consistency, also give the treat or star after the nap. Often a big glass bowl filled with treats on top of the refrigerator, where it is visible to the child, will enhance motivation.

Either the treat or a token to be exchanged for the treat is given immediately upon awakening. Later, the treats can be placed in a 'treat bowl' to delay gratification, and later the child will substitute heightened self-esteem for the treats. One caveat: this method is guaranteed to fail if the treats are insufficiently motivational.

Let's take a moment to look more closely at the difference between rewards and bribes. I am sensitive to the fact that some people will claim that it is wrong to give something to a child to make a behaviour occur – that it is like a bribe. The simple answer is that we smile, hug and praise our children when they perform in a socially desirable way. This is how a child learns to share toys and develop manners and desirable social habits. But our social rewards simply aren't powerful enough to change the behaviour of a strong-willed two- or three-year-old who is dead set on fighting sleep for the pleasure of your company. Opponents to giving rewards come up with theoretical objections, but the fact remains that when rewards are used in the context in which I am describing them, they work.

Actually, rewards are only half the story here. Think of what your child loves to do around the house. Exclude creative activities such as reading, painting or building things. Think of somewhat passive things, such as watching videotapes, DVDs or television; playing with the computer; or perhaps playing with some favourite dolls or trucks. Choose one activity and call it the 'privilege'. So, after you recite the sleep rules, you say 'John, remember to follow the sleep rules so that when you wake up you can choose a treat and play with your trucks.' All the trucks are put in a box in the cupboard. If he follows the rules, after he wakes up you say, 'Thank you for following the sleep rules. Here, choose a treat. And here are your trucks to play with.' Or, if he did not abide by the rules, say, 'You did not follow the sleep rules, so no treat and no trucks to play with until you follow the rules.' If John decides he doesn't care about his trucks, then restrict some other privilege next time in addition to the trucks.

When a child refuses to comply with sleep rules during the day when a nap should be taking place, and anytime a problem behaviour occurs at night, employ the silent-return-to-sleep strategy. Put a bell on his doorknob so you know when he is leaving his room. One very cute and bright girl ripped up three sleep rules posters before she got the message. Then she started to tell friends, with great pride, that she now sleeps by the rules!

What we are simply trying to accomplish is to encourage behaviours (described as sleep rules) that are compatible with allowing the sleep process to happen and to discourage behaviours (such as singing, calling and running around) that are incompatible with sleeping.

When you employ sleep rules or the silent return to sleep, do not be surprised if your child's behaviour gets worse for a short time. It's as if he is putting forth more effort to get back to the old way.

PRACTICAL POINT

Problems may get worse before they get better during a retraining phase.

Also, we know from many studies that when you think you have finally solved a problem, it will resurface sooner or later. This is called a '*response burst*', either because your child is testing to see if the rules still apply or because you have slipped a little regarding consistency in enforcing the rules or maintaining a healthy sleep pattern. Don't be dismayed. Stick to what worked and usually the problem will subside for good.

Refusal to Take Naps

Playtime in the park or shopping together is so much fun; who wants to take a nap? Ask yourself whether napping is your *child's* problem or *your* problem. Some parents simply find it too inconvenient to hang around the house to enable their child to get his needed daytime sleep. But reflect on how inconvenient it is to drag a tired child around while shopping.

Please review the first chapter of this book if you feel that naps are not that important.

Let's consider two common problems regarding naps: (a) resistance for one nap and (b) no naps.

Resistance for one nap: This often occurs after a special event, such as a holiday or party. There was so much excitement the day before, the children don't want to miss anything again! Sometimes this becomes apparent because of unappreciated chronic fatigue due to an abnormal sleep schedule, brief night-sleep duration or sleep fragmentation. If these problems are present, work on them as you work on day sleep.

The trick to solving the problem of resisting a nap is judging when your child is tired but not overly tired. This is usually after being up about three or four hours. If the interval is too short, the child may not be tired enough. If the interval is too long, she may be overtired and not able to fall asleep easily.

Keep a sleep chart, log or diary; pick a time interval that you think is right, and put your child down in the cot at that time. *You* are controlling the nap time. Spend however much time you want – ten, twenty or thirty minutes – hugging, kissing, rocking and nursing to soothe your child. Then down is down – leave him alone for one full hour.

If your child has been quite well rested up to now, the crying may be brief. But if your child has a history of chronic fatigue, prepare yourself for a full hour of crying. Here's one mother's account of how her fourteen-month-old daughter responded.

'She Woke in the Morning Smiling . . . We Were Reassured That She Loved Us'

My daughter was fourteen months old, ate poorly, resisted naps, woke two or three times in the night, needed to be rocked to sleep and was tired all the time. My husband and I were exhausted, angry, resentful and blaming each other for the situation we were in.

We were ambivalent, scared, concerned and sceptical about letting our daughter cry, as the treatment plan recommended. We thought she would feel unloved and worthless if no one responded to her.

After only one episode of crying, she learned how to lie down and fall asleep on her own! It was very difficult listening to her crying, but when she woke in the morning smiling and kissing us good morning, we were reassured that she loved us. Now she naps regularly, sleeps through the night, eats better, plays better and is able to play in her cot before going off to sleep on her own.

The more rested the child is, the sooner you'll see improvement. A very tired child might require several days of training before he relearns how to nap.

Your goal is to establish an age-appropriate nap routine so the child comes to associate being left alone in a certain place and a familiar soothing routine with feelings of being tired and taking a nap. No more playtime, no more games, just sleep. If the child is young, then every day at about 9:00 A.M. and 1:00 P.M. the parents should put their child down to nap; older children may be put down only in the afternoon. I call this 'nap structuring'; we are trying to use natural sleep rhythms to help the child sleep best. After one hour, if there is no nap, then we go to the next sleep period, but a little earlier.

Parents who would rather hold their child in a rocking chair or let her catnap in the pushchair are robbing their child of healthy sleep. This lighter, briefer, less regular sleep is less restorative – it's not as effective in returning your child's energy and attentiveness to its best levels.

No naps: If your child is a young two-year-old, you might simply establish a pattern as described under 'Resistance for one nap' and sticking with it, especially if the duration of not napping wasn't too long. But if you have an older two-year-old who hasn't napped for a long time or is very tired because of unhealthy sleep habits in general, try the methods described on page 313 for how to re-establish naps in the older child.

Q: *My problem is not that my child refuses to nap or resists naps, but that her nap schedule is very irregular. What's wrong?*
A: If your child is well rested, it may be that you are in fact very sensitive to her need to sleep and place her in an environment conducive to sleep when she needs it. Differences in daily activities produce differences in wakeful intervals and differences in the duration and timing of naps. Perhaps you have unrealistic expectations regarding the regularity of naps according to clock times. If your child is very tired, however, she might be crashing at irregular times when she is totally exhausted. A common problem here is a slightly too-late bedtime. Early bedtimes appear to regularise and lengthen naps.

Q: *My problem is that my baby takes such long naps that we don't have much time to play together. Are long naps a problem?*
A: There may be a problem if your child snores or mouth-breathes when asleep. These are symptoms of respiratory allergies or large adenoids or tonsils (see Chapter 10). Another possible problem is that the bedtime is too late and the long naps are attempts to compensate for the lost sleep. In the long run, this compensation will fail because the too-late bedtime causes cumulative sleep deficits.

Getting Up Too Early

Getting up too early is another major problem in toddlers. The first question to ask is: how early is too early? If your child gets up at 5:00 or 6:00 A.M. and is well rested, perhaps this pattern is not changeable. You may wish to try encouraging her to sleep later by making the room darker with opaque shades. Getting everyone together in a family bed at that hour may also allow all of you to get some more snooze time. Often families have established the habit of giving the baby a bottle at this early hour, after which she returns to sleep for a variable period of time.

While bottles given early in the morning may help the child return to sleep, be aware that if the baby is allowed to fall asleep with a bottle of milk, formula or juice in her mouth, the result is decayed teeth. This will not occur if the bottle contains only water. Unfortunately, many parents go to their child at 4:00 or 5:00 A.M. with a bottle of milk and then let the baby feed herself.

Treatment for the well-rested child who has the early-morning-bottle habit is to first switch to juice, and then gradually, over about a week, dilute the juice more and more, until it is only water. Once the child is drinking only water, place a water bottle at either end of the cot and point them out to her at bedtime.

One mother used to allow her child to watch a videotape every morning as soon as she woke up. This allowed the mother to have some free time to take care of herself. Her child woke up earlier and earlier in order to enjoy the videotape. Stopping the routine of watching videotapes in the morning was part of the solution.

If your child wakes up too early and is not well rested, work hard to establish a healthy sleep pattern. In the morning, don't go to her until the wake-up hour.

REMEMBER

Getting up too early may be caused by going to sleep too late. Earlier bedtimes often prolong night sleep and prevent early wake-ups.

For a three-year-old child, we can try a variation of controlling the wake-up hour using *stimulus control*. We previously used a timer as a signalling device at bedtime. Now we are going to use a digital clock. Place a digital clock in her room and set the alarm for 6:00 or 7:00 A.M., which may be *after* the expected spontaneous wake-up time. Draw a picture of the clock face showing 6:00 or 7:00 – the time that corresponds to when the alarm will go off. You do not respond to her cries before this wake-up time. Then, at the wake-up time *you* have picked, you bounce into her room, exclaim how the clock matches the picture, shower her with affection, open the curtains, turn on the lights, bring her into your bed or give a bath. Be dramatic, wide-eyed and happy to see her. Point out the numbers on the digital clock and on the picture of the clock and exclaim, 'Oh, see, it's time to start the day!' The child learns that the day's activities start at this time. The pattern on the digital clock acts as a cue, just as a green traffic light tells you to start moving. Before the wake-up time, the child has her water bottles but no parental attention.

Resistance to Falling Asleep/Night Waking

The last major problem centres on enforcing the bedtime hour and on waking at night. Time cues can also be used as stimulus control to enforce the bedtime hour. Use a digital clock and say, 'Oh, look, it's seven o'clock [say 'seven, zero, zero'], time for your bath.' After the bath, hugs, stories and kisses, say, 'It's now seven-thirty [seven, three, zero], time to go to sleep.' Then turn out the lights and close the door. No returning or peeking. The child learns that after a certain hour, no one will come to play with him, so he falls asleep and stays asleep until the morning. He learns to amuse himself with cot toys or other toys in his room until the wake-up time.

If your child has had a long history of resistance to falling asleep or of night waking, then read the earlier chapters and work on establishing a healthy sleep pattern in general. Prepare yourself for some long or frequent bouts of crying as you extinguish the habit. A fade procedure probably won't work if your child is chronically tired and has long-standing disturbed sleep; he'll outlast you. The following published account of a cold-turkey strategy in a twenty-one-month-old boy shows that it is effective, that the improvement occurs over several days and that the treatment has *no ill effects*. This account was published in a professional journal for psychologists, so please forgive the dry style of writing.

Case Report: The Elimination of Tantrum Behaviour

by Carl D. Williams

This paper reports the successful treatment of tyrant-like tantrum behaviour in a male child by the removal of reinforcement. The subject child was approximately twenty-one months old. He had been seriously ill much of the first eighteen months of his life. His health then improved considerably, and he gained weight and vigour. The child now demanded the special care and attention that had been given him over the many critical months. He enforced some of his wishes, especially at bedtime, by unleashing tantrum behaviour to control the actions of his parents.

The parents and an aunt took turns in putting him to bed both at night and for the child's afternoon nap. If the parent left the bedroom after putting the child in his bed, the child would scream and fuss until the parent returned to the room. As a result, the parent was unable to leave the bedroom until after the child went to sleep. If the parent began to read while in the bedroom, the child would cry until the reading material was put down. The parents felt that the child enjoyed his control over them and that he fought off going to sleep as long as he could. In any event, a parent was spending from one half to two hours each bedtime just waiting in the bedroom until the child went to sleep.

Following medical reassurance regarding the child's physical condition, it was decided to remove the reinforcement of this tyrant-like tantrum behaviour. Consistent with the learning principle that, in general, behaviour that is not reinforced will be extinguished, a parent or the aunt put the child to bed in a leisurely and relaxed fashion. After bedtime pleasantries, the parent left the bedroom and closed the door. The child screamed and raged, but the parent did not re-enter the room. The duration of screaming and crying was measured from the time the door was closed.

The child continued screaming for forty-five minutes the first time he was put to bed. The child did not cry at all the second time he was put to bed. This is perhaps attributable to his fatigue from crying.

By the tenth occasion, the child no longer whimpered, fussed or cried when the parent left the room. Rather, he smiled as they left. The parents felt that he made happy sounds until he dropped off to sleep.

About a week later, the child screamed and fussed after the aunt put him to bed, probably reflecting spontaneous recovery of the tantrum behaviour by returning to the child's bedroom and remaining there until he went to sleep. It was necessary to extinguish this behaviour a second time.

No further tantrums at bedtime were reported during the next two years.

It should be emphasised that the treatment in this case did not involve aversive punishment. All that was done was to remove the reinforcement. Extinction of the tyrant-like tantrum behaviour then occurred.

No unfortunate side- or after-effects of this treatment were observed. At three and three-quarters years of age, the child appears to be a friendly, expressive, outgoing child.

Q: *Does this mean that after my baby falls asleep I can never peek, never go in to soothe or comfort him?*
A: No. Only during the period when you are establishing a new sleep pattern is it important to avoid reinforcement. After your child is sleeping better and becomes well rested, there is nothing wrong with going in to check on him at night.

Q: *I took his older brothers out of their bedroom so his crying wouldn't disturb them. When can they go back into their old bedroom?*
A: Allow several days or a couple of weeks to pass before making changes. The more rested the baby becomes, the more flexible and adaptable he will be. Changes then will be less disruptive.

Q: *My two-and-a-half-year-old son understands what I'm saying; why can't I discuss these problems with him?*
A: You want to avoid discussions or lectures at the time the problem is taking place because your reasoning calls attention to the problem and thus reinforces it. Instead, choose some

low-key playtime to voice your concerns regarding his lack of cooperation. But when there *is* some cooperation, make sure to praise the *specific behaviour*: 'Thank you for staying in bed' or 'Thank you for trying to sleep'. Praising the child ('Thank you for being a good boy') does not tell him exactly what it is that you want him to do again.

Q: *My fifteen-month-old child shows separation anxiety during the day, and at night she wants me to hold her and sit with her on the sofa until she falls asleep. How can I leave her alone at bedtime, when she is most anxious?*

A: Separation anxiety, stubbornness or simply exhibiting a preference for parents' company over a dark, boring room might separately or in combination cause your child to behave this way. Please understand that it is normal for children to feel some anxiety and learning to deal with anxiety and not be overwhelmed by it is a healthy learning process. Let's not use separation anxiety as an excuse for our own problems in dealing with a child's natural disinclination to cooperate at bedtime.

If there has been long-standing ambivalence or inconsistency regarding putting your child to bed at night, then the naturally occurring separation anxiety will only aggravate or magnify the problem. The same could be said of the naturally occurring fears of darkness, death or monsters that children often express around age four. In order to deal with separation anxiety or fears at night, we must understand that all children experience them, and that they can learn not to be overwhelmed by them at the bedtime hour with the help of the consistent, calm resolve of their parents. The routine of a set pattern in a bedtime ritual reassures the child that there is an orderly sequence: Sleep will come, night will end, the sun will shine again and parents will still be there, smiling.

Some children go to bed later than I recommend and get up later in the morning. This may fit the parents' lifestyle and they might not appreciate that this is not healthy for their child. One recent study examined children at eighteen months and again at three years and noted that those children who went to bed at a late hour not only woke up late in the morning, but they also had longer naps compared to those children who went to bed earlier. However, neither the late wake-up time nor the longer nap compensated for the reduced sleep time caused by the late bedtime. In other words, late bedtimes cause less sleep. In addition, sleeping out of phase with your natural rhythms, like shift workers or when crossing time zones, is as unhealthy as jet-lag syndrome.

PRACTICAL POINT

Don't hide behind excuses; there will always be one handy! Some families use extreme fussiness/colic (birth to six months), teething (six to twelve months), separation anxiety (twelve to twenty-four months), 'terrible twos' (twenty-four to thirty-six months) and fears (thirty-six to forty-eight months), one after another, to 'explain' why their child wakes up at night and has trouble returning to sleep by himself.

Summary

Previously, the terms *sleep/wake organisation* (duration and time of occurrence of the sleep period) and *sleep quality* (consolidated or fragmented sleep and the duration of different stages of sleep) were introduced. Now add two more terms to the vocabulary. *Temporal control* means establishing age-appropriate sleep/wake schedules. In other words, the time when you do your soothing to sleep coincides with the naturally occurring biological rhythms of sleep. *Stimulus control* means that you are trying to avoid behaviours that disrupt sleep or are incompatible with sleep and promote behaviours that allow the sleep process to surface both at sleep onset and throughout the night.

Action Plan for Exhausted Parents

Months Thirteen to Fifteen: 1 per cent have three naps, 43 per cent have two naps, 56 per cent have one nap

- Earlier bedtimes usually help the child get through the transition to a single afternoon nap.

Months Sixteen to Twenty-one: 23 per cent have two naps, 77 per cent have one nap at eighteen months; 12 per cent have two naps, 88 per cent have one nap at twenty-one months

- If you have only a morning nap, try to delay its onset by shifting it slowly towards midday. Try a ten- to twenty-minute delay every few days.

Months Twenty-two to Thirty-six: 5 per cent have two naps, and 95 per cent have one nap at twenty-four months; 0 per cent have two naps, 91 per cent have one nap, and 9 per cent have no naps at thirty-six months

- If your child refuses to nap but still needs to nap, experiment with earlier or later bedtimes to help him get more rest.
- If your child climbs out of his cot, practise a 'silent return to sleep' (see page 320), whereby you always promptly return him to the cot without any talking. If this fails, consider buying a crib tent (see page 323).
- Around age three, consider sleep rules (see page 325) to help keep your child in his cot or bed.
- If your child gets up too early, use a digital clock to provide a visual cue that signals the start of the day.
- If your child has fears, spend extra time soothing to sleep and return once during the night for reassurance; use a timer to control the duration of the middle-of-the-night soothing.

CHAPTER 8

Preschool Children

Most children between three and six years of age, according to my survey, still go to sleep between 7:00 and 9:00 P.M. and awaken between 6:30 and 8:00 A.M. As previously discussed, I think these bedtimes are too late for many children. Going to bed too late may cause bedtime battles, night waking or early morning wake-ups, or it may mess up the nap schedule. One mother described her son as turning into a 'total monster' at 4:00 P.M. every day because he was going to bed too late, waking up tired and taking a morning nap, which prevented an afternoon nap and so caused cumulative sleepiness by late afternoon. Another mother described her child's new early bedtime as 'a rescue manoeuvre to get back the old good pattern he fell out of'.

Years Three to Six: Naps Disappear

On their third birthday, most children (91 per cent) are still napping every day. At age four, about 50 per cent of children nap five days each week, and by age five, about 25 per cent of children are napping about four days each week. Naps are usually gone by age six unless it is the family custom to nap at weekends. In Japan, it is customary to have naps in nursery school, and in one study of 441 children three to six years of age, the naps caused the children to go to sleep later at night. Between ages three and four, the length of the nap varies between one and three hours, and between ages five and six the length is one or two hours. Normally, naps gradually decrease in duration; some parents try to eliminate the nap in order to enable their children to participate in organised activities. This may or may not be a problem, depending on the child's sleep needs and the remainder of the sleep schedule. For example, some children might seem to need a nap but the nap makes it difficult for them to fall asleep even when tired in the evening. If the parents eliminate the nap and the child goes to bed extra early and/or sleeps extra late in the morning, then there might not be any problems. This flexibility is mainly apparent in children who have been good sleepers in the past; serious sleep problems and disturbed sleep usually do not develop in these children.

Major problems, however, occur when parents push their children too soon into too many preschool, nursery school, or other scheduled activities. The children are overprogrammed, and naps get scheduled out before the child is ready.

> **PRACTICAL POINT**
>
> **A missed nap is sleep lost forever.**

Some parents provide partial compensation for their children's increased mental and physical stimulation by shifting bedtime to an earlier hour. Working parents may not accept this solution, because it reduces their playtime with their children. When you sign your child up for courses, classes or activities, another solution to prevent sleep deficits is simply to enforce a policy of 'declared holidays': once or twice a week the child stays home and naps, or he engages in less-structured, low-intensity, quieter activities.

The Sleep-Temperament Connection

I studied a group of sixty children when they were about four months old and again when they were three years old. At both ages, children with easy-to-manage temperaments slept longer than children with difficult-to-manage temperaments. Easier children were more regular, approaching, adaptable, mild, and positive in mood than the more difficult children. Which came first, the temperament traits or the sleep?

I don't think sleep habits, temperament and fussing or crying are independent; rather, I believe they are all interrelated. However, we name and measure items such as sleep duration, temperament traits or fussiness in the same way we might describe different features of a rose: its colour, its smell, or its texture. But the rose is still a rose and a baby is still a baby; even though we give names to different features, none of them could exist without the whole.

It seems to me that after about four months of age, parenting practices such as loving attention during wakeful periods and encouraging good-quality sleep during sleep times can modulate or influence those features we call temperament. For example, easy infants who stayed easy slept a total of 12.4 hours (day and night sleep combined), but those easy infants who became more difficult slept less, 11.8 hours. So to help keep easy infants easy when they arrive at toddlerhood, protect their sleep.

What about those difficult infants? Some of them remained difficult and slept only 11.4 hours, but others became easy and slept 12.0 hours. I think part of the reason why these difficult infants mellowed into easy three-year-olds is because they were handled in a more structured and regular fashion, learning more social rules and becoming better rested.

Adaptability, which is the ease with which children adjust to new circumstances, was the only trait that showed individual stability over the three-year study. But this does not mean that a fussy baby will always have a fussy personality. Temperament traits are not like fingerprints, which are completely biologically based, unchanging over time and unique identifiers. Temperament traits are more like hair. Our hair has a biological basis, but it changes over time; texture, length, curliness and colour can change naturally or at our will. How we care for our hair affects its health and appearance. And how we care for our children, including how we care for their sleep, influences temperament.

You shouldn't be surprised if your colicky three-month-old has a difficult temperament at four months, but this doesn't predict anything for the future, not even for five months. A fussy nature may persist when colic and parental mismanagement cause enduring post-colic sleep deprivation, and it may improve when the child develops healthier sleep habits. You cannot change the fundamental personality of your child, but you can modulate it.

Evidence that social learning, temperament and sleep habits go together comes from my nap study. Among the children I studied were three between the ages of two and three who stopped napping during a period of marital discord or problems with carers. And when they stopped napping, they underwent what looked like a personality transplant! Fatigue masked their sweet temperaments. But after resolution of the conflicts, all three resumed napping and continued to nap for years. The resumption of napping restored their original or 'natural' temperament.

Re-establishing naps will be discussed later. But it is noteworthy that stressful events that tend to disorganise home routines, such as the death of a parent, divorce, a move to a new home, the birth of twin siblings, or the death of a sibling, did not cause any napping problems in 90 per cent of the children during the study. It appears that when parents and carers maintain nap routines, children continue to nap, despite disruptive and stressful events.

After the publications of my original discovery on the association between sleep patterns and temperament – in infants in 1981 and in toddlers in 1984 – many other studies in preschool children confirmed my findings. In adults, sleep loss has been shown to affect mood more than cognitive or motor performance; we all get a bit irritable when we are tired, but we can still learn and perform reasonably well. For children it may be a different story, because the developing brain may be more sensitive to sleep loss than the mature brain. Evidence to support this suggestion comes from animal studies, which have shown that less light was needed to affect the sleeping and behaviour of young animals. In other words, the developing brain may suffer more, and in more ways, than the adult brain from the harmful effects of insufficient sleep.

Q: *Is it ever too late to see benefits from better sleep quality?*
A: No. It is never too late to help *healthy* children sleep better. In addition, some neurologically impaired children can be helped to have fewer seizures by becoming better rested. Other children have neurological diseases or medicine requirements, which directly disrupt sleep. And finally, recent research suggests that children who have been so severely traumatised by abuse or neglect beginning in infancy might not respond to ordinary sleep training like healthy children.

The Sleep-Behavior Connection

Many research studies have shown more daytime behavioural problems in preschoolers who are poor sleepers. In particular, 'externalising' problems such as aggression, defiance, noncompliance, oppositional behaviour, acting out and hyperactivity were associated with less sleep. When parents listed the types of daytime behaviour problems their children were expressing, it became apparent that the less sleep they had, the longer the list! (There was no association between sleep and 'internalising' problems such as anxiety or depression.)

So sleep duration is clearly a factor associated with behaviour problems. Still, we do not have absolute scientific proof on whether (1) less sleep directly causes daytime behaviour problems, (2) parenting or biological forces cause both the daytime behaviour and night-time sleep problems, or (3) daytime problems cause the night-time problems. However, recent research by Dr John Bates on 202 four- to five-year-olds shows that sleep does have a direct effect on daytime behaviour in children, in support of the first theory. My impression is that parents who are somewhat regular, consistent and structured –

in terms of both meeting the child's need to sleep and helping the child learn social rules – enable the child to have fewer behaviour problems. In contrast, circumstances such as a parent who works late and keeps the child up too late in order spend time with her produce an overtired child; then behavioural problems will be more frequent.

Another study of preschool children noted that the poor sleepers who had more behavioural problems did not get up more frequently than good sleepers, but that the poor sleepers were unable to soothe themselves back to sleep unassisted. They always disturbed their parents' sleep. I think the ability to return to sleep unassisted to avoid fragmented sleep (and to avoid upsetting parents!) is learned behaviour. So, in addition to longer sleep, consolidated sleep helps avoid behaviour problems.

Regular bedtimes also seem to be important, maybe even when the total amount of sleep is not quite enough. There were fewer school adjustment problems in one study where a regular bedtime was maintained by the parents. Although it is possible that better parenting practices might have caused both a more regular bedtime and a better adjustment to school, the researchers studied the families and concluded that there was a more direct link between sleep patterns and school adjustment. Again, we have the same conclusion: better sleep quality produces fewer daytime problems. (More about regularity of sleep times later.)

New research on five- and six-year-old children in Japan and Germany has shown a connection between short sleeping hours and *obesity*. In the Japanese study, the later the bedtime, the greater the risk for obesity. In both studies, the shorter the duration of sleep, the more likely the children were obese. The researchers controlled for many of the variables, such as parental obesity, physical inactivity, long hours watching TV and so forth. Maybe these overtired children felt stressed and dealt with it by eating. We know that American society is becoming more overweight; maybe our modern lifestyle is causing us to become more overtired.

Preventing and Solving Sleep Problems

Three-year-olds may no longer have tantrum behaviours, but they may call parents back many times and clearly express their feelings of love for their parents or fears of the dark.

Here are some simple ways to help your child settle down for day or night sleep. Consider them to be a sleeping routine for preschool children. Choose from this list those items that work best for your child and do them at all sleep times.

- **Slow down activity**
- **Close physical contact**
  - **Gentle massage or mild stretching**
  - **Cuddle up with the child in a chair**
  - **Nestle or snuggle in her bed**
- **Quiet voices**
  - **Imagine a fun event**
  - **Tell a story, talk about your family**
  - **Read a book**
  - **Sing or hum a song**
  - **Chat about the day**
  - **Say goodnight to everyone and everything in the room**
  - **Play a favourite tape, maybe grandparents singing or saying goodnight, sounds of nature**
- **Comfortable room**
  - **Photos of family and pets**
  - **Favourite stuffed animals or dolls**
  - **Night-light or torch**
  - **Fairy or guardian angel for protection**

Four-year-olds might be helped to sleep better if you try the following:

- **Make a schedule and post it in his room: time for bath, time for sleep routine, lights off. (Regularity helps but the times might include a range because not all days are the same.)**

Try to engage or enlist cooperation by doing something together such as singing, reading out loud or doing artwork.

During the day, you might only request a quiet time of one hour or so. Please don't think that it is all right to have a late bedtime, or late wake-up time, and a regular nap. In a recent study of 1,105 three-year-old Japanese children, it was observed that half fell asleep at 10:00 P.M. or later. For all children, the later they went to sleep, the later they woke up in the morning and the longer they napped. However, the later bedtime was associated with less total sleep compared to those with an earlier bedtime. The later wake-up time and longer nap did not compensate for the later bedtime. Let's look at the problems that may occur with night- and daytime sleep habits and some of the strategies we can use to deal with them.

Night Sleep

Here's one mother's account of how hard it was to ignore her three-year-old at night.

'Mum, I Need a Hug and Kiss Good Night'

My daughter Chelsea is almost three years old. Putting her to bed has always been an ordeal. At eighteen months of age she started to climb out of her cot anywhere from seventy-five to a hundred times a night. The problem seemed to be solved with the advent of a 'big bed'. She now sleeps through the night. However, having her stay in bed and fall asleep is still an ordeal.

I have yelled and screamed. I have used gates and locks on her door to physically keep her in her room. I have used treats as an incentive for positive reinforcement of desired behaviour. Unfortunately, the only consistent behaviour has been my inconsistency.

If Chelsea knows that I will put a gate on her bedroom door if she leaves her room, even once, then she will gradually conform and stay in her room. But there is a catch! She eventually will start to challenge my inconsistent behaviour. One night she will appear in the living room and say, 'Mum, I need a hug and kiss good night.' As a parent, do you deny your child such a loving request and lock her in her room? So you give her a hug and kiss and send her off to bed again. Then the next night she wants water, and before long she's out of bed three or four times a night for hugs and kisses, water, Band-Aids, scary noises – you name it! Within a week, saying goodnight and falling asleep takes an hour or more. Then we have to start all over again.

My dictionary defines the word *consistent* as 'free from self-contradiction; in harmony with'. I long for the night when I'm in harmony with Chelsea.

As this mother said, 'Unfortunately, the only consistent behaviour has been my inconsistency.' In other words, when a behavioural approach fails with older children, it almost always is not a failure of the method, but rather a failure of the resolve of the parents to implement it.

In an English study of children about three years of age, psychiatrists examined children who displayed difficulty in going to bed, night waking, or both. Parents were counselled to keep a sleep diary for a week and establish goals for the child that included sleeping in his own bed, remaining in his bed throughout the night and not disturbing his parents during the night. The treatment consisted of identifying the factors that reinforced the child's sleep problem and then gradually withdrawing them or temporarily substituting less potent rewards. It was a 'fade' strategy, not a 'cold-turkey' approach.

Here's an example of how subjects gradually reduced reinforcement: (1) father reads story to child in bed for fifteen minutes; (2) father reads newspaper in child's bedroom until child falls asleep; (3) child is placed back in bed with minimal interaction; and (4) father gradually withdraws from bedroom before child is asleep.

Another example: (1) parents alternate, but respond to child; (2) parent gives no drinks but provides holding and comforting until crying stops; (3) parent only sits by the bedside until child is asleep; and (4) parent provides less physical contact at bedtime.

PRACTICAL POINT

At every stage of reduction of parental attention, expect the problem to get worse before improvement begins. That's because the child will put out extra effort to cling to the old style.

In the English study, 84 per cent of the children improved. Not surprisingly, the two factors that most likely predicted success were both parental: the absence of marital discord and the attendance of both parents at the consultation sessions. Also, when one problem – such as resistance in going to sleep – was reduced or resolved, other problems – such as night waking – rapidly disappeared. And although half of the mothers in this study had current psychiatric problems requiring treatment, this did *not* make failure more likely.

I think this study points out the importance of working with professionals who can provide guidance that is directed towards changing the child's behaviour without dwelling on current psychological/emotional problems within the mother or father. The exception, of course, is when these problems are directly related to marital discord or the parents' ability to maintain a behavioural management programme.

Another study from England included children who took at least an hour to go to bed, who woke at least three times a night or for more than twenty minutes at a time, or who went into their parents' bed. Treatment started with the parents recording the present sleep pattern in a sleep diary. A therapist worked with the parents to develop a programme of treatment based on gradually reducing or removing parental attention, adding positive reinforcement for the desired behaviour, making bedtime earlier and developing a bedtime ritual. Target behaviours were identified, and an individual treatment programme was developed for each child. Also, mothers were evaluated for psychiatric problems. Mothers who showed psychiatric problems were more likely to terminate treatment, which again points out how stressful treatment can be. But for those families who completed four or five treatment sessions, 90 per cent showed improvement. The authors concluded:

> The evidence that children's night-time behaviour could thus change so radically, often within a surprisingly short time, suggests that parental responses were extremely important in maintaining waking behaviour. . . . A rapid achievement of improved sleep pattern with reduced parental attention would be unlikely if anxiety in the child or *lack* of parental attention were causing the sleep difficulty . . . Parents needed help in analysing goal behaviour into graded steps so they could achieve successes. Once some success was obtained, the morale and confidence of the parents rose and they were reinforced in their determination to persist by the more peaceful nights.

MAJOR POINT

The rapid improvement of sleep patterns produced by reduced parental attention tells us that neither lack of parental attention nor anxiety in the child was causing the sleep difficulty.

I have seen this over and over again; when you see even partial improvement, you gain confidence and you no longer feel guilty or rejecting when you are firm with your child.

Often it appears that the child is listening to the treatment plan in the office, because they often sleep better that very night, as if they knew something was going to be different. I think they are responding to the calm resolve and firm but gentle manner in their parents, which tells them that things are going to be different.

Another sleep strategy appropriate for three-year-old or older children is called 'Day Correction of Bedtime Problems'. The idea here is that because everyone is tired and less able to cope with the stress of bedtime battles or night-waking problems at the end of the day, daytime behaviour should be tackled first. The following instructions explain this strategy in detail. Under item number 3, 'Relaxed', the author says, 'Perhaps the easiest way to teach self-quieting, during the day, is by allowing your child to self-quiet during naturally occurring times of frustration.' In my conversation with Dr Edward Christophersen, a prominent child psychologist, he clarified this statement by explaining that you do not always rush to help a child struggling with a puzzle or accomplishing some task. When there is something that is slightly bothering him, it is sometimes better to leave him alone to learn to deal with it. Dr Christophersen's observation is that some mothers need to be taught to disengage or ignore some of the child's low-level distress. He does not mean you should ignore your child when he comes home from school crying or has had a very frightening experience. In one study, when children learned how to cope with frustration during the day, they were observed to settle themselves better at bedtime and later at night when they awoke.

*Day Correction of Bedtime Problems**

There are three important components to getting a child to go to sleep at night. The child must be:

1. **Tired**
2. **Quiet**
3. **Relaxed**

When these three components are in place, children who have adequate 'self-quieting skills' will be able to go to sleep rather easily.

---

* From *Beyond Discipline: Parenting that Lasts a Lifetime*, 2nd ed., by E. R. Christophersen (Shawnee Mission, Kans.: Overland Press, 1998), pp. 127–128. Copyright 1998 by Edward R. Christophersen. Reprinted with permission.

1. Tired. The easiest way to make sure that your child will be tired when he or she goes to bed is by getting him or her up at the same time every day and by getting him or her an adequate amount of exercise during the day – vigorous exercise that requires a good deal of energy. For an infant include several long periods of time when he or she is on the floor and can see what you are doing, but the infant must hold his or her head up in order to really see much. For almost any child, twenty minutes of good exercise each day, after a nap, is usually adequate.

2. Quiet. You can elect either to quiet down the entire house or quiet down your child's room. Quieting down your child's room by closing the door and keeping it closed is probably the easiest. . . . You might need to turn on the furnace or fan as a masking noise for the first few nights.

3. Relaxed. Children can relax only if they have learned self-quieting skills. Self-quieting skills refer to a child's ability to calm himself or herself, with no help from an adult, when the child is unhappy, angry, or frustrated. Whereas older children (at least age six years) can be taught relaxation procedures, infants and toddlers need to practise self-quieting skills in order to know what works for them. Perhaps the easiest way to teach self-quieting during the day is by allowing your child to self-quiet during naturally occurring times of frustration.

Self-quieting behaviours. The baby who goes to sleep with help from one of his or her parents by nursing, rocking, or holding learns only adult transition skills and needs an adult present in order to fall asleep. The baby or toddler who goes to sleep alone cuddling a stuffed animal, holding his or her favourite blanket, or sucking his or her thumb learns valuable self-quieting skills that can be used for many years to come.

How they feel. Children who go to bed easily and sleep through the night uninterrupted get a good night's sleep. They will feel better during the day, just as the adults in their household will feel better during the day. It may take from several nights to one week to teach a child the skills he or she needs for going to sleep alone, but this is one behaviour that the child will be able to use for the rest of his or her life.

These three components described here have the added advantage that they can be taught during the day, which removes many of the fears parents have about handling behaviour problems at bedtime. Even parents who choose cosleeping can allow their infant or toddler the opportunity to fall asleep on their own, with the parent joining the child at the parents' regular time for retiring. In this way, the infant or toddler gets the perceived advantages of cosleeping and the known advantages of learning self-quieting skills.

* * *

Q: *How important are regular bedtimes?*
A: In general, the bedtime should reflect your child's needs. With decreasing naps and increasing physical activity, your child's night-sleep needs may increase. Therefore, the bedtime often needs to be earlier not later simply because he is older. To maintain orderly home routines such as meals and baths, you might want to keep the bedtime within a narrow range.

Dr John Bates's study on 204 four- to five-year-olds examined in great detail the home environment, behaviour at preschool and sleeping patterns. The researchers noted that the more variable bedtime, as well as the lateness of bedtime, predicted poor adjustment in preschool, even after considering the roles of family stress and family management/discipline practices. This study provides evidence that sleep problems directly cause behavioural problems in children at preschool. Other research suggests that when older children are overtired, they learn to bother their parents no longer, but instead, they bother their teachers.

Regularising the sleep/wake schedule has also been shown to reduce daytime sleepiness and promote long-lasting improvements in alertness for well-rested young adults. It appears that regularity itself improves the ability of sleep to reverse daytime drowsiness. But some children are so excited at the end of the day, they have trouble unwinding whether they are overtired or not. Hot lavender bubble baths (described in the next chapter) may help make the transition to sleep easier.

Some previously well-rested children who slip into a night-waking mode need only gentle reminders to return to sleep. My wife used to teach the 'dolphin game' to one of our sons. She would read a story about how the dolphin swims deep in the water but sometimes has to come up for air before returning to a deep swim. Then she told our son to pretend that he was a dolphin at night and that it was perfectly all right to come up from sleep, but that he had to go back by himself. It worked.

Some previously very overtired children are so unmanageable at night that the family resources are stretched to the limit. In such cases the idea of more extreme measures may come up.

Q: *Do I ever lock my child in her room?*
A: Let's say that you've already tried other sleep strategies, patient reasoning, threats and criticisms. You've wracked your brains for something that might work, but all methods have failed. Also, let's assume that you are not working with a therapist to reduce reinforcing behaviours gradually. What's left to be done? Maybe the answer is a stiff door hook that, when locked, holds the door in a slightly open position but prevents opening or completely closing. The door is held locked in a slightly open position to protect the child's fingers from a crush injury. Completely closing and locking the door may be an overwhelming degree of separation for either you or the child.

By doing this you establish the unambiguous message that leaving the room after a certain time is unacceptable. The child learns that you mean business. The usual result is that after a night or two the child negotiates to stay in bed, and does, even if you do not lock the door. Also, you avoid the repeated prolonged stresses of your trying physically to separate from a child who is clinging to you, or of trying to pull the door closed while your child is in the room trying to pull the door open.

Take your child with you to the shop when you purchase the lock, and make your child watch you install the lock on the door. Often this observation alone will cause a change in your child's behaviour. In fact, for many families who once had a well-rested child, they never actually had to use the lock, because the child knew on the first night that this was the beginning of a new routine.

Simply locking the door solves nothing if your child is going to bed too late, getting up too late, not getting the nap he needs, taking a nap too late in the afternoon, having a very irregular bedtime or talking to you through the closed door. You will still have an overtired child. No quick fix, whether a locked door, or, worse, drugs to make your child sleep, will make an overtired child less tired.

Sleep rules, as described on page 325, are often helpful. Rewards are frequently used to encourage the child to cooperate. They must be items the child really wants. One mother rewarded cooperation by placing a sweet under a special doll after her child had gone to sleep; part of the motivation was the excitement of discovery in the morning when the child looked for her treat. Paper stars on a chart may be used, but by themselves might not be sufficiently motivating. One strategy that often works is withholding a favourite wholesome food and giving it only as reward for cooperation. Other rewards might be small toys, surprise trips or wholesome snack foods. By using a timer, you can give measured amounts of extra time for games, stories, TV or free play as rewards. As the new behaviour becomes a habit, the expectation of a specific reward is usually forgotten and the child's heightened self-esteem seems to substitute for the pleasure of the reward.

Now, let us consider the fifth sleep rule for the older children.

This rule is for older children who like to get up too early, leave their room and bother their brother, sister or parents. Set a clock radio, a CD player on a timer or an alarm clock – placed under a pillow

SLEEP RULE No. 5

Do not leave your room until you hear the music (or the birds, or the alarm).

to muffle the loud noise – to the time it is all right for your child to leave her room. Some children who have never slept well and have just turned three might completely disregard all five sleep rules and trash their room or simply stay up late playing in their room with the lights on. These children might have to be placed in a cot with a crib tent for a while, or maybe the light bulbs have to be removed to keep the room dark.

Q: *Why can't I just keep my child up later at night to see if he will sleep in later in the morning?*
A: If your child has been well rested up to now, then slowly try a later bedtime. If you move it too late, he might just become more overtired and have difficulty falling asleep and staying asleep in the morning. If your child has always been a problem sleeper and overtired, a later bedtime will only make matters worse.

Q: *My child is scared at night and I don't want to leave her alone.*
A: Try to spend extra time soothing her to sleep, buy a fairy or guardian angel to protect her, or go around the room catching all the monsters and put them in a bag that you take out of the room. Maybe give her a bell that she can ring once at night when she is scared, and you then respond promptly and use a timer for a measured amount of middle-of-the-night soothing. This could be a *sixth sleep rule*: if you are scared, ring the bell and I will come, but I will come only once. Tell her not to abuse ringing the bell. Ringing the bell many times would violate the sleep rule.

PRACTICAL POINT

Always reward even partial cooperation: small rewards for small efforts, bigger rewards for more cooperation. Rewards are best given in the morning after awakening or immediately following a nap.

Day Sleep

You may conclude that life is impossible if your child does not take a nap, but it is also impossible to get him to nap. You've worked at sleep schedules, night wakings and resistance to sleep, and things *are* better, but he also really needs a nap. Not necessarily a long one, but no nap at all is no good.

Some parents have successfully re-established naps as a routine even when the naps have been absent or sporadic for several months. The method involves taking a nap with your child (at least initially): Take her into your own bed, dress yourself for sleep and nap together. The idea is to make this a very comforting, soothing event. Try to be fairly regular according to clock time. Use a digital clock as a cue, and be consistent with the routine of biscuits and a glass of warm milk or reading from a favourite book. Try to fall asleep yourself.

Tell your child what is expected of him. If he sleeps with you, then A occurs; if he rests quietly next to you but doesn't fall asleep, then B occurs. You decide what kind of reward A and B will be. If he doesn't cooperate at all and jumps on the bed or runs around the room, then you might restrict or withdraw some pleasurable activity or privilege. If you are able to get him to nap with you, then eventually you'll want to try to shift him into his own room for a nap. This should be done in a graded or staged fashion. You might decide that the next step is for the child to be in his bed and you're in the room resting as long as needed. Rewards are now given *only* for this new behaviour. This process of reinforcing successive approximations to the desired target behaviour is called 'shaping'.

Preschool children who slept well when they were younger might develop problems because too many activities interfere with napping or, as discussed in Chapter 10, because allergies interfere with sleep at night. Reorganising daytime activities or managing allergies may provide a rapid solution. On the other hand, preschool children who have not previously slept well may have ingrained habits or expectations that are not easily changed. Parents should seriously consider working with a professional if they think their child is so tired that he might not do well in school.

One recent study of 499 children from ages four to fifteen showed that sleep problems at age four years predicted behavioural and emotional problems, such as depression and anxiety, in adolescence. So, although your older overtired child may not bother you as much as he did when he was younger, that does not mean that the problem has gone away.

No Apparent Solution

Parents with older children have more scheduled activities to attend and they are more likely to have more than one child requiring attention. What happens if the parent is a shift worker, or works in a bakery or restaurant, or travels a lot for her job, or has irregular hours built into the job like some physicians? It is hard to be with your children when they participate in an important scheduled school or sports event. I have met some mothers and fathers who are absolutely dedicated to their children and try very hard to strike a balance between the time requirements of child care and their work outside the home. Usually there is a sharing of responsibilities regarding putting the children to sleep at night. However, what do you do if both parents have work schedules that make it difficult to be home reasonably early at night for bedtimes? To further complicate matters, one parent alone cannot easily manage different bedtimes for two or more children. To make it even more of a problem, what if the parents are blinded by their love for their children and cannot see that the late afternoon tiredness, headaches or developing academic problems are connected to unrelenting mild sleep deprivation in their child? For some parents, it appears impossible to change his or her lifestyle or work schedule in order for their children to have a reasonably early bedtime. When the children were much younger, as infants and preschoolers, morning times were available to enjoy being together as a family, but now mornings are a frantic blur trying to get ready for out-of-the-house activities. So the night is the only quiet and relaxed time the family has together. These factors converge into a too-late bedtime. The solution is apparent, but not easy.

Action Plan for Exhausted Parents

- Naps begin to disappear after the third birthday. Some children are so busy during the day, they need a slightly earlier bedtime. Be careful to not overschedule activities.
- Day correction of bedtime behaviour (page 349). For example: your son is on the floor in the family room playing with blocks. He is a little frustrated with stacking and becomes agitated or upset. You are pretty certain that he can accomplish this by himself. You ignore his distress. You pick the easiest situations to ignore and ignore them first. The older your child is the harder this will be. Do not ignore your child if he is scared by a dog or returns home from school crying.
- Review sleep rule 5 (see page 353) to reward your child for staying in his room until a certain time in the morning.
- Review shaping (see page 355).
- Sleep will improve your child's mood, behaviour and performance, don't sell it short. If the bedtime is always too late, do the best you can to make it regular.
- It is far better to lock the door at night than it is to get angry at and possibly harm your child.

CHAPTER 9

Schoolchildren and Adolescence

The list of new concerns for older children is long: school assignments, organised after-school activities, individual lessons, parties, more homework, dating, driving cars, drugs, and alcohol. Health habits may appear to be less important to parents than the development of children's academic, social, athletic, or artistic skills. But as you will see, the contribution of healthy sleep habits to a child's well-being does not diminish with age.

Years Seven to Twelve: Bedtime Becomes Later

School-age children are sleeping less and less as the bedtime hour gradually becomes later and later. Most twelve-year-olds go to sleep around 9:00 P.M.; the range is from about 7:30 to 10:00. The range for total sleep duration for most twelve-year-olds is about nine to twelve hours. These data, from a large survey I performed of middle-class families, are in close agreement with the data from an ongoing study at Stanford University. Researchers there have shown that the prepubertal teenager needs nine and a half to ten hours of sleep in order to maintain optimal alertness during the day.

If healthy sleep habits are not maintained, the result is increasingly severe daytime sleepiness.

Difficulty Falling Asleep

In one survey of about 1,000 children, where the average age was between seven and eight years, about 30 per cent of the children resisted going to bed at least three nights per week. This was the most common sleep complaint of the parents. About 10 per cent of the children had difficulty falling asleep once they were in their beds. Many took up to an hour to fall asleep on more than three nights per week. Some children both resisted going to bed and had difficulty falling asleep, and these children had a host of other problems: fears, anxiety, night wakings, need for reassurance, closeness of parents, complaints of fatigue and a *history of difficulties of not being able to successfully self-soothe.*

PRACTICAL POINT

As your preteen grows older, he will need *more* sleep, not less, to maintain optimal alertness.

If your child resists bedtime and does not have difficulty falling asleep, then treatments such as an earlier or more regular bedtime and the other strategies described later in this chapter and in previous chapters are likely to help. But if your child also has difficulty falling asleep, has never slept well and exhibits chronic mild anxiety-related symptoms, then consulting a child psychologist or other mental health professional may be needed.

This study also confirmed other observations that night wakings in early childhood tend to persist. Persistence of sleeping problems is a theme in many reports, and it is only ignorance among some professionals that leads to the advice 'Don't worry, he'll outgrow the problem.'

Two other sleep surveys of about 1,000 pre-adolescents, one each from Belgium and Taiwan, show additional findings. School achievement difficulties were encountered significantly more often among poor sleepers compared to good sleepers. For those children on a college path, the more academic pressure they felt, the fewer the hours slept. So it's a global concern: young children who have difficulty sleeping become older children with more academic problems. But children who are academically successful risk not getting the sleep they need!

Recurrent Complaints

Many children in this age range complain of aches and pains for which no medical cause can be found: abdominal pains, limb pains, recurrent headaches and chest pains. Children who suffer from these pains often have significant sleep disturbances. Stressful emotional situations thought to cause these complaints include real or imagined separation of or from parents; fear of expressing anger that might elicit punishment or rejection; social or academic pressures; or fear of failing to live up to parents' expectations.

These are real pains in our children, just as real as the tension headaches adults get when they work too hard or sleep too little. All laboratory tests or studies during these episodes of tension headache will have normal results. All tests will also show normal results in children who have similar somatic complaints. Unless there is a strong clinical sign pointing towards organic disease, performing laboratory tests to rule out obscure diseases should be discouraged, because of the pain of drawing blood, the risks of irradiation, the expense and, most important, because of the possible result of creating in the child's mind the notion that he is sick. Also, a slightly abnormal test result might lead to more and more tests, all of which, in the end, are likely to show basically normal results.

Adolescence: Not Enough Time to Sleep, Especially in the Morning

Surveys of the sleep habits of teenagers show that the gradual decline in total hours of sleep flattens out around age thirteen or fourteen. In fact, many fourteen- to sixteen-year-olds now actually require more sleep! Research has shown that most teenagers would probably be much better rested if they were allowed to sleep longer in the morning. Starting school or sports early in the morning often causes teenagers to have to nap in the afternoon, which interferes with going to bed at a reasonable time.

In a study of about ten thousand Japanese junior high and high school students, 50 per cent napped after school at least once a week. Because the late naps made the bedtime later, the result was shorter sleep at night. This probably caused less sleep overall. My impression is that it would be better not to nap, to go to bed earlier, and wake up much earlier to do the unfinished homework. I think doing homework late at night, after a brief nap, is much more inefficient than very early in the morning after many hours of sleep.

PRACTICAL POINT

Many teenagers over age fifteen require more sleep than in previous years to maintain optimal daytime alertness.

Excessive tiredness, daytime sleepiness or decreased daytime alertness develops in many adolescents – there simply are not enough hours in the day to do everything. The time demands for academics, athletics and social activities are enormous. Even without worrying about sex, drugs, alcohol and loud music, parents worry that their teenagers may become burned out from lack of sleep.

PRACTICAL POINT

Social pressures and early start times for schools cause reduced sleep times and chronic sleep deficits.

Chronic sleep deficits were observed in 13 per cent of teenagers in a Stanford University study that included over 600 high school students. These poor sleepers attributed their sleep problems to worry, tension and personal, family, and social problems. The students appeared to be mildly depressed. Of course, we don't know which came first, disturbed sleep or the mood changes. Perhaps both the mood changes and the sleep disturbance develop from the same endocrine changes that occur naturally during adolescence. But healthy lifestyle habits, including sensible sleep patterns, might prevent or lighten the depression seen in so many adolescents. Here's how the Stanford sleep researchers defined chronic and severe sleep disturbances in adolescents:

1. **Forty-five or more minutes required to fall asleep on three or more nights a week**

or

2. **One or more awakenings a night followed by thirty or more minutes of wakefulness occurring on three or more nights a week**

or

3. **Three or more awakenings a night on three or more nights a week**

So, if your teenager has this kind of sleep pattern, don't consider it a 'normal' part of growing up.

In New Zealand, as in California, about 10 per cent of teenagers had sleep problems. They appeared anxious, depressed and inattentive, and they had conduct disorders more often than those without sleep problems. Anxiety and depression were also common symptoms of poorly sleeping teenagers in Italy, where about 17 per cent of all teens met research criteria for sleep problems.

Solid research, published in 1991, has documented that students' sleep time has decreased one hour over the past twenty years. The evidence is clear, whether it's from Belgium,

Taiwan, China, South Africa, New Zealand, or Italy, that teenagers are increasingly at risk for becoming overtired.

In two separate studies of sleep restriction in children ten to fourteen years of age, the researchers either limited the night sleep to seven hours for three days or five hours for a single night. Although routine performance was maintained, higher cognitive functions such as verbal creativity and abstract thinking were impaired. This highlights an important point, that our children can and do perform quite well even when mildly sleep-deprived as long as they are not too challenged academically to write or be creative.

Thus, mild sleep deprivation is often trivialised or overlooked because more routine memorisation tasks and athletic performances are successfully accomplished.

Another experimental sleep restriction study was performed on eleven- and twelve-year-olds. Comparisons were made between sleeping ten hours on six nights versus six and a half hours on six nights. The sleep restriction caused measured inattentiveness, irritability, noncompliance and academic problems. A separate survey study of 3,136 children between ages eleven and seventeen showed that 17 per cent were having non-restorative sleep just as in the Italian study.

In Israel, starting times in school were examined in children ten to twelve years of age. One group started at 7:10 A.M. at least two times a week and the other group always started school at 8:00 A.M. The children in the early start time group had less total sleep, more daytime fatigue and sleepiness, and complained more about difficulties in attention and concentration compared to the later start time group. Dr Mary Carskadon, a pioneer in adolescent sleep research, points out that earlier start times for school is a fairly recent development and its impact on sleep deprivation for older children is only now being appreciated.

Dr Carskadon had also identified *irregular sleep times* at night to be a significant problem independent of short sleep duration. Her research showed that the more irregular the bedtime hour, the more impairment of grades, the more injuries associated with alcohol or drugs and the more days missed from school. Previous research among preschool children also focused on the importance of bedtime regularity regarding school adjustment behaviours.

Teenage behaviour can be stressful for parents; however, if you start early, as did the family in the following report, some of the sleep issues are more manageable.

With Privilege Comes Responsibility

As the parents of five children ranging in age from eight to fifteen, my husband and I still incorporate the wisdom of Dr Weissbluth with the sleep routines established in our home many years ago.

We started learning the sleep process fifteen years ago with our oldest daughter, Trisha. Dr Weissbluth taught us how to recognise her fatigue and get her to sleep before she became over-tired. When her sister, Julia, was born, we thought she would show the same signals and enjoy the sleep routine we had set up for Trisha. We were so wrong. Although her routine was different the method was the same. Identify fatigue and put to bed before she became overtired. By the time our fifth child was born we felt like pros.

My husband and I noticed each child, as toddlers, had a 'cue' that would signal nap time or bedtime. One son would start to run his fingers through his hair, one would rub his eyes and another would climb onto the nearest lap. Again, letting us know it was time to rest. At this age actions speak louder than words.

The learning has not stopped. As the children age, we adjust their sleep habits, yet remain cognisant of the fact that overtired children are not happy, productive people. This has proven especially true with teenagers. Sometimes the privilege of staying up late will have an adverse affect on their lifestyle. An overtired and grumpy teen may not do so well in a sporting event or an exam. Emotions run high during these years, and we find it is best to have the child well rested in order to face the daily challenges of a growing body. As parents we try to convey the idea that with privilege comes responsibility. Teens need to learn to act responsibly to themselves (this includes a healthy diet as well as a good sleep routine). Although we do allow flexibility in the bedtime routines on special occasions and during school breaks, we always just naturally slide back into a routine.

Dr Weissbluth once told me that when a child says he is bored it is usually fatigue. If my children mention that they are bored, I suggest they take a nap.

Sleep in our home is as important as good eating habits, regular exercise and good moral behaviour.

In addition to difficulties falling asleep and staying asleep, there are other abnormal sleep patterns and problems that begin in pre-adolescence or adolescence.

Delayed Sleep Phase Syndrome

Do you notice that your teenager is going to bed later and later? Eventually she might consider herself to be a night person. You may have heard of 'owls' and 'larks', and if you yourself are an owl, you might consider this tendency of your teenage daughter to delay going to sleep as normal. But what may be occurring is the development of an inability to fall asleep at a socially and biologically appropriate time. Alternatively, a biological process associated with the development of puberty might cause a shift to a later bedtime. If this is the case, then the late bedtime is not the problem; rather, it's the too early start of the school day that's causing problems.

In delayed sleep phase syndrome, the child has no difficulty falling asleep or staying asleep, but only when sleep onset is delayed, maybe to 1:00, 2:00, or 3:00 A.M. When she tries to go to sleep earlier, she can't. On weekends and holidays, she'll sleep later, so her total sleep time is about normal. But on school days it's always a struggle to get her up for those early classes.

As a consequence, schoolwork suffers and the child's mood

swings widely – the long-term result of brief sleep on school days and a chronically abnormal sleep schedule. As I'll discuss in the 'exercise' section of Chapter 11, some teenagers try to combat the fatigue with internal stimulation (anger or elation) or external stimulation (sports or exercise).

Kleine-Levin Syndrome

This is a rare condition, but it may be mistaken for other psychiatric or neurological illnesses. The major features include excessive sleepiness, overeating and loss of sexual inhibitions. The exact cause of this problem is not known, but if you notice dramatic abnormalities in sleeping, eating, or other behaviours, do not simply assume this is a teenage 'phase'. Other uncommon disorders involving abnormal sleeping might be associated with changes in temperature sensitivity, thirst or mood.

Fibromyalgia Syndrome

Fibromyalgia syndrome is an uncommon sleep problem that occurs mostly in preteen and teenage girls, and sometimes in their mothers. Children with fibromyalgia syndrome feel fatigue and diffuse pain. They 'feel tired all the time' or they 'hurt all over'. The pain occurs on both the right and left sides of the body, and above and below the waist. In addition to this diffuse aching pain, they have specific tender points that, when pressed, cause much more intense localised pain.

All of these girls have disturbed sleep. For many years, their parents may have noticed these girls moving around a lot during sleep. This restlessness, or 'motor agitation', causes the sheets and blankets to be thrown all about and is a characteristic feature of fibromyalgia syndrome. Further, they usually awaken in the morning feeling tired or 'unrefreshed', as if they had not had a good night's sleep. The non-restorative sleep is another characteristic feature of children with fibromyalgia. Some children also have night awakenings. Other symptoms include morning stiffness, morning fatigue, headaches, lack of energy, a sense of sleepiness during the day, negative mood and depression. These children are disabled because of their chronic pain; they cannot comfortably participate in the activities most teenagers enjoy.

Interestingly, the pattern of restless sleep with the sheets and blankets strewn about or night waking is usually not recognised by the child as a problem because it is long-standing. Because she has always slept like this, the child or parents often think it is 'normal' for her. These children do *not* complain of sleeping poorly; instead, they complain of fatigue and pain. The physician's evaluation usually reveals the sleep disturbance.

The fatigue and pain may cause the child to miss school, not participate in social activities and avoid sports. This may lead to lower self-esteem and a 'deconditioned' body, both of which superficially resemble the symptoms of depression. Remember, children with fibromyalgia syndrome are most often preteen or teenage girls, and many of the symptoms may be misattributed to changes associated with adolescence.

Because the cause of fibromyalgia syndrome is not known, there is no specific cure or treatment. But the good news is that improvement tends to occur over time in response to treatment. Rheumatologists in paediatric centres specialise in treatment with exercise programmes, and sometimes they prescribe anti-depressant medications. This can help these children get through difficulties that disturb their sleep, such as final exams. Most children improve after about two years of treatment.

Curiously, there is a predicable sequence of improvement. First, the sleep disruption improves. Second, weeks later, the skeletal muscle pain symptoms start to improve. When the sleep disturbance does not improve, it is much less likely that the other symptoms will decrease. This observation that sleeping better needs to precede improvement in fatigue and pain reduction suggests that poor-quality sleeping might cause the other symptoms. Furthermore, among adults who suffer with this disease, the poorer the sleep, the more extreme the pain. This again suggests that there is a causal link between disturbed sleep and the other symptoms of fibromyalgia.

Chronic Mononucleosis

Infectious mononucleosis is caused by a virus. Children as young as fourteen have been identified as having a chronic condition, following the acute infection, characterised by disabling daytime sleepiness. Because of the daytime sleepiness, the child's school performance deteriorates. Not surprisingly, misdiagnoses of depression are sometimes made among these children. The correct diagnosis is made only after blood tests confirm the viral infection.

Preventing and Solving Sleep Problems

Let's look at the two major areas of concern for children in this age group, namely, falling asleep and maintaining a healthy sleep schedule. In treating these sleep problems, we attempt to break the self-perpetuating sequence in which sleep disturbances cause hyperarousal, which further interferes with sleeping well.

Falling Asleep

Working with a therapist, older children can learn to sleep better through relaxation training techniques similar to those used by adults. The attempt is to reduce the level of arousal, therefore permitting the sleep process to surface. Here are a few techniques:

1. ***Progressive relaxation* is a method whereby you tense individual skeletal muscle groups, release the tension and focus on the resulting feeling of relaxation.**
2. ***Biofeedback* involves focusing on a visual or auditory stimulus that changes in proportion to the tension within skeletal muscles. Both progressive relaxation and biofeedback techniques can help reduce muscle tension and thus make it easier to fall asleep.**
3. ***Self-suggestion* to produce relaxation involves repeating suggestions that your arms and legs feel heavy and warm.**

4. ***Paradoxical intention* is based on the idea that trying hard to spontaneously fall asleep might create a vicious circle, which can be broken by focusing on staying awake.**
5. ***Meditative relaxation* procedures vary, but simple instructions to focus on the physical sensation of breathing seem to help some people fall asleep.**

Stimulus Control and Temporal Control

Stimulus-control treatment tries to make the bedroom environment function as a cue for sleep. Spending lots of time in bed watching television, reading or eating directly competes with sleeping, and therefore these activities must be discontinued. *Temporal control* means establishing a regular and healthy sleep schedule.

Richard R. Bootzin, a psychologist specialising in insomnia, incorporates the elements of stimulus control in the following instructions he developed.

STIMULUS-CONTROL INSTRUCTIONS

1. **Lie down intending to go to sleep *only* when you are sleepy.**
2. **Do not use your bed for anything except sleep – that is, do not do homework, read, watch television, eat or worry in bed.**
3. **If you find yourself unable to fall asleep, get up and go into another room. Stay up as long as you wish and then return to the bedroom to sleep. Although you should not watch the clock, you should get out of bed if you do not fall asleep immediately. Remember, the goal is to associate your bed with falling asleep *quickly*! If you are in bed for more than about ten minutes without falling asleep and have not got up, you are not following this instruction.**
4. **If you still cannot fall asleep, repeat step three. Do this as often as necessary throughout the night.**
5. **Set your alarm and get up at the same time every**

morning, irrespective of how much sleep you got during the night. This will help your body acquire a consistent sleep rhythm.

6. **Do not nap during the day.**

Dr Rosalind Cartwright, a pioneer adult-sleep researcher, teaches a variation of Richard Bootzin's stimulus control that has helped some children fall asleep more easily.

1. **Do something that is pleasurable for a limited amount of time, using a timer set for fifteen to twenty minutes. Do anything you want, but not in your bedroom.**
2. **Take the hottest lavender bubble bath you can tolerate for fifteen to twenty minutes. This is for relaxation, so don't read a book or listen to music while you're in the tub. The bath helps prevent the storm of thoughts and worries that strike the brain like meteorites when the protective shield of activity, sports, or homework is down.**
3. **After the bubble bath, immediately get into bed. Don't start any other activities – no books, no music, no telephone calls. Close your eyes and try to sleep.**

If these instructions do not provide help, consider encouraging your child to get involved in sports programmes, to increase the amount of physical exercise he gets. If this fails and your child still can't sleep well and appears exhausted, too tired, and not interested in outside activities, ask yourself whether the problem might not be depression.

Children do get depressed, and some stupid, risk-taking 'accidents' in overtired teenagers are really deliberate suicide attempts. If this is a concern of yours, seek outside help immediately. Start with school social workers, your physician or local suicide prevention centres.

Maintaining a Healthy Sleep Schedule

As already discussed, some teenagers suffer from what we call delayed sleep phase syndrome. This occurs when teenagers are unable to fall asleep at a desired conventional clock time but have no difficulty falling asleep long after midnight. On holiday, they sleep a normal duration, do not wake up at night and feel refreshed in the late morning or midday, when they awaken. The problem lies in the disrupted sleep schedule that often develops during the school year, when sleeping late is not possible.

Treatment is called 'chronotherapy', or resetting the sleep clock. Let's say your child can easily fall asleep at 2:00 A.M. The therapy consists of forcing him to stay up until 5:00 A.M. and then letting a natural sleep period follow. (Obviously, we don't do this during the school year!) The next time sleep is allowed to start is at 8:00 A.M. the following day and at 11:00 A.M. the day after that. In other words, you are allowing sleep to occur about three hours later every cycle. Over the next few days, sleep begins at 2:00, 5:00, 8:00, and finally 11:00 P.M. Now, keeping careful watch over clock time, *always* try to have the child go to sleep at 11:00 P.M. You have shifted the sleep clock around to a more conventional time, and usually this can be maintained by sustaining a regular night-time sleep schedule.

Drugs and Diet to Help Us Sleep

Drugs don't solve sleep problems. Diphenhydramine or other antihistamines are often used to induce sleep in children. The common situation is for these drugs, or others, to be thought of as a temporary, short-term measure, 'just to give everyone a break'. It sounds great – get your strength back to muster up enough courage to try to correct problems caused by your own mismanagement – but I have observed many times that those parents who demand drugs most strongly are those who are least likely to change their behaviour, so the basic sleep problems continue. No study has shown that sleep-inducing drugs are really useful and safe for children. Diphenhydramine has been shown *not* to be an effective hypnotic in adults. Hypnotic drugs such as phenobarbital can actually cause sleep disturbances, daytime fussiness and irritability.

PRACTICAL POINT

Don't depend on drugs to solve your child's sleep problems.

Other drugs that can interfere with good sleeping include non-prescription decongestants, such as Sudafed and caffeine. So let's sleep better by not taking any drugs. An important exception might be drugs used by an allergist or paediatrician to help a child breathe more easily at night if he is suffering from allergies.

Dietary changes that are known to make some people sleepy include high-carbohydrate meals and foods high in the amino acid tryptophan. It is possible that the contents of a nursing mother's diet affect the carbohydrate content of her breast milk, and this may indirectly influence the levels of tryptophan in the baby. In one study of infants, tryptophan caused the babies to begin quiet sleep twenty minutes earlier and active sleep fourteen minutes earlier. But the total amount of sleep time was not affected. So giving tryptophan to infants or other children will probably not make them sleep longer. Furthermore, tryptophan administration in adults has been associated with severe diseases, even though tryptophan is a naturally occurring amino acid. Melatonin is another naturally occurring chemical that has been popularised as a sleep aid. The safety and effectiveness of melatonin have not been established for infants or children.

The effects of high-carbohydrate or high-protein meals in adults show differences between the sexes and differences based on age. There is no scientific data on nutrition in children that could be translated into a sleep-promoting diet. Eliminating refined sugar, because of the commonly held belief that this makes children hyperactive, also does not appear to have any effect on sleep patterns.

Another report suggested that cow's milk allergy could cause insomnia. But the results of the study could have been caused by a placebo effect, because the parents knew when they were giving a cow's milk challenge and when they were eliminating cow's milk from the diet. Dietary challenges and elimination diets are best performed when both the parents and the researchers, at the time of the challenge, are ignorant of whether the child is or is not receiving the substance in question. Only then can bias or wishful thinking be reduced.

Many school-age children have difficulty falling asleep because they worry about their grades, test scores, appearance or sports skills. Anxiety about not doing well academically or athletically might lead to impaired performance. This is called 'performance anxiety'. Impaired sleeping likewise occurs when there is too much worrying or nagging about not getting enough sleep. Worrying too much about not sleeping well creates anxiety or stress, interfering with the relaxation needed to successfully perform the task, which is to fall asleep. Ask your general practitioner to help you approach a child psychologist for information about the solution, which is called 'relaxation training'. If your child, at any age, appears to need more sleep, and he wants to sleep but cannot easily fall asleep, please consider working with a professional to help your child learn to relax and avoid performance anxiety.

PART III

Other Sleep Disturbances and Concerns

Special Sleep Problems

Specific sleep problems may occur at different ages, and it would be useful to read the earlier sections to determine whether your child's sleep pattern is appropriate for his age. Some specific sleep problems, such as sleepwalking, sleep talking or night terrors, appear to occur more frequently when children have abnormal sleep schedules. Most of these common problems are bothersome to the family but are not harmful to the child.

However, one problem, severe and chronic snoring, may be hazardous to a child's health. Please read the section on poor-quality breathing even if your child has no specific sleep problems or you think he does not snore. Snoring is sometimes not appreciated as a problem because the child has always snored, or because allergies developed when the child was older – an older child is usually in his own bedroom and the parents are unaware of how much snoring is occurring every night because they do not go into his bedroom after he has fallen asleep.

Sleepwalking

Between the ages of six and sixteen, sleepwalking occurs about three to twelve times each year among 5 per cent of children. An additional 5 to 10 per cent of children walk in their sleep once or twice a year. When it starts under age ten and ends by age fifteen, sleepwalking is not associated with any emotional stress, negative personality types, or behavioural problems. Research has shown that there is a substantial genetic factor to sleepwalking, as it was found that the behaviour is more common among identical twins than fraternal twins.

Sleepwalking episodes usually occur within the first two to three hours after falling asleep. The sleepwalk itself may last up to thirty minutes. Usually the sleepwalker appears to be little concerned about his environment. His gait is not fluid and his movement not purposeful. In addition to walking, other behaviours such as eating, dressing and opening doors often occur.

Treatment consists only of safety measures to prevent sleepwalkers from falling down stairs or out of open windows. Try to remove toys or furniture from your child's path, but don't expect to be able to wake him. Rousing him won't hurt, but usually the child wakes spontaneously without any memory of the walk.

Sleep Talking

Sleep talkers do not make good conversationalists! They seem to talk to themselves and respond to questions with single-syllable answers. Adults appear annoyed or preoccupied. Children often repeat simple phrases like 'get down' or 'no more', as if they were remembering important stressful events that had occurred that day.

Between the ages of three and ten years, about half of all children will talk in their sleep once a year. Older studies have suggested that sleepwalking and sleep talking tended to occur together and were more common in boys; however, newer studies do not support this association.

Night Terrors

Your child utters a piercing scream, and you rush into his room. He appears wild-eyed, anxious, frightened. His pupils are dilated, sweat is covering his forehead and as you pick him up to hug him you notice his heart is pounding and his chest heaving. He is inconsolable. Your heart is full of dread, and it almost seems as if some evil spirit has gripped your child. After five to fifteen minutes, the agitation and confused state finally subside. This is night terror.

Night terrors, sleepwalking and sleep talking all occur mainly during non-REM sleep and usually within two hours of going to sleep. They usually do not occur when we dream (during REM sleep); they are not bad dreams. In fact, children have no memory of them once they are awake.

Night terrors usually start between four and twelve years of age. When they start before puberty, they are not associated with any emotional or personality problems. Night terrors have nothing to do with seizures, convulsions or epilepsy. Night terrors appear more often when a child has a fever or when sleep patterns are disrupted naturally, such as on long trips, during holidays, or when relatives come to visit. Recurrent night terrors are also often associated with chronically abnormal sleep schedules.

Enabling them to get more sleep is the way of treating overtired children who have frequent night terrors. I have observed that night terrors disappear when the parents moved the bedtime earlier by only thirty minutes.

Drug therapy is not warranted for most children with night terrors, sleepwalking or sleep talking problems. Most children should be allowed to outgrow these problems without complex tests (such as CT scans), drug treatments or psychotherapy.

Nightmares

In old English mythology, a nightmare was thought to be a female spirit or monster that beset people and animals at night, coming upon them when they are asleep and producing a feeling of suffocation.

I myself have had nightmares of suffocation, strangulation, breathlessness, choking, being crushed or trapped, drowning, entrapment and being buried alive – but only when I sleep on my back or have an alcoholic drink before going to bed. My wife says that at these times my breathing sounds like a diesel truck with a bad motor. When she pokes me to get me up, the nightmare ends and I breathe normally again. You see, my nightmares occur when my upper airway is partially blocked, and this obstruction happens only when I sleep on my back or drink alcohol before bedtime. Occasionally, I have less dramatic dreams of breathlessness while running, flying (without a plane, of course) or being chased. If my wife does not awaken me, I wake up to breathe, but I have no dream recall. Maybe some children have similar nightmares when they have bad colds or throat infections that partially obstruct their upper airway.

The child with a nightmare can be awakened and consoled, in contrast to the child with a night terror, which spontaneously subsides. About 30 per cent of high school students have one nightmare a month. Adults who have more frequent nightmares (more than two per week) often have other sleep problems: frequent night awakenings, increased time required to fall asleep and decreased sleep duration. They appear more anxious and distrustful, and experience fatigue in the morning.

But nightmares in most young children do not seem to be associated with any specific emotional or personality problems. However, two recent reports in children, one for five to eight years of age, and the other for six to ten years of age, concluded that anxiety issues or other psychological problems are associated with nightmares. Analysis – guesswork, really – of dream content in disturbed children who have been referred to psychologists or psychiatrists should not be generalised to normal populations of children with the assumption that normal anxieties or fears represent a mental or emotional problem. We really do not know the exact value or limitations of dream interpretation. If you think your child is having a nightmare, shower him with hugs and kisses and try to awaken him.

What do you do if the child comes into the parents' room, sometimes several times a night, complaining of nightmares?

If you strongly suspect that your child is not feigning nightmares just to get extra attention at night, consider consulting a child psychologist or psychiatrist.

Head Banging and Body Rocking

My third son banged his head against the cot every night after we moved into a new house. Actually, he struck his shoulder blades more than his head against the headboard of his cot. My solution was to use soft cushions to pad both ends and both sides completely. Now when he banged away there was no racket, no pain and no parental attention. After a few days he stopped. Other parents are not so lucky.

About 5 to 10 per cent of children will bang or roll their heads before falling asleep during their first few years. This usually starts at about eight months of age. Boys behave this way more than girls. No behavioural or emotional problems are seen in these children as they develop, and they certainly have no neurological problems. Body rocking before falling asleep also occurs in normal children.

All this rhythmic behaviour usually stops before the fourth year if there are no underlying neurological diseases. Your paediatrician can diagnose these uncommon conditions if they are present.

Bruxism

Teeth grinding, or bruxism, during sleep is common in children. At the Laboratory School at the University of Chicago, about 15 per cent of the students were reported by their parents to have a history of bruxism. In the age range of three to seven years, the percentage of bruxists was about 11 per cent; between eight and twelve years, it was 6 per cent, and between thirteen and seventeen years, the percentage dropped to about 2 per cent.

Teeth grinding does not occur during dreams or nightmares. Furthermore, there is no association between emotional or personality disturbances and teeth grinding. No treatment is needed for bruxism in children.

Narcolepsy

The major characteristic of narcolepsy is excessive abnormal sleepiness. It appears as if the child has a sudden sleep attack while engaged in ordinary activities such as reading or watching television. The child with a mild form of narcolepsy may drift into a state of excessive drowsiness; the child with a more severe form might fall fast asleep in the middle of a conversation.

Narcolepsy is less common under the age of ten. When it begins in older children it may be mistaken for lack of concentration or inattentiveness.

Other features of narcolepsy seen in older children are *cataplexy*, a muscular weakness triggered by emotional stress; *sleep paralysis*, a passing sensation of inability to move when drifting off to sleep; and *hypnagogic hallucinations*, visual or auditory experiences that occur as sleep begins.

Poor-Quality Breathing (Allergies and Snoring)

If you've ever suffered through a head cold, I'm sure you'll agree that when you can't breathe easily during sleep, you can't sleep easily either. In turn, this makes you sleepy during the day, which can affect your mood and performance. When the cold finally disappears, you feel like your old self again and your mood improves, as does your performance. Some children experience the same type of disrupted sleep *every night* because of allergies or snoring. Let's look at them both.

Allergies

Allergies are frequently suggested as a cause of the typical signs and symptoms characterising snorers. Here's a list of symptoms from one study of children with difficulty breathing during sleep, conducted at the Children's Memorial Hospital in Chicago.

Snoring
Difficulty breathing during sleep
Stopping breathing during sleep
Restless sleep
Chronic runny nose
Breathing through mouth when awake
Frequent common colds
Frequent nausea/vomiting
Difficulty swallowing
Sweating when asleep
Hearing problem
Excessive daytime sleepiness
Poor appetite
Recurrent middle-ear disease

Perhaps the 'chronic runny nose' and the 'frequent common colds' are due to allergies.

Allergists have long associated food sensitivities or sensitivity to environmental allergens with behavioural problems, such as poor ability to concentrate, hyperactivity, tension or irritability. Terms such as 'tension-fatigue' syndrome or 'allergic-irritability' syndrome are used by allergists to describe children who exhibit nasal or respiratory allergies, food allergies and behavioural problems. It is possible that allergy causes behavioural problems in children by producing swollen respiratory membranes, large adenoids or large tonsils, which partially obstruct breathing during sleep. The difficulty these children experience in breathing during sleep causes them to lose sleep and thus directly causes fatigue, irritability and tension.

Also perhaps due to allergies, large adenoids or tonsils can partially or completely obstruct breathing during sleep as well as cause hearing problems or recurrent ear infections. So, either because of the actual enlargement of the tonsils or because of the underlying allergies that cause swelling of the membranes in the nose and throat, these children suffer from frequent 'colds' – runny nose, sneezing, coughing and ear problems.

Snoring

Two of the world's leading sleep researchers, Dr Christian Guilleminault and Dr William C. Dement, published a landmark paper in 1976 that was the first careful study of how impaired breathing during sleep destroys good-quality sleep in children. At Stanford University School of Medicine, they studied eight children (seven boys and one girl, ages five to fourteen years), all of whom snored. All eight children snored loudly every night, and snoring had been present for several years. Snoring started in one child at six months, and while the snoring in most children was originally intermittent, it eventually became continuous. Here's how their symptoms were described.

Daytime drowsiness: Five of the eight children experienced excessive daytime sleepiness. The report noted that 'the children, particularly at school, tried desperately to fight it off, usually with success. To avoid falling asleep, the children tended to move about and gave the appearance of hyperactivity'.

Bed-wetting: All the children had been completely toilet trained, but seven started to wet their beds again.

Decreased school performance: Only five of the eight children had learning difficulties, but all the teachers reported lack of attention, hyperactivity and a general decrease in intellectual performance, particularly in the older children.

Morning headaches: Five of the eight children had headaches only when they awoke in the morning; the headaches lessened or disappeared completely by late morning.

Mood and personality changes: Half the children had received professional counselling or family psychotherapy for 'emotional' problems. The report noted that 'three children were particularly disturbed at bedtime; they consistently avoided going to bed, fighting desperately against sleepiness. They refused to be left alone in their rooms while falling asleep and, if allowed, would go to sleep on the floor in the living room'.

Weight problems: Five of the children were underweight, and two were overweight.

Overall, we have a picture here of impaired mood and school performance, which deteriorated as the children grew older or as the snoring became more continuous or severe. Sleep is definitely not bliss for these children!

But was this a new discovery? Not really. As I will discuss further, most snoring children have enlarged adenoids, which medical texts written as early as 1914 acknowledged can disrupt sleep and cause behaviour problems. As one early textbook noted:

> Restlessness during the night is a prominent symptom; the patient often throws the covers off during the unconscious rolling and tossing which is so characteristic. . . . Daytime restlessness is also a characteristic sign. The child is fretful and peevish, or is inclined to turn from one amusement to another . . . the mental faculties are often much impaired . . . difficult attention is very often present. The child is listless and has difficulty in applying himself continuously to his play, studies, or other tasks, of which he soon tires. He has fits of abstraction.

Interestingly, increased motor activity or physical restlessness during sleep, distractibility and reduced attention span are also characteristic features of children who have been diagnosed as 'hyperactive'.

Another study, this one done in 1925, showed enlarged adenoids and tonsils as a physical cause of poor sleep. Even a major paediatric professional journal cited 'difficulty in breathing, such as seen with extreme enlargement of the adenoids' as a common cause of 'infantile insomnia' as far back as 1951. In truly severe cases of enlarged adenoids and tonsils, affected children appear to be mentally retarded, have impaired growth and suffer from heart disease.

In one study of children who had documented difficulty

breathing during sleep, the following problems were observed in addition to snoring:

'Breath holding', 'stopping breathing' during sleep
Frequent night-time awakening
Breathing through an open mouth
Sleeping sitting up
Excessive daytime sleepiness
Difficulty concentrating
Bed-wetting
Decreased energy, poor eating, weight loss
Morning headaches
Hyperactivity

Some parents have also described to me their child's apparent 'forgetting to breathe' during sleep. Their child's chest is heaving, but during those moments of complete airway obstruction airflow is stopped. These periods are called 'apnoea'. With only partial airway obstruction, though, excessively loud snoring throughout the night is the result. In either case, it's the poor-quality sleeping that's the culprit, causing daytime sleepiness, difficulties in concentration, school and behavioural problems, decreased energy and hyperactivity . . . even though the total sleep time may be normal!

Why, then, has kids' snoring particularly been ignored? Are there more snorers around today? Perhaps yes, because although surgical removal of tonsils and adenoids is much less common today, it was for years a very popular procedure for recurrent throat infections; it also happened to 'cure' snoring in children. And perhaps yes, because the air we breathe is increasingly polluted and our processed foods increasingly allergenic; this may cause reactive enlargement of adenoids or tonsils in more children.

Whatever the causes of snoring, we've seen so far that children who snore aren't getting the best-quality sleep. Now we see that generally they aren't getting the best quantity either. One study of snorers at Children's Memorial Hospital in

Chicago also showed that children with documented obstruction of breathing generally slept less than normal children. At about age four, average night-sleep duration was only eight and a half hours in affected children, compared to ten and a quarter hours in normal children.

In another study I performed, also at Children's Memorial, the affected snoring children were somewhat older, about six years of age, and their total sleep duration was about half an hour less than that of normal kids. They also had night wakings that lasted longer, went to bed later, and took longer to fall asleep after going to bed. These affected children exhibited snoring, difficult or laboured breathing, or mouth-breathing when asleep. Parents described problems such as overactivity, hyperactivity, a short attention span, an inability to sit still, learning disabilities or other academic difficulties in their snoring children. And as we have seen, a chronic sleep deficit of only half an hour per night might cause impaired intellectual development.

Even in infants, snoring might be a problem. I studied a group of 141 normal infants between four and eight months of age. In these infants, 12 per cent exhibited snoring and 10 per cent exhibited mouth-breathing when asleep. These snoring infants slept one and a half hours less and awoke twice as often as infants who did not snore.

In another study of infants about four months of age, cow's milk allergy was thought to be the cause of brief night-sleep durations and frequent awakenings. Other studies have suggested that an allergy to cow's milk protein can cause respiratory congestion.

PRACTICAL POINT

Although snoring reflects difficulty breathing during sleep, it is not related to sudden infant death syndrome ('cot death').

The night waking in these snoring infants and the restless light sleep in older children probably represent protective arousals from sleep. As we learned earlier, these arousals mean that the child awakens or sleeps lightly in order to breathe better. When awake, the child breathes well, but the brain's control over breathing is blunted during sleep stages. So, to prevent asphyxiation, the child awakens frequently, cries out at night and has trouble maintaining prolonged, consolidated deep-sleep states. Here, the crying and waking at night and resistance to falling asleep are caused by a valid medical problem, not a behavioural problem, not nightmares, not a parenting problem.

Not all children who snore a lot have all of the problems listed above. Differences among snorers can probably be explained by differences in severity and duration of the underlying problems. Also, I have encountered many monster snorers with minimal problems because they habitually take very long naps or have been able to go to bed much earlier than their peers. In other words, there are snorers and there are snorers! Some, like myself, have never been studied, and except for occasional nightmares – like the ones of asphyxiation, drowning or strangulation I have when sleeping on my back – do not suffer adversely from snoring. Other snorers are not so fortunate because their snoring is more severe, a result of enlarged adenoids or tonsils.

PRACTICAL POINT

All children snore a little, and frequent colds or a bad hay fever season might cause more snoring, which usually does no harm. Consider snoring a problem when it gets progressively worse, is chronic or continuous, disrupts your child's sleep and affects daytime mood or performance. About 10 to 20 per cent of children snore frequently.

The reason attention has been focused on the problem of enlarged adenoids and tonsils is that sleep researchers have proven that breathing is actually disordered during sleep. This is an important point, because when the child opens his mouth, the tonsils do not necessarily look enlarged. In fact, the adenoids and tonsils may cause partial airway obstruction in some children during sleep only because the neck muscles naturally relax and the airway thus narrows. In other words, the real problem in some children might not be enlarged adenoids or tonsils, but rather too much relaxation in the neck region during sleep. This relaxation of the muscles in the neck may permit enlarged tonsils or adenoids to swing towards the midline, causing a partial or complete blockage of the flow of air. If snoring appears to be disrupting your child's sleep, consult your GP. Your child's doctor may have to do some tests to determine how serious the problem really is.

The term 'sleep-related breathing disorders', or SRBDs, was coined to describe those children who had snoring or heavy or loud breathing while sleeping, or who appear to have trouble struggling to breathe while sleeping, or who make a snorting sound and wake up. One research study conducted in 1997 directly connected SRBDs to attention deficit hyperactivity disorder (ADHD). They calculated that about 25 per cent of children with ADHD would have their symptoms eliminated by correcting their habitual snoring or SRBD. In 1998, two studies showed that SRBD was associated with extremely poor academic performance in first grade (improvement occurred upon removal of tonsils and adenoids) and also that SRBD was associated with difficulties with behavioural sleep disorders such as fighting sleep at night or bedtime battles. By 2002, the terminology had changed to 'sleep-disordered breathing', or SDB, but the message was the same. Inattention, hyperactivity, behavioural and emotional difficulties are more common in children with SDB. Again, surgical intervention helped these children.

Locating the Problem

Try to suck through a wet paper drinking straw. You can't; it collapses. When we inhale, active neuromuscular forces keep our neck from collapsing like a wet straw. Sometimes things don't work well during sleep and the neck muscles lose their tone. Sometimes the major problem involves the tongue, which may not stay in its proper position during sleep and flops backwards, causing upper-airway obstruction.

Think of this as a neurological problem involving the brain's control over our muscles while we sleep. The result is that the airway is not kept open during sleep. If it's a neurological problem, then consider the possibility that there are other associated problems involving the brain: difficulty concentrating, poor school performance, excessive daytime sleepiness or hyperactivity. If the major problem involves the tongue or neck muscles, removing the tonsils or adenoids might not help. So it is obviously important to determine the cause of the problem before considering surgery.

Children who snore and have many of those problems associated with poor breathing during sleep often have abnormal X-rays of the neck when viewed from the side. The most common abnormality is enlargement of the adenoids or tonsils. A simple X-ray might tell the entire story. But some children who snore might have normal X-rays and will require studies designed to document airway obstruction; it is important to pursue this before clinical problems develop.

Studies that have been used to document obstructive breathing problems during sleep include actual measurements of respiratory flow through the nose, skin oxygen levels and the carbon dioxide concentration in the air exhaled during sleep. Another type of sleep study, using fluoroscopy, may visualise the level of obstruction. CT scans during sleep also have been used to measure the cross-sectional area at different levels of the airway to determine the anatomical location of the airway narrowing.

Electrocardiograms are useful because, in severe instances,

the right side of the heart shows signs of strain. This strain can lead to pulmonary hypertension in long-standing cases.

Pulmonary hypertension also occurs with massive obesity, as in Pickwickian syndrome. This is named after Dickens's *The Pickwick Papers*, in which an extremely fat boy is pictured as standing motionless, barely awake and feebly snoring. Massive obesity itself apparently causes difficulty breathing.

Finding the Answers

If the tonsils or adenoids are causing significant airway obstruction, they should be removed. Sometimes a surgical procedure to correct an abnormal nasal septum solves the airway problem. Tracheostomy, or creating a breathing hole in the neck, is occasionally needed when the obstruction is due to

OBSTRUCTIVE SLEEP APNOEA

SNORING, DIFFICULT BREATHING OR
MOUTH-BREATHING WHEN ASLEEP

↓

DISTURBED SLEEP

ABNORMAL SLEEP SCHEDULE
BRIEF SLEEP DURATIONS
SLEEP FRAGMENTATION (PROTECTIVE AROUSALS)
NAP DEPRIVATION
PROLONGED LATENCY TO SLEEP

↓

BEHAVIOURAL, DEVELOPMENTAL AND ACADEMIC PROBLEMS

REVERSIBLE

FIGURE 8: POOR-QUALITY BREATHING CAUSES PROBLEMS

airway closure or narrowing not caused by enlarged adenoids or tonsils. During the day, the hole is closed and covered by a collar. Oral devices are now available that keep the tongue from flopping backwards, when that's the major problem.

Weight reduction to correct obesity and management of allergies may be crucial nonsurgical treatments in some children. The management of allergies might include a trial of a diet without cow's milk, making the bedroom dust-free by using efficient air purifiers, reducing the level of mould spores in the air by using dehumidifiers, or getting rid of pets. Nightly administration of decongestants or antihistamines are sometimes needed to reduce the allergy symptoms. Often, intranasal steroid sprays are used to keep the nasal airway open; this treatment avoids the side effects of oral decongestants. A 'snore ball', which is a small glass marble or half of a small rubber ball sewn to the pyjamas or attached with a Velcro strap in the midback region, will prevent a back snorer from sleeping on his back.

Enjoying the Cure

When treatment restores normal breathing during sleep, the loud snoring, daytime sleepiness, morning headaches and other problems either disappear or are greatly reduced. Sleep patterns return to normal, and electrocardiogram abnormalities disappear. These changes are rapid and dramatic. For example, in one report, a thirteen-month-old boy was assessed as having the developmental level of an eleven-month-old baby before surgery, but five months after surgery, his developmental level had jumped past his real age, to the level of a twenty-month-old!

Remember, sleep deficits may directly cause behavioural, developmental or academic problems. These problems are *reversible* when the sleep deficits are corrected (see Figure 8).

One word of caution: if the problem has been long-standing, then once children are cured of their snoring or their allergies are under control, bad social or academic habits or chronic stresses in the family or school will still require the continuous attention of professionals, such as psychologists, tutors or family therapists. The treated child is now a more rested child, however, and is in a better position to respond to this extra effort.

Hyperactive Behaviour

Educators and parents have used different terms to describe children with hyperactive behaviour, but the current popular diagnosis is *attention deficit hyperactivity disorder*, commonly called 'hyperactivity'. Hyperactivity in children is not usually thought to be related to snoring or severe allergies, although children suffering from ADHD, snoring problems or allergies all have similar academic problems and characteristically poor sleep patterns.

Yet restless sleep, or increased amounts of movement during sleep, has been documented in hyperactive children. Could these turned-on school-age children be cranked up from chronically poor sleep habits that started in infancy?

I studied a group of boys whose ages were between four and eight months. Only boys were included, because most hyperactive school-age children are boys. The infant boys in my study also had active sleep patterns – they moved throughout the night in a restless fashion, with many small movements of the hands, feet or eyes. They also had difficult-to-manage temperaments: they were irregular and withdrawing, had high intensity, were slow to adapt and were moody. This temperamental cluster is thought to be common among hyperactive children as well. The results of my study showed that infant boys with more difficult temperaments and active sleep patterns also had briefer attention spans. Perhaps their motors were racing so fast, day and night, that they couldn't sleep quietly at night or concentrate for prolonged periods when awake during the day.

Another study I did involved preschool children at age three. It also showed that children who had increased motor activity when awake had a physically active sleep pattern. A child with active sleep patterns was more likely to be described in the following terms, taken from a questionnaire used to help diagnose hyperactivity:

Restless or overactive
Excitable, impulsive
Disturbs other children
Fails to finish things he starts – short attention span
Constantly fidgeting
Inattentive, easily distracted
Demands must be met immediately – easily frustrated
Cries often and easily
Mood changes quickly and drastically
Temper outbursts, explosive and unpredictable behaviour

Figure 9 summarises my research suggesting how a transformation could take place from an extremely fussy/colicky/difficult temperament baby with brief sleep durations to a hyperactive school-age child. The upward-pointing arrows before certain terms mean that high ratings for rhythmicity signify irregularity and high ratings for persistence signify short attention spans. These infant traits are replaced by hyperactivity and increased intensity as the child becomes more fatigued. As an infant, the child would have been negative in mood and less easily adaptable due to brief sleep durations, and would have remained so at three years.

Such children never learned how to fall asleep unassisted and had accumulated a chronic sleep loss, which caused chronic fatigue. As discussed in Chapter 3, this long-lasting fatigue turned such children 'on', making them more active night and day, and interfered with learning.

Learning may suffer, then, in children who do not sleep well because they breathe poorly during sleep or sleep too little, and who in turn suffer from chronic fatigue that causes hyperactivity. Figure 10 summarises this entire cycle. It shows how crying and sleeping problems present at birth can trigger parental mismanagement. Parental mismanagement or breathing problems during sleep can in turn cause disturbed sleep, elevated levels of neurotransmitters and a more aroused, alert, wakeful, irritable child. This turned-on state directly causes even more disturbed sleep because of heightened arousal levels. It also may indirectly cause parents to misperceive their child as not needing much sleep: 'Johnny just won't stop – he certainly doesn't seem to be running out of steam.'

All of these factors in combination – the fatigued child who is too alert to sleep well, plus irregular, inconsistent parents who also are tired and anxious – conspire to produce a child who may find it difficult to concentrate, may seem hyperactive or may have behavioural problems that make him difficult to manage. These school and behavioural problems make the parents even more anxious, and the cycle continues on and on. Of course, there may be other causes for school problems or hyperactivity, but disturbed sleep appears to be onc that is both preventable and treatable.

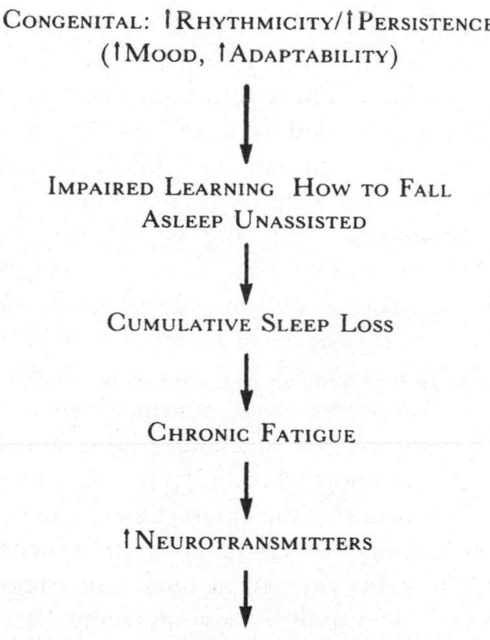

FIGURE 9: TRANSFORMATION OF TEMPERAMENT CHARACTERISTICS ASSOCIATED WITH BRIEF SLEEP DURATIONS

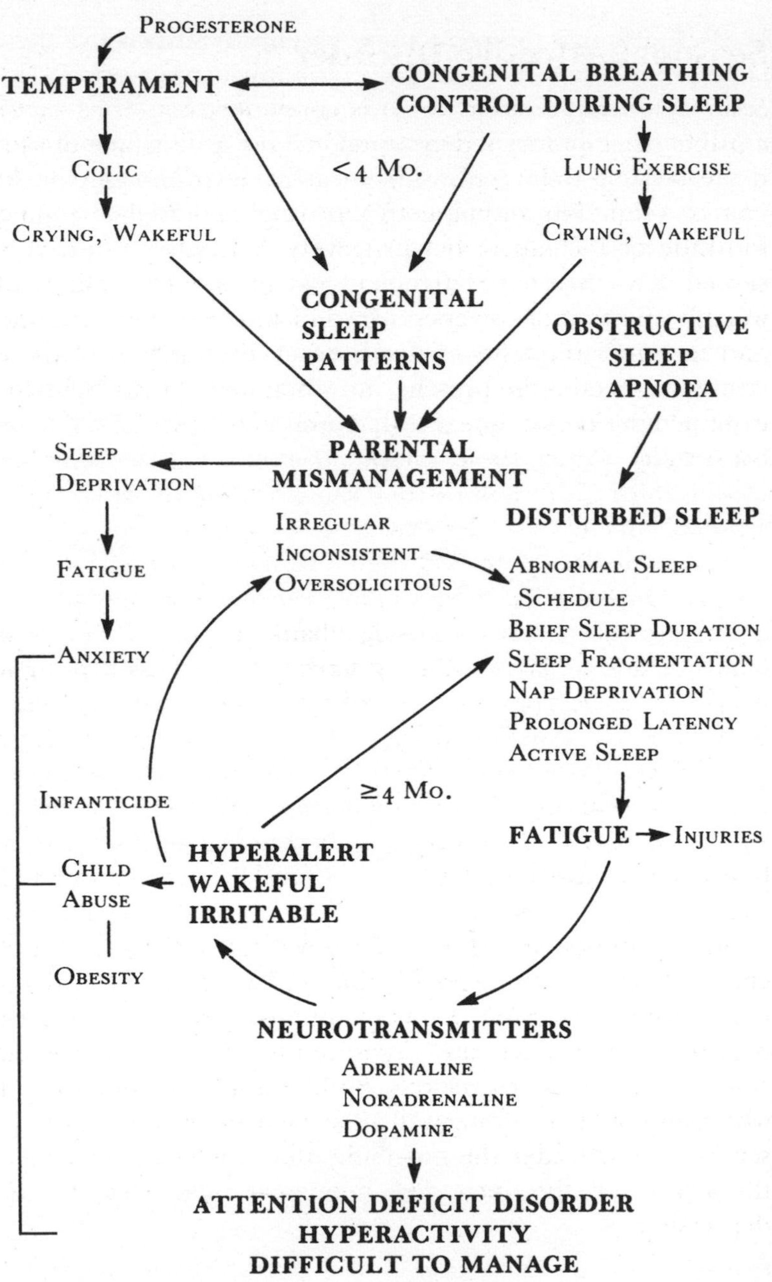

Figure 10: Disturbed Sleep

Seasonal Affective Disorder

Seasonal affective disorder (SAD) is commonly known as *winter depression*. Symptoms of depression include feeling blue or sad; decreased interest or pleasure in activities; dramatic weight gain or weight loss, or failure to gain weight normally; sleeping too little or too much; behaving very restlessly or in a very slowed-down manner; fatigue or loss of energy; feelings of worthlessness; indecisiveness or difficulty in concentrating; and recurrent thoughts of death or suicide. Not all of these symptoms need to be present, but when many occur daily for extended periods of time, the diagnosis of depression has to be considered. When these symptoms tend to occur only or mainly during the months of October and November, then seasonal affective disorder may be the problem.

The reduced amount of daylight during winter, with its short days and long nights, seems to cause the depressive symptoms, and treatment may include using a bank of special fluorescent lamps behind a plastic diffusing screen. The intensity of light needed, the duration of the light treatment and the risks bright-light treatment may pose for the eyes are currently being investigated. Light therapy has been shown to be effective in children, but it's not like taking penicillin for a strep throat, so if you think your child might have SAD, your best bet is to ask your GP for a referral, for evaluation and treatment.

Survey studies have shown that between 2 and 5 per cent of children between the ages of nine and nineteen fulfil diagnostic criteria for SAD. More symptoms appear in northern regions, where days are significantly shorter in winter, compared to southern regions. So if you have an older child who seems not to be doing well after the first few months of the school year, consider the possibility that it is not the teacher, the coach or the increased homework load, but winter depression.

Bed-wetting

Bed-wetting during sleep occurs in about 20 per cent of children at age four and 10 per cent at age five. By the age of ten, it occurs in about 5 per cent of children. The exact cause of bed-wetting is not known. It is not caused by emotional problems. It tends to occur more often in boys and has a tendency to be inherited. Paediatricians or paediatric urologists may offer bladder-training strategies or other treatments, but it is difficult to prove that one treatment works best, as most children outgrow the problem. Restricting fluids before bedtime does not work.

I find that moisture alarms are an effective treatment for bed-wetting. These alarms wake the child as he begins to urinate. This seems to disturb the sleeping brain, and so to prevent such an abrupt arousal from the alarm in the future, the brain controls the bladder better and prevents urination.

Sometimes the alarm does not rouse the child, so the parent has to be able to hear the alarm in order to wake the child. The reason the child might sleep through the alarm is that bed-wetters appear to have very deep sleep. Even though older research suggests that bed-wetters are not more difficult to awaken than children who are not bed-wetters, this deep sleep may be a major part of the problem for some children.

In my experience, some children with too-late bedtimes or severe allergies causing difficulty breathing through the nose appear to be overtired during the day and wet at night. When they are helped to sleep better, they often appear to be better rested during the day and drier at night. The most dramatic 'cures' of bed-wetting sometimes occur when enlarged adenoids or tonsils are removed. Now the child breathes easier during sleep, sleeps better and becomes drier.

Special Events and Concerns

As if growing up were not hard enough, there are inevitable events that might significantly disrupt your child's healthy sleep habits. Other special concerns, such as frequent injuries, may well be the result of unhealthy sleep habits. Here are some examples:

Changes with Daylight Saving Time

When you move the clock time an hour earlier or later, continue to sleep your child according to the new time. If her bedtime has been about 6:30 P.M., and you moved the clock forward an hour so her old 6:30 is now 7:30 P.M., still put her down to sleep at the new clock time of 6:30 P.M. The reason you can ignore the time change is because a lot of social cues in the family such as active or quiet times, meals, bathing, outdoor play time is adjusted with the time change, and these social cues help regulate your child's sleep schedule.

New Sibling

If you are expecting another child, it is best to maintain as much regularity as possible during the pregnancy and not move your young child to a bed until the new baby is about four months old, if then. Towards the end of the pregnancy, the mother is more tired and the older child becomes aware that her mother has less energy or patience. Receiving less attention or not as prompt a response is something that she will have to get used to. So don't kill yourself putting forth a heroic effort; it will only delay your older child's learning to adapt to the inevitable: a decrease in parental attention. When the newborn is about four months old, the developing biological rhythms in the baby permit a new and stable social rhythm in the household. The older child now knows that there are approximate times when her mother is feeding the baby or putting it to sleep. The stability of these events makes the older child feel more secure.

If you need to move the older child from a cot to a bed, consider leaving the cot up and empty for a while before the younger child is shifted to it. The parents' understanding is that she is graduating to a 'big kid's' bed, but the child might not have the same opinion. Prepare yourself for the possibility that, either because of fearfulness in the big bed or because the child now realises she can easily get out of bed to explore the house, you might have to return her to the cot. Sometimes a crib tent is necessary because your child is curious about the new baby at night but you do not have the energy to repeatedly do the silent return to sleep (see Chapter 7). Don't be inhibited because of a fear that you are causing a 'regression' or sense of failure in your child. Under these circumstances, the baby might have to go to a portable cot, another cot if the children are close together in age, or maybe some temporary larger substitute for the bassinet.

Twins, Triplets and More

Let's face it: having a baby is a blessing and a bother. With two or three babies at the same time, the blessings are two- or threefold, but the bother is about ten or twenty times as great! The reason why the bother is so much greater is that you can't clone yourself. When one child is awake and wants to play but the other needs to be put to bed, or when one baby needs to be fed at the same time as the other needs to be changed, you've got a problem. Not everyone has family members or hired help to give them a break, and even if you are lucky in this regard, there are still times when both the mother and father are exhausted from not getting enough sleep. However, if you plan ahead and if the father is actively involved, as described in the story of Caleb and Ezra, then the duration of your sleep-starved state will be shorter.

Caleb and Ezra

As much as it gave us great joy, the news that we were having twins shocked us as well. We hadn't had children yet, so how our lives would work with one baby was a big question, but two seemed to raise to an unimaginable degree the level of responsibility and the sheer amount of labour we anticipated. Eventually the shock faded, giving way to excitement tempered by trepidation, and we began facing the many tasks we had to do.

We had our share of endless nights, during which someone was up every hour with one fussy fellow or another – or both didn't fall back to sleep without being walked back and forth. In a sleep-starved daze, we both covered many miles during those nights. To keep track of who fed whom, Jen and I drew two clock faces, one for each boy, on which we would record the time we retrieved either Ezra or Caleb, how many ounces of formula he consumed, and what time he went back down. To maintain our sanity – or as a record of its fragility during these sleep-drained hours – we would amuse each other with humorous notations on the clocks.

During the day the boys would sleep with regularity; up for an hour or so and down for several. One thing we experienced in full force, when the boys were around six weeks old, was heart-rending, inconsolable, nonstop crying at the end of the day, starting around 6:00 P.M. and sometimes lasting until as late as 10:00 P.M. before the exhausted babies would relent and drift off to sleep. During their fifth and sixth months, they began to sleep through the night. On the rare occasion when we did hear one of them cry or yell out during the night, we would resist the urge to react, and within a few minutes the baby would soothe himself back to sleep. We took advantage of their ability to soothe themselves to catch up on our sleep, too – even with the rest, two babies are a lot of work and we need all the energy we can muster.

One of our concerns, specific to having twins who sleep in the same room, has been about one baby waking the other. When our boys were about seven and a half months old, Ezra was waking Caleb up consistently. We consulted with Dr Weissbluth, who instructed us to keep a twenty-four-hour chart for each baby over the course of a week. We recorded, in half-hour increments, whether the boys were asleep, awake and crying, or awake and happy. With this information, Dr Weissbluth was able to tell us that we should put Ezra and Caleb down for naps at 9:00 A.M. and 1:00 P.M., and that it was time to eliminate their third nap of the day. This approach smoothed out their sleep pattern.

Overall, we have simply had to revise our expectations of how much time we have available and what we can accomplish. Adhering to a schedule that dictates the amount of time the children will be awake has circumscribed our activities. This would be true for anyone who chooses to abide by Dr Weissbluth's approach to sleep. But with twins, it's even more pronounced: since the multiplied tasks of child care place a greater demand on our time, there's even less time left for the extras. We had adjusted to this in various ways, but the sacrifices we've had to make during these months have very clearly been worthwhile. We never cease to hear people comment when we go out: 'Oh, look, twins!' and 'They're so cute' (which I, of course, can confirm). More than that, we constantly hear remarks to the effect that the boys are so well behaved and remarkably calm.

Raising 'multiples' requires an extra degree of forethought, communication, planning and sheer work. Two parents for whom sleep is an enchanting memory have to struggle to find the energy it takes to do all the work, mental and physical, necessary to take care of twins. Having had this experience, it's clear to me that training a child to sleep well is an extraordinarily crucial component to child rearing, especially when you're having more than one.

Here is an account from a family where the twins initially were overtired.

Nikolai and Aleksander

Nikolai and Aleksander, our identical twin boys, were born six weeks early. For the first few weeks, the boys slept soundly and cosily together in their cot. We had been instructed by the hospital to wake them at night for feedings, which we did happily. As they gained weight and their actual due date neared, they became more and more alert, much to our delight. Perhaps due to their early sleepiness, it didn't even occur to Mike and me to put the boys on any kind of schedule, or to protect the sleep. We both just assumed they would fall asleep when they were tired. When Nik or Aleks started to cry after two or three hours of wakefulness, we chalked it up to fussiness. When they took only a few very brief naps a day, we assumed they weren't sleepy children, and that most babies were like that. We told our friends and family that the boys could barely sleep an hour or two at a time at night, and they advised us to keep them up during the day so they would be tired at night. When that didn't work, we relied on reports that things would improve when they hit the three-month mark. We took the nights in shifts – I would sleep from 8:00 P.M. to 1:30 A.M., and then take over so Mike could get some rest – and gritted our teeth, waiting for the day they would be three months old, at which time they would embrace naps and bedtimes with sweet smiles and contented sighs.

Not only did that day never come, but the older Aleks and Nik got, the worse their sleep patterns became. They could manage to sleep a couple of hours if they were cuddled up on Mike or me, but they did not sleep in their cot for longer than twenty minutes at a time. When I asked their paediatrician about it at their four-month check-up, he told me it was normal for infants to have such short, erratic sleep. When I left his office, I knew he was wrong. I sought out Dr Weissbluth and his book, and was amazed by what I read! I had been doing all the wrong things with my children – keeping them awake for several hours at a time, rushing in to rescue them from their beds at the slightest peep, allowing them to 'snack' on poor-quality pushchair, swing or car seat sleep all day! Was it possible that my kids *did* need sleep, and I just hadn't been providing the right conditions for it? I felt horribly guilty for torturing my poor boys!

We began trying to help Nik and Aleks improve their sleep habits immediately. It seemed logical to attempt to get the boys on the same sleep schedule. We decided temporarily to have the boys sleep in separate rooms, which was a difficult decision for me to make. I had very strong feelings about keeping the boys together from the time they were born. I felt they would feel safer, more secure and comfortable if they could sleep together. I think I wanted them to continue what I considered to be an idyllic, symbiotic existence inside the womb. I still feel strongly about sleeping twins together, and wish that our circumstances hadn't forced our hand in this matter.

Our boys were incredibly overtired when we began to employ Dr Weissbluth's ideas and, as a result, they were overly sensitive to outside stimuli. The slightest floorboard creak would wake them from sleep with a jolt, and they would scream at the top of their lungs. As one can imagine, if small household sounds woke them so easily, the ear-piercing wails of a brother would do the same. Having two screaming babies was inordinately stressful, and made it virtually impossible for them to settle down and fall back asleep. We didn't have much room in our apartment, so we chose to let Nik, who slept more soundly, sleep in our room in his cot, while Aleks stayed in his own room.

Mike and I continued our nightly 'shifts' as we instituted Dr Weissbluth's plan and set out to improve our children's sleep habits. I spent many difficult nights questioning myself and feeling bad for 'making' my children cry. Although we saw improvement immediately, it took several weeks before Aleks and Nik had completely adjusted to the new sleep routine. I believe it really took them months to get over those first months of so little sleep. The transformation was slow, but nearly miraculous. Our sweet, dear boys, who had probably been getting no more than eight to nine hours of irregular sleep a day, were now sleeping up to sixteen and eighteen hours a day! I often wonder if I ever would have figured out on my own that my sons, who initially seemed to need so little sleep, were actually in need of the absolute opposite.

As the months passed, I began to see that Nik and Aleks were way at one end of the sleep continuum – they needed, and continue to need, a lot more sleep than the average child. Around the time they were a year old, they were actually falling asleep at around 4:30 or 5:00 in the afternoon, and sleeping until about 6:30 in the morning! Then they would take a nap at around 8:30 for one to two hours, and a nap at noon for another one to two hours. They didn't give up their third nap until just before their first birthday. Our realisation that they required so much sleep was a revelation – we had finally found the 'key' to unlock their sunny, curious, exuberant personalities. Having kids with such high sleep needs, however, hasn't been easy. On the contrary, it's been a real pain in the neck to protect their sleep so vigilantly. Before they were about two and a half years old, missing one nap would send our family into a tailspin – three to four days of fragmented night-time sleep, resistance to their regular naps, grumpiness, and so on. I can count on my hands the number of times we allowed them to miss a nap or stay up late before they turned three. The cost of such a move was so great that few things were worth the price.

When Aleks and Nik were thirty months old, Michael and I were preparing for the birth of our youngest son. My in-laws purchased two beautiful 'big boy' beds for the twins, and we excitedly set them up and let them loose. The twins had escaped from their cots on a couple of occasions, but had responded well to reprimanding. They were capable of sleeping safely in the twin beds, but did not seem able to follow instructions to stay in them. Looking back, I realise that attempting to make the move so early was a mistake. Bedtime became a circus, complete with two wild monkeys, jumping and running around their rooms each night. After two months of little improvement, one night they fell silent almost immediately after their bedtime routine. I was hopeful that all the bribes, cajoling and scolding had finally worked, but I went in to check on them anyway. I walked in to find Nik standing on his bed, snapping the wood blinds from his window in half, carefully sliding them out of their frames and handing them over to Aleks. Aleks was sitting quietly, stacking my broken blinds on his bed. We dismantled the beds and put their cots back up the next day.

We set the twin beds up again soon after the boys turned three.

The first few nights were successful, but things began to deteriorate soon after. Even in their pitch-dark room, Aleks and Nik would run around their room, empty their dressers, jump on their beds and stay up one to two hours past their normal bedtime. Within a few weeks they were engaging in the same kind of behaviour at nap time, and Mike and I knew we had to make a change. This time, it was easy for me to make the decision to separate them. The difficulty was where to put them! We settled on putting Aleks to bed in our room. After their bedtime stories, Nik stays in his room, and we take Aleks to our bed where he sleeps until we're ready to go to bed. At that time, we carry Aleks back into his room. While the situation is not ideal, it has been very successful for us. At three years of age, the boys fall asleep between 7:00 and 7:30, wake up around 7:00 A.M., and take one nap a day from 1:00 to 3:00 P.M. Aleks is incredibly cuddly and happy to return to his bed each night, and it doesn't seem to affect his overall sleep habits. After feeling so strongly about keeping the twins in the same bedroom, I would be the first to give them their own rooms now if our house provided it. At this stage in their lives, I think it would be healthy for them to have a few hours to themselves after playing together all day. In addition, the separation relieves them of the pressure to perform for each other.

Tomas arrived when the twins were thirty-two months old. I never realised how difficult it was to have twins until he arrived! It's such a relief not to panic at every cry, for fear of waking the 'other' baby. Of course, I have to admit that Tomas has made it really easy on us. He is even-tempered, sweet and happy. He was practically sleeping through the night within a week of coming home from the hospital. In the first few months, we could tell when he was sleepy, as it would be the only time he'd cry. Now that he's nearly six months old, he continues to be patient and calm. I'm careful to maintain his nap schedule and to put him to bed early at night, and he wakes up happy and content, cooing and smiling. His sweet, gentle demeanour makes me wonder what Nikolai and Aleksander would have been like at his age if I had incorporated Dr Weissbluth's ideas immediately after they were born!

There is ample evidence that genetics contribute significantly to shaping our sleep patterns. Identical twins sleep more like each other than fraternal twins. So there are limits on what we can do to modify their schedules if we attempt to synchronise them. As discussed previously, the regularity of the mother's activity/rest cycles and her sleeping and eating patterns before the babies are born may substantially contribute to the regularity or irregularity of her babies.

With twins, triplets, or more, the major principle is to start sleep training *early*.

Early sleep training means starting around the time the babies are born, or around the time of their due date for children born early (many twins or triplets arrive before their due date). The first principle is to *avoid the overtired state*. Try to put your babies down for a nap, using Method A (see page 235), after a wakeful period of one or two hours. If they get overtired, it is harder for them to fall asleep. The more rested they are, the more adaptable they become later, and the more successful you will be in synchronising their sleep schedules when they are older. Because the clock machinery is not really well developed during these first few weeks, you can't set their clocks to thc samc 'timc'.

Counting from the due date, over the next six weeks, you will notice more and more fussiness and wakefulness; by six weeks of age, it is mostly concentrated in the evening hours, about 7:00 to 10:00 P.M. During these increasing spells of agitated or fussy wakefulness, do whatever you can to calm and comfort your babies. Remember, you can't spoil your babies, so during these spells do all the holding, hugging, nursing or whatever works to keep your infants comfortable.

The next step in early sleep training, at about six weeks after the due date, means trying to *control the wake-up time* in the morning with the goal of partially synchronising the babies' sleep/wake cycles. The earlier we start the process and the more rested our children are, the more likely it is we will succeed.

So, around six weeks after the due date, when one baby awakes in the morning, you declare that the day is starting and night sleep has ended. This will usually occur between 5:00 and 8:00 A.M. At that time, awaken the other baby or babies. Remember, we are doing this at a few weeks of age to help synchronise their sleep schedules, but this manoeuvre of controlling the wake-up time may also be applied to older twins and triplets. If you are experienced parents, you might want to try to control the wake-up time when the children are much younger. If you are good at reading the babies' cues and you have identical twins, then you might be able to synchronise their schedules when they are very young.

After both children are up in the morning, the next step is to keep the following interval of wakefulness ultra-short. We are going to try to put both children down for the first nap – together, in the same room or cot – after only *one hour* of wakefulness. Try as best you can to change, feed and soothe them back to sleep within a total time of one hour. This means that you will probably have no time to play with them during this brief morning wakeful period. During this hour of wakefulness, if there is bright natural sunlight, open all your curtains and expose them to this light, because exposure to *bright morning light* helps to set the sleep/wake clock.

Let's stop for a quick review: start early, avoid the overtired state, use Method A, control the wake-up time, allow a very brief interval (only one hour) of wakefulness, and exposure to bright light.

Now comes the hard part, especially if you are an inexperienced parent. Our hope is that your children will be able to learn some self-soothing skills even at this very young age. The most important point is to put your babies down to sleep after several minutes of soothing whether or not they are in a deep sleep state. This simply means that your children may be fully asleep, completely awake, or in a state between wakefulness and sleep at the time when you put them down.

If one or both babies cry as you walk away, leave them alone – but look at a clock so that you will know when they have been alone for five to ten minutes. Here are two common scenarios: your babies cry very hard for a few minutes, then cry quietly for several minutes, and then fall asleep. Or possibly your babies cry hard for several minutes and do not appear to be able to fall asleep. Of course, one child may go one way and the other child another way. Your goal is to get and protect the morning nap for one or both children.

If your baby does fall asleep, don't be surprised if the duration of the nap is brief; naps tend to lengthen only at twelve to sixteen weeks of age, counting from the due date. Within any subsequent two-hour interval, try to put both children back down for a nap. This is because most young babies do not comfortably tolerate more than two hours of wakefulness.

If your baby does not fall asleep, rescue your baby or babies. You now have two choices. First, you may sense that after several minutes of hard crying your baby will now be able to fall asleep, so you repeat the process of soothing back to sleep. Or else the crying was so stressful for all of you that you will quickly go out for a walk, enjoy playing with and comforting your baby, and try this manoeuvre again another day. Remember, you want to give your babies the opportunity to learn how to soothe themselves to sleep. You are practicing *consistency* in how you soothe the baby to sleep and *timing* to avoid the overtired state.

If you had only one child, you might decide to always hold or nurse that child until he or she was in a deep sleep state and then either put the baby down alone or sleep with the baby in your bed or sofa (Method B, see page 236). The simple truth is that you cannot be consistent with Method B if you have twins or triplets. So stick with Method A. Because the process of falling asleep is learned behaviour, your babies will learn faster if you are consistent in how you soothe them to sleep.

At night, an early bedtime is helpful because it regularises and lengthens naps. Here, too, consistency in the style of soothing to sleep is helpful.

If you have older twins or triplets, between four and fifteen months of age, control the wake-up time, expose them to bright light in the period after they wake up and practise consistency in how you soothe your babies to sleep. Now your goal is to put them down for naps at about 9:00 A.M. and 1:00 P.M., and not to let them sleep at other times during the day. Expect your babies at fifteen to twenty-one months of age to need a single nap between noon and 2:00 P.M.

Here is the story of one mother who started sleep training her twins at eleven months of age.

Caroline and Laura

As a new mum, I was very reluctant to let my babies cry when they reached the four-month mark. Although my rational side (smaller every day, due to sleep deprivation) believed that children would sleep better if they learned to soothe themselves to sleep, I was filled with anxiety that I might be doing the wrong thing . . . they would be emotionally scarred, feel abandoned or at a minimum be in pain and need our care. My husband, convinced that life must get better, had to force me to stay in our bedroom while the girls learned to soothe themselves to sleep. They cried for only about fifteen minutes, but it seemed like days.

They cried less each day for three or four days and rarely cried at nap time after they learned to soothe themselves to sleep. I no longer spent hours every day rocking them to sleep. What a relief. We also found that sleep begets sleep . . . the better they napped, the better they slept at night.

I now have six-month-old Peter, who has been a joy in every way, starting with the fact that he was not part of a set. With two 'guinea pigs' before him, I don't need to try all the tried-and-true sleep remedies. I now know what works and what doesn't. When he was fourteen weeks old, I started him on a 9:00 A.M. and 1:00 P.M. nap schedule with a 6:00 P.M. bedtime. Starting a predictable schedule at fourteen weeks was much better than waiting for eleven months for some organisation in my chaotic household. When he was four months old, I let him learn to soothe himself to sleep. He cried on only four different occasions, for no more than ten minutes each time. Starting a schedule and self-soothing are proving much easier at such a young age.

The plan to have the babies asleep and awake at about the same time may initially fail, because there is a strong genetic component that influences how long babies sleep, how regular are the times when they need to sleep, and how self-soothing they are when put down to sleep. Therefore, you may be more successful in synchronising sleep schedules with identical twins than with fraternal twins. But even identical twins can have their own personality! Prepare yourself for the possibility that one twin may be a good sleeper (self-soothing, long sleep durations, regular sleep patterns) and the other twin is the opposite.

As I mentioned, in the beginning, place your babies together in the same room, or even the same cot. Many of these babies seem to enjoy touching each other and sometimes appear to help the other one sleep by stroking, petting or even putting a hand or finger in the mouth of the other. Later, if it becomes apparent that one twin or triplet is interfering with the sleep of another, then you have to try to separate the 'bad sleeper' from the 'good sleeper'. Sometimes this is easier said than done because of the number of rooms in your house. Be creative. You might temporarily put one child in your bedroom for naps, or perhaps you have a large walk-in cupboard, or maybe there is some attic or basement space where you can create a nest for naps. This temporary separation might be needed until the 'bad sleeper' settles down to a regular nap pattern, which usually evolves between twelve and sixteen weeks after their due date. Also, please do not be surprised if the twins do a flip-flop and the one who had been a 'good sleeper' becomes a 'bad sleeper' and vice versa. The truth is that during the first few months, there is a lot of shifting around in daytime sleep patterns. All children sleep better during the day around three or four months of age, so be patient.

When I discussed the problem of trying to synchronise sleep schedules when one twin naps better than the other with mothers and fathers at a support group for parents of twins, some said they would wake up the good sleeper, go out to have fun and then put them both down together for the next sleep period. The risk is that the good sleeper might become over-tired because the child's needs are not met. Other parents let the good sleeper finish the nap and later put them down together. Here, the risk is that the bad sleeper becomes very overtired from being up too long. The mother of Ezra and Caleb, currently two excellent sleepers, really summed up the majority sentiment when she said, 'You just have to compromise.' Sometimes letting the good sleeper snooze a little longer before waking him up is all it takes to produce some regularity in the sleep routines.

Here's the conflict: you want to avoid the overtired state *and* you want to synchronise their sleeping patterns. Sleep logs, as described on pages 118 and 221, are very helpful to get a handle on how to strike a good compromise.

Each family with twins and triplets has its own strengths, resources and stresses; please consider reviewing your situation with other parents of twins and triplets or your paediatrician before sleep problems develop.

Moving

The only thing worse than moving is moving with children. You pack, they unpack. You clean up, they make a mess. Here is one account of how moving upset a child's routine.

'Nicholas Knew This Was the Time to Really Try It On'

Nicholas had an established sleep pattern before we moved, but after . . . !

Bill and I started packing up the flat about two months before we moved; Nicholas's response to this preparation was to change his sleep pattern. But we weren't too worried, since we assumed it would change back once we were moved and settled. It didn't. We moved when he was about eight months old. Well, by the time Nicholas was nine months, I needed another chat with Dr Weissbluth to discuss Nicholas's frequent night wakings.

My husband was with my father for the opening of trout season that weekend, and Nicholas knew this was the time to really try it on with me.

Nicholas had had a cold for weeks. Thursday night he cried from 7:00 until 11:00 P.M. I went in several times to try to calm him. I knew that what I should be doing was turning off, or down to a whisper, the intercom and letting him work it out, but I thought the cold had something to do with it. Dr Weissbluth said the cold *did* have something to do with it – plain and simple. Nicholas needed more sleep to shake it, but just as important was the routine Nicholas had to learn (again). The doctor made me promise not to go in the room at all until between 5:00 and 7:00 A.M.: 'Load him up with a layer cream and hugs and kisses and close the door.' The first night the crying stopped after about an hour and a half, but by Saturday Nicholas cried for only five minutes. Now he will perhaps play for at least a few minutes, then before I know it, his head is down and we have a quiet, happy baby twelve hours later!

Your general goal is to maintain as regular and consistent a pattern as possible when preparing for and following a move. Resist the temptation to drag the baby to the home improvement store or garden shop when he should be sleeping. If your child is young, say less than a year old, quickly re-establish the bedtime rituals and sleep patterns that worked best before the move. Be firm, and after allowing a day or two for adjustment to the new surroundings, ignore any protest crying that may have evolved from the irregularity and inconsistency during the move. If your child is older, say a few years, go slower. Fears of newness, excitement over novelty, and uncertainty regarding further changes may cause new problems of resistance to naps, difficulty falling asleep at night, or night waking. Be gentle, firm and decisive. Reassurance, extra time at night, night-lights and open doors have a calming or soothing effect. Be somewhat consistent in controlling this extra comfort so that the child does not learn that it is completely open-ended. For the older child, consider using a kitchen timer to control the amount of extra time you are going to spend with her. The timer helps the child to learn to expect that mum or dad will leave for the night after a predictable time period. Place the timer under a pillow or cushion to muffle the sound.

Anxiety or fear in your child regarding a move is natural, normal and not something that should unduly alarm you. After several days, start a deliberate process of 'social weaning' to encourage a return to your old, healthy sleep habits by gradually reducing the duration on the timer. This should usually take no more than several days in most instances.

Holidays and Crossing Time Zones

Think of a holiday with your child as sort of a semi-holiday. After all, you may spend a lot of time baby-sitting among the palms on sun-drenched beaches. I have spent many hours building simple sand castles, trying to keep one eye on the castle architecture and the other eye on a nonswimmer jumping over small waves. This intense concentration is not very relaxing!

Try to flow with your child; be flexible, forget schedules, try to have as much fun as possible and don't worry much if your kids become tired. Irregularity and spontaneity are part of what makes holidays fun.

When you cross time zones, you might suffer the ill effects of jet lag. You are conditioned to sleep when it is dark, but activity/rest cycles and feeding habits also get messed up when you cross time zones. Children seem to be more sensitive to light, especially morning light, than adults are, so use this to help defeat the jet lag. The day after you arrive, or the next day for a very long trip – both at your destination, at the beginning of the trip, and home when the holiday is over – wake your child at the usual wake-up time.

Scenario one: You leave your home very early in the morning because of holiday traffic and the extra time required because of airport security. You arrive at your destination, and it is now very late at night. By the time you claim your luggage, rent a car, drive to your hotel and get settled, everyone is exhausted. It's been a long day! So everyone sleeps in late the next morning. If your child is napping, the late morning wake-up causes the nap(s) to be later. Therefore, wake up your child after a one- to two-hour nap in order to protect a reasonably early bedtime. The following morning, either wake up your child at his routine time to re-establish his regular sleeping schedule, or repeat the process of shortening the nap to more gradually get the bedtime to its regular early time. If your child is not napping, over the next day or days control the wake-up time by waking your child earlier either a lot or a little until you get to your normal wake-up time.

Scenario two: You arrive at your destination and get settled in by mid-afternoon or early evening. The day after you arrive, wake up your child at the usual time. That is, if you usually get up at 7:00, rouse your child at 7:00 local time, no matter what the time difference. Try to expose him to bright morning light. Continue with the schedule as if you had not taken a trip, using local time for naps and the night sleep. Naturally, there will be some irregularity, no matter how hard you try, so assume that when you return home, your child may be overtired.

Once you're home, it's boot camp again – back to the basics, with all the regular routines. Repeat the strategies described above. Within a few days, if you are firm, consistent and regular, your child will learn quickly that the holiday is over. If your child was well rested prior to this holiday, expect only one difficult recovery day of protest crying. Trying to gradually soothe your child back to her previous good sleep routine over several days often fails because the child fights sleep in order to enjoy your company.

You may avoid having a 're-entry' problem by carefully planning ahead, as Claire's parents did.

Claire's First Holiday

Having spent our previous holidays as young marrieds, jaunting lightheartedly to Hawaii, the Canadian Rockies, England, Europe and New England without an itinerary or reservations, it was with some trepidation that my husband, Tom, and I launched off on our first holiday as new parents with our eight-month-old daughter in tow. We chose a family-oriented beach resort (only one time zone away), which was conveniently located near a major city of historical interest that we had never visited. We decided to spend our money on above-average accommodation, knowing that with an eight-month-old we would be spending more time there and might as well make ourselves comfortable. We selected a two-bedroom/two-bath flat with a kitchen and large living/dining area, which ensured that Claire's naps and bedtimes wouldn't interfere with our activities and vice versa.

Our daily schedule certainly was not as hectic as when we were just a couple, but we did manage to relax more and have a great deal of fun. We tried to preserve Claire's two-nap-a-day schedule and approximate bedtime hour, but we wanted to be flexible, too. A typical day for us would begin with breakfast at the flat followed by a walk on the magnificent beach looking for shells and pebbles. Because the sand is firmly packed there, we could push Claire's pushchair right along on the beach, which allowed us to venture farther than if she'd been in the backpack. About midmorning we'd return to the flat for Claire's nap. One of us would lounge on the sundeck while Claire was sleeping, while the other would be free to go swimming, shopping, cycling or whatever.

After lunch – either a picnic by the park/playground near the flat or a meal at the snack bar by the pool – we'd pack up the car and head to a nearby attraction. Claire would promptly fall asleep in her car seat for her afternoon nap, a habit we never practised back home, and be ready to go again after we reached our various destinations about an hour or so later.

We ventured out to dinner with Claire on several occasions, picking one of the resort's family-oriented restaurants and arriving early (both before the larger crowds and to be closer to her typical suppertime). After another walk on the beach, we'd follow Claire's bedtime routine and put her to sleep at about her normal hour in the rented full-size cot in her own room. We then had time to enjoy some wine, read, catch up on our conversation or plan the next day's activities.

Yes, it was quite a different style of holiday for us! But the new scenery was fascinating, and with some advance planning (like arranging the cot rental and packing a special box with Claire's walker, backpack carrier, and favourite toys), we all were able to enjoy our first holiday as a family.

Frequent Illnesses

Night wakings routinely follow frequent illnesses. First, let's have a clear understanding of what is happening. Videotapes of healthy young children in their homes at night show that many awakenings occur throughout the night, but the children usually return to sleep without any help. Fever can alter sleep patterns and can cause light sleep or more frequent awakenings. So it is not surprising that a painful illness with fever, such as an ear infection, causes an increased number of night wakings. These more frequent and prolonged arousals often require your intervention to soothe or calm the child back to sleep. Your child might now begin to associate your hugging, kissing or holding at night with returning to sleep. This learning process might then produce an alteration in the child's behaviour or expectations that continue long after the infection passes. Now we have a night-waking pattern.

Actually, awakening at night is *not* the problem. As we have seen, spontaneous awakenings are normal, as are increased awakenings with fever. Naturally, parents should go to their sick children at night. The real problem once the child is healthy again and not bothered by pain or fever is his learned difficulty in returning to sleep unassisted.

How can you reteach your child to develop her own resources to return to sleep after awakening? Remember, parents are teachers and we teach health habits, even if the child might not initially cooperate or appreciate our efforts. Here are three options:

Option one: You might decide that since children are frequently ill and you can't let your child down when he needs you, you will always respond and you will simply wait for the child to 'outgrow' this habit. The problem with this option is that the awakenings initially tend to become more frequent, because your child learns to enjoy your company at night. After all, who wants to be alone in a boring, dark, quiet room in the middle of the night? Eventually, months or years later, the child sleeps through the night and the parents can congratulate themselves for always having attended to their child's crying at night. You have, however, paid a price. Parents following this course of action often become sleep-deprived or chronically fatigued, and occasionally feel resentful towards the child for not appreciating their dedicated efforts. In addition, the sleep fragmentation and sleep deprivation often produce a child who is more irritable, aroused, agitated and hyperexcitable because the child is always fighting chronic fatigue and drowsiness.

Option two: You might try to go to your child at night only when she is really sick and to leave the child alone at night when she is healthy. This is a strategy that often fails, because you may often be uncertain whether an illness is serious or just a minor concern. After all, at 7:00 P.M., you might decide that your child has only a minor common cold and that you are going to ignore her crying, but by 2:00 A.M. you begin to worry about the possibility of an ear infection. Is it still reasonable to ignore the crying? What usually occurs is intermittent reinforcement: you sometimes go to your child and sometimes do not. This behaviour generally teaches your child to cry longer and louder when she awakens at night, because she learns that only loud and persistent crying will bring her parents. Quiet or brief crying often fails to get the parents' attention.

Option three: Work closely with your paediatrician to devise a reasonable strategy whereby frequent visits or phone calls permit a clearer distinction between non-serious common colds and more distressing or disturbing illnesses. Generally speaking, the child's playfulness, sociability, activity and appetite during the day are good clues; common colds do not cause much change in your child's behaviour when awake. Then, in a planned and deliberate fashion, your child is left alone more and more at night, so that she learns to return to sleep without your help. When an acute illness develops that is associated with high fever or severe pain, of course, do whatever comforts the child best, both night and day. But when the acute phase of this illness is over, start again to give her less and less attention at night. Remember, most children sleep through most common colds; with your paediatrician's help, you can learn to distinguish between 'habit crying' that occurs with a common cold and the more painful crying that is associated with a serious and painful acute infection.

Research has shown that sleep loss itself can cause impairments in our immune system, which is the body's defence mechanism to prevent infections. So it's a vicious circle: illnesses might disturb sleep, and not sleeping well makes us more vulnerable to becoming sick.

Mother's Return to Work

Some adults develop sensitivity to children's needs and appreciate the benefits of regularity, consistency and structure in child care activities. Some do not. The quality of the carer is what is important, not whether the person is or is not the biological parent.

> **PRACTICAL POINT**
>
> **Write down specific instructions for sleep rituals so that the baby-sitter, the nanny or the day-care provider knows what soothes your child best.**

Do not assume that when the mother returns to work outside the home, your child's sleep habits will suffer. Keep data: track the schedule of naps when she is cared for by someone else, ask the nanny to keep a sleep log so you know exactly what is going on, watch for signs of tiredness in the early evening that might suggest nap deprivation.

Sometimes a nanny is a very nurturing person who wants to hold your baby all the time. But at some point you'll want to be able to use Method A, which means putting your child down for naps after soothing whether or not she is asleep. If the nanny refuses to do this, then your child will not be able to learn to soothe herself to sleep.

PRACTICAL POINT

To help your child sleep better during natural room changes such as holidays, moves or taking her to your workplace, try to build an environment of familiarity by using certain cues only for sleeping:

The same bumper pads
The same music box
The same stuffed animal or blanket
A spray of perfume, used only at sleep times

The child will then learn to associate these sensations with falling asleep, and this will help reduce the disruptive effect of the novelty of any new surroundings. None of these items, however, will work in the absence of regularity and consistency of parent care.

Please don't let your guilt about being away so much during the day cause you to keep the child up too late, to reinforce night wakings for sweet nocturnal private time with your baby, or to induce nap deprivation at weekends when you cram in too many activities. And don't let household errands, chores or non-essential social events rob you and your child of unstructured, low-intensity playtime. The most common mistake is to keep your child up past the time of tiredness; your child needs sleep just like she needs food. Don't withhold sleep any more than you would withhold food.

Home Office

Parents who work at home are closer to their children throughout the day, and some parents have a similar situation when they are able to take their baby to their workplace. The general problem is that some parents try to schedule their child's sleep around their work. In the beginning, with a newborn baby who naturally sleeps a lot, parents sometimes have the illusion that it will be smooth going. This is especially true if you have an easy-temperament baby. Unfortunately, the ebb and flow of the baby's developing sleep rhythms cannot be moulded to fit a work schedule. An exception might be made if both parents are working together and there is always one available to attend to the baby.

Let's say that you have a home office and have hired someone to assist you with the care of your baby. Please do not expect to work, care for your baby, and breast-feed on any regular schedule. Your baby can smell you; she will know you are there! When she is hungry and wants to be fed, even though she might not see you, she senses your presence and expects you to feed her – now, not later. If you decided to feed formula instead of breast milk, then others will be able to help out more with the feedings. Expect to make lots of compromises between your needs, the baby's needs and the expectations of the person helping you care for your child.

One thing you can do to make it easier is to start early to respect your child's need to sleep, and be very careful to avoid the overtired state. Starting as soon as you come home from the hospital is the best. The reason for starting early is that a well-rested baby is more adaptable to schedule changes that might occur when you try to coordinate baby care and working in your home office. Second, if you are breast-feeding, introduce a single bottle per day of expressed breast milk or formula at about two weeks of age. It does not have to be at the same time each day. If you do this, your baby will be able to take a bottle. If you wait a longer time to introduce a bottle, your baby may decide that he will take only the breast, and you lose some flexibility. The single bottle will not confuse your baby or cause weaning to occur.

Here is one mother's account of how starting a bottle early and establishing a schedule really helps.

'Mummy Works at Home'

In some ways, working from home proved to be much more challenging that I had expected. The hardest part of being at home was hearing my new baby cry and realising that my caregiver was unable to quieten her as quickly as I could. The urge to go to Katherine was incredibly strong, and many times I had to force myself to stay at my desk and allow the caregiver to find her own way of comforting the baby. While I knew intellectually that she needed to bond with Katherine, it was very hard to fight the maternal instinct.

I also found that the noise a two-year-old makes carries quite easily up two flights of stairs and through two closed doors! My oldest child, Caroline, became an unexpected participant this way on many phone calls with my clients and co-workers. I quickly learned to plan important phone calls around nap times, or go into the office on busy days to avoid the distraction.

It's not easy being a parent; it's harder when you have to work outside the home. The home office option is not available to everyone, but with planning and an attitude of flexibility and willingness to compromise, many mothers and fathers find the rewards are more than worth the effort.

Even when children outgrow naps, the home office is a possibility. Charlie's mother describes the lifestyle of a parent who works out of her home.

New Arrangement

I've had a home office for five years, ever since my son Charlie was born. Before Charlie entered our lives, I had a fast-paced job at a public relations agency, which I thoroughly enjoyed. But as my maternity leave progressed, I lost my appetite for going back to the gruelling hours that were expected at the office. What kind of time or energy would be left for my son? Not surprisingly, the agency didn't have much sympathy for my point of view. I was lucky, however, because my biggest client suggested I work for them from home, and they were willing to accept a part-time arrangement. I know full well how fortunate I am; in fact, I wish I had a pound for every person who has told me that I have the best of both worlds.

From my perspective as a home-office veteran, there are many, many benefits. For example, working from home allowed me to nurse my son for thirteen months. A home office set-up also makes it much easier to establish good sleeping habits for your child. First, you have more opportunity to get tuned in to your baby's need for sleep, especially during that first year. When he gets tired, you're able to pick up signals – which can be subtle – and you can put him down before he gets overtired. It used to amaze me how much sleep my son needed once he got past that newborn, semi-colicky period; a couple of hours awake, and then it was back to bed. He took three naps a day until he was nine months old.

I sympathise with parents who don't get home from work until 6:00 P.M. and then, quite naturally, want to spend time with their children. Early bedtimes have to be tough. But if you're already home, you can give your child dinner at a reasonable hour and get him to bed when he's ready to sleep, not when it's convenient for you. When our son was going through the transition period from two naps to one, he needed to go to sleep by 6:30 P.M. at the latest. Instead of all of us gobbling down our food, I gave Charlie an early dinner, and when my husband got home, he would give him a bath. My husband and I would eat later in peace and quiet. This was only a temporary period, and in a few months, we were back to eating dinner as a family again, which we felt was important.

For most of the time that I've had a home office, I've had a baby-sitter come in two or three days a week. On the days that she's off, I'm on my own. I used to relish nap time because I could get so much accomplished. When Charlie was taking two naps, I would have uninterrupted blocks of one to two hours, both in the morning and in the afternoon. A friend of mine used to warn me darkly that this two-naps-a-day stuff wouldn't last, and, of course, it didn't. But I've also discovered a side benefit to working at home, which is that you tend to become very productive. No meetings, no interruptions from colleagues, no hanging around in the break room. When I am in my office, I work.

I routinely work at night, after Charlie goes to bed. He is asleep by 7:30 P.M., which pretty much leaves the whole evening. That's another benefit of early bedtimes! Sometimes I have to work very late to make a deadline, and then I'm tired the next day, but I'm willing to pay this price.

Home offices are not a perfect arrangement. You miss out on the office gossip, so you have to make an effort to stay connected. Another problem is that things come up unexpectedly, and I have to scramble if my baby-sitter isn't here. Yet the best thing about a home office is the flexibility. I used to think that I'd probably go back to work when Charlie got a little older, but now I'm not so sure. I like being able to participate in his school activities, and I like being here when he gets home. My home office represents freedom and I can't imagine trading that in, even for a regular paycheque.

Some parents try to set up a mini-nursery or nest in their offices or stores for their babies to sleep. The truth is that it is difficult to answer phones or do business with clients at the same time your baby needs your attention. Perhaps for a few months, your child might seem to fit in, but it will become increasingly more difficult as he becomes more social, more alert and more needy for your attention. Again, an exception might be when both parents are working together, so that one is always available for the baby.

Dual-Career Families

When both parents are working outside the home, the major problem is that the child tends to be put to sleep too late. Sometimes this occurs because, by the time the child is picked up from day care and brought home, it is already past the child's biological time for night sleep to start. Occasionally this is further complicated by the day-care facility not being able to maintain a routine and environment conducive to good-quality day sleep. At other times, both parents return home late from work and they naturally want to play with their child before feeding, bathing and bedtime.

If the child goes to sleep past the time of biological sleep onset, then the child gradually becomes overtired. If the child is young, naps might be extra long in order to partially compensate for going to bed too late. Later, the older child begins to outgrow naps, and then the problems associated with the too-late bedtime begin to develop. But research has clearly shown that even with a fixed amount of sleep deficit, the child's irritability, fussiness and short temper do not stay fixed; rather, they increase. Everything gets worse, but this process may develop very slowly. Eventually bedtime battles and night waking emerge, perhaps for the first time. Many parents assume that there is some other problem, such as teething pain, separation anxiety, insecurity from the mother returning to work, the 'terrible twos', nightmares or the stress of a move or new sibling. Parents often do not see that the child has simply, slowly become overtired because several months before, the bedtime was allowed to become later.

MAJOR POINT

Constant sleep deficits cause increasing amounts of impaired functioning during wakefulness.

Q: *When should my child go to sleep at night?*
A: Before she becomes overtired.

If you think your child might be overtired in the late afternoon or early in the evening, try putting her to sleep twenty minutes earlier than is your current custom. If she falls asleep at this earlier time, then you will know that you have been putting her to bed too late. After several days, consider moving her bedtime another twenty minutes earlier if she still looks overtired. Remember, the way your child behaves or appears to you is more important than any recommended sleep duration or bedtime for 'average children'.

The most common inhibiting fear in putting your child to bed early are that he will start the day too early and he will love you less because you are spending less time with him. Not true! Because sleep begets sleep, if your child becomes better rested, he will be better able to fall asleep and stay asleep. He will not get up earlier and earlier because of an earlier bedtime. You will prevent or correct bedtime battles and night waking for attention. Naps will tend to become longer and more regular if your child goes to bed earlier. One common scenario is that because of a too-late bedtime, the child takes a too-long morning nap, which causes him to be extremely tired by 4:00 or 5:00 P.M. A temporarily very early bedtime will often shorten the morning nap so that the child is able to take a restorative afternoon nap between noon and 2:00 P.M. and subsequently be able to stay up a little later.

REMEMBER

Sleep begets sleep. It's not logical that earlier bedtimes allow children to sleep in later in the morning, it's biological.

Q: *I miss my baby so much during the day, why can't I spend more time with her at night? The only time I have to love my baby is late at night. Won't she miss me?*

A: If she becomes overtired, her company will not bc much fun. She will not enjoy or benefit as much from your social interaction because both of you will become increasingly fatigued. Her evolving bedtime battles and night waking will eventually produce an overtired family. At the price of seeing her less at night, she will stay better rested, more charming, more sweet, and you will mutually enjoy each other's company more in the morning and at the weekends.

Sometimes parents have to allow the sitter or the parent who comes home early to bathe, feed and dress the child for bed; immediately after the arrival of the parent who comes home late, the child is quietly soothed to sleep. With our busy lifestyles, it may be difficult to coordinate a work schedule with a child's biological needs. If this is the case for you, your baby's needs must come first. You would not withhold food when the body needs it because it is inconvenient to feed your child, and you try to anticipate when your child will become hungry in order to feed her before she becomes overly hungry. Similarly, try not to withhold sleep when the brain needs it, and try to anticipate when your child will become tired before she becomes overtired.

Occasionally it happens that, during the week, a sitter or day-care centre is protecting and maintaining naps, but at weekends everything falls apart. Dual-career families might try to do too much playing with their children at weekends to compensate for being with them less during the week, or they may simply not respect the child's need to nap because there are so many errands that have to be done. Either way, these children are often so overtired that they appear to be in pain. Every paediatrician gets some of these calls Monday morning because the parents often believe there is a painful ear infection. Severe *sleep inertia* can cause a child to awaken from a nap, which might be extra long, and scream as if in severe pain. Also, *night terrors* are often more common when children become severely overtired. On busy weekends, you should not feed your baby on the run; you need to find a quiet time to feed. Same thing for naps; don't nap on the run.

Adoption

Infants' sleep patterns are influenced by powerful biological or genetic forces when they are very young, but as they become older, their sleep patterns begin to reflect more of the social circumstances of their family and their culture. The child's biological sleep needs may or may not be met by their experiences. The following story illustrates how experienced parents were able to help their new child learn to sleep better, even though she hadn't slept well for nine months.

'Within About a Week or So, She Was on a Reasonable Schedule'

With our son, we had followed Dr Weissbluth's method from the start and Charlie developed excellent sleep habits. As a kindergartner, he's no longer napping, but per Dr Weissbluth, it's lights off by 7:30 P.M., and he's fine. As an infant and a toddler, Charlie very much needed consistent nap times and an early bedtime. Without that structure, he tended to fall apart. There was absolutely no question that Carina, our adopted daughter, would follow the 'Weissbluth method', too. She just didn't know it yet. As it turned out, there was plenty we didn't know yet either.

The big moment finally arrived, and we met Carina. (No, I didn't fall in love immediately.) At the time, she was nine and a half months – old enough to be wary of strangers, which is what Bill and I were. She clearly preferred her foster family, as we had anticipated and understood. They got to the hotel about an hour and a half later than originally planned, and I naively asked if they were late because she was napping. Well, no, that wasn't the reason; in fact, she hadn't had a nap that day.

We arrived back home late that night, and for the first time in her short life, Carina slept in a cot. She cried for a little while, but she managed to sleep pretty well, probably out of sheer exhaustion. The next day was a blur. We called Dr Weissbluth, who arranged for Carina to have a battery of tests performed right away at Children's Hospital. Blood and stool tests are typically recommended for international adoptions, and we were concerned about the parasite issue. The good news is that she turned out to be perfectly healthy, and the lab could find no signs of parasites.

The next day we paid a visit to Dr Weissbluth's office, and he advised us how to get Carina on schedule. Put her down at 9:00 A.M. for a morning nap, he said. Ideally, she should sleep an hour and a half. If she cries, pick her up after an hour. After lunch, try again. Put her down at 1:00 P.M., and if all goes well, she'll sleep until 2:30 P.M. If not, don't let her cry more than an hour. Bedtime should be between 6:00 and 7:00 P.M.

That sounds pretty simple. It wasn't. Carina didn't like her cot, she didn't like her room; she just didn't want to be alone. And she let us know it – vociferously. The trick was keeping her awake until bedtime. I'd learned from Charlie that those little catnaps can wreak havoc with sleep schedules.

Then, once Carina went to bed, there was no guarantee she would stay asleep. Bill and I were so tired and so tense, and we kept asking each other if one of us should go back into her room. But we honestly didn't think it would help, and besides, Dr Weissbluth had said to leave her alone. She finally stopped crying at about 2:45 A.M.

The next night was much better, and believe it or not, within about a week or so, she was on a reasonable schedule. It wasn't perfect. Sometimes she would take a good morning nap, and then her afternoon nap would be restless. Sometimes she would wake up in the middle of the night. But as time went on, her sleep rhythms seemed to consolidate, and she became much more predictable.

We thought all our problems were solved until we went through a period where she was waking up in the middle of the night. I was convinced that she was missing her foster father and that she was grieving for everything she had left behind in Guatemala. I felt so tormented by this that I went into her room and snuggled with her. This did not help at all. In fact, one night after I had supposedly soothed her, she cried for two more hours. I gave up on sleep and went downstairs to cut out coupons from the Sunday paper.

I mentioned my 'grieving' theory to Dr Weissbluth, who politely discounted it. He said that when babies wake up in the middle of the night, they are in a twilight state between sleep and waking. They aren't likely to be grieving or doing much else. Obviously, if a baby has an ear infection, she might be in pain, but this wasn't the case here. He suggested putting her to bed fifteen minutes earlier – at 6:45 P.M. instead of 7:00 P.M. Even with all our good efforts, Carina might still be overtired. Well, no one ever said that it was easy being a parent.

Carina has been with us now for nearly four months. She takes good naps in the morning and in the afternoon, and she sleeps about twelve hours at night. She is very happy to get into her cot and snuggle into her special corner. Occasionally she will wake up in the middle of the night, but we have learned to leave her alone. We have also learned to recognise the noises she makes when she's settling back to sleep, and these are very different from cries of pain or hunger.

Have these healthy sleep habits produced a happy child? You bet. Carina is a joy to be around. As we've all come to know each other better, she has become much more affectionate. She is clearly crazy about Charlie, and he is very proud to be a big brother. As for me, I fell in love. And despite all my trepidation, it really didn't take that long.

Injuries

Injuries occur to children of all ages. Some can – or should – be prevented, but some cannot. Examples of preventable injuries include leaving a four-month-old infant alone on a changing table from which she falls, poisonings occurring when safety seals are not used or medicines are left lying around, or electric shocks from uncovered wall sockets. A nonpreventable injury is truly an accident – for example, those resulting from an earthquake or a lightning bolt.

The truth is, though – and I realise this sounds harsh to

many parents' ears – that most so-called childhood accidents are really preventable injuries that occur because of parental neglect or the lack of parental forethought. These injuries can be one consequence of home routines that create tired children – and tired *families*.

But is there such a thing as an accident-prone child? To determine if traits within a child can cause him to suffer frequent injuries, various studies have examined babies before injuries start to occur. (After a child has had several injuries, a 'halo' effect develops and adults are more likely to perceive traits in the child – clumsiness, lack of self-control, and so on – that 'explain' why he has had so many injuries.)

One study included two hundred babies who were evaluated between four and eight months of age. Some of the infants were difficult to manage. As we saw earlier, these infants were called 'difficult' because they were irregular, low in adaptability, initially withdrawing, and negative in mood. During the next two years, difficult babies were much more likely to have cuts requiring stitches than were babies with the opposite or easy-to-manage temperaments. This study showed that during the first two years of life, about one-third of the difficult children had cuts deep or severe enough to require stitches, while only 5 per cent of easy babies had similar cuts.

Remember also my data: at four to eight months of age, difficult babies slept about three hours less than easy babies, and at age three, the difference was about one and a half hours. By age three, the briefer the sleep, the more active, excitable, impulsive, inattentive and easily distracted the child appeared – the perfect description of an accident-prone child. Little wonder, then, that these tired children fell more often, sustaining deep cuts.

Obviously, for both the 'difficult' kids and all other children, chronic fatigue can lead to more injuries, such as cuts and falls. More sleep is the remedy.

Another study that supports this fatigue-injury connection included more than 7,000 children who were one to two years old. Researchers compared children who frequently woke up at night with those who slept through the night. Among the night wakers, 40 per cent had injuries requiring medical attention, compared to only 17 per cent of the good sleepers. The parents of the children who were night wakers reported that they immediately went to their child when they heard a cry in order to prevent further crying. There was a tendency for the mothers of night wakers to feel more irritable in general and 'out of control'. One sign of family tension was that these mothers felt unable to confide in their husbands; the association of marital difficulties with disturbed sleep has been mentioned in many studies.

Maybe the parents who don't supervise sleep patterns so that the child can have his sleep needs met are the same ones who don't supervise children at play in order to protect their physical safety. The message is clear: if your child is often injured, it's not necessarily because he is careless or clumsy – he may be exhausted instead.

I have seen many children who were so overtired that they fell down only a stair or two or fell from a very low height. But because they hit their head and were later noted to be sleepy or wobbly, the parents worried about a head injury or concussion. What these children needed was more sleep, not a CT scan!

Falls from bunk beds can be serious, but most can be prevented by always using side rails in the upper bed and removal of the bed ladder when not in use.

Overweight, Exercise and Diet

Difficult-to-manage children fuss and cry a lot. One way to respond to their demands is to put food in their mouths. This certainly quietens them. Coincidentally, their fussiness might also have some evolutionary value, ensuring their survival in times when food is scarce. This was shown to be the case among the Masai of East Africa during drought conditions in 1974. But in a study conducted in a white, middle-class Pennsylvania paediatric practice, the more difficult babies tended to be fatter babies. Perhaps this connection between fussiness and being fed sets the stage for obesity in later years.

In my own paediatric practice, fat babies are almost always overtired babies. That's because their mothers have incorrectly attributed their babies' crying to hunger instead of fatigue. These mothers are always feeding their babies, then telling me that their babies can't sleep because they're always hungry! The major point here? Overfeeding the crying child to keep him quiet could cause unhealthy obesity.

This overfeeding habit may actually begin innocently enough in some children at three to four months of age, when nutritional feedings in the middle of the night give way to recreational feedings. Later, the bottle or breast is used as a pacifier and the frequent sipping and snacking causes excessive weight gain. Please try to become sensitive to the difference between nutritive and non-nutritive feeding. Overdoing milk or juice bottles is a common way babies learn to not 'like' eating solids. After all, they are getting calories, so they have no appetite to motivate them to eat solid foods when they are older. For children between five and seven years, we now have direct evidence that the more tired the child is, the more likely it is that he will be overweight or obese.

Q: *If I give my child a bottle at naps or at bedtime, will I make him fat? When should I not include a bottle in the bedtime ritual?*
A: Sucking or sipping a bottle before falling asleep comforts most babies and even older children. There is no harm in doing this and there is no particular age when you should stop as long as (a) you prop the baby, not the bottle, so he drinks in your arms, (b) the rate of weight gain is not too fast, and (c) frequent or prolonged feedings are not part of a sleep problem.

The effects of exercise on sleep are hard to prove, even though most people assume that muscular fatigue induced by exercise will produce better sleep. Another possibility is that exercise reduces anxiety. However, strenuous exercise, especially common among teenagers, might mask an under-lying problem of chronically insufficient sleep. The chronically or severely overtired adolescent is sometimes described as living in a 'twilight zone': frequent episodes of drowsiness, 'micro-sleeps', lethargy, depression, apathy, cognitive impairment and proneness to accidents. Counteracting measures that fight the fatigued state are internal stimulation (heightened emotionality such as anger or elation) or external stimulation such as exercise. So, exercise may be helpful, but it will not solve an underlying sleep problem.

Diet should influence sleep, because food provides the chemical building blocks for the brain's neurotransmitters. But studies in infants and adults do not show support for any strong link between sleep and diet.

Child Abuse

Let's get one ugly fact out in the open: when we are very, very tired of hearing our baby cry to fight sleep at night, we would like to shut her up. We don't act on our feelings; we don't harm our baby. But at night-time, the thought might have occurred to us: 'What if I weren't in so much control, might I . . . ?'

The tired, difficult-to-manage infant whose howling at night will not stop can become a target for abuse or infanticide. Crying is the behaviour that seems to trigger child abuse in some parents, and crying at night instead of sleeping is the historical set-up for infanticide.

So when your baby gets miserable late at night, with desperate, angry or relentless screaming when she should be asleep, and you feel like a tightly wound spring, don't be surprised if you feel you want to 'punish her' or 'shut her up for good'. If you and your child don't get the sleep you need, you may have experienced these intense feelings of anger, resentment or ill will towards your child.

Contact the following organisations, social workers at local hospitals or your paediatrician if you feel the need for help.

NSPCC
0808 800 5000

Parentline Plus
0808 800 2222

It's difficult to see how we can help solve sleep problems when we ourselves are extremely sleep-deprived. This is the time to call for help.

Atopic Dermatitis and Eczema

Atopic dermatitis is a chronic skin condition that causes severe itching. Itching of the skin can cause restlessness during sleep because a lot of the scratching goes on during light and REM sleep. As a result, children wake frequently throughout the night. Some studies have shown that these children have difficulty waking up for school, difficulty staying awake in the afternoon and major discipline problems. However, one study that used sleep lab recordings and videotapes during sleep of atopic children showed that the sleep abnormalities of frequent arousals actually did not occur with the act of scratching. This study was performed when the skin condition was in remission, so it is possible that, during flare-ups, there might be more intense itching that interfered with sleep consolidation. If your child is often scratching his skin, the best idea is talk to your paediatrician or ask for a referral to a dermatologist.

CHAPTER 12

Competent Parents, Competent Child

Karen Pierce, M.D.

The role of parent is the most rewarding job and also the most challenging one. A complex relationship develops when parents devote themselves to meeting a child's needs. Maturation does not proceed as effortlessly as one thinks. The hard work of rearing children gradually improves parents' competence, which, in turn teaches that same competence to their child.

Why is a child psychiatrist writing a chapter in a book about sleep? When my first child was about five months old, I was in a toy shop. A distraught mother came to me, frantically asking, 'Do you know a child psychiatrist? My paediatrician just told me to let my five-month-old cry to train him to sleep through the night. Will I damage his self-esteem if I let him cry?' We both had a good laugh when she found out that I *was* a child psychiatrist. I took the opportunity to commiserate but pointed out that my training was not needed for this task. Setting limits and teaching a child self-soothing are part of every parent's job. Doing this job does not cause psychological harm. Instead, setting limits promotes growth.

Loving our children includes introducing and teaching them to live with frustration. Saying no to a child becomes just as important as loving her unconditionally. There is a popular misunderstanding that loving parenting means unconditional acceptance, without rules. This is not the case. We must start training children in infancy. This is not easy! But early training will help later on, when you try to teach your child in other areas, such as bike riding, homework and social skills.

Here is a story from a parent of one of Dr Weissbluth's patients illustrating how difficult it is to set limits even though it is frustrating for both parents and children not to have them. As the mother writes, 'We don't want to break her spirit.'

'One More Story'

'One more story, Mummy,' your two-year-old pleads. What parent doesn't feel conflict when they hear those words? Books are good, you think; books are educational. And your child is on your lap, and she's warm from her bath and her hair smells sweet, and she's letting me hold her hand!

Can you love your child too much? Never, and yes. If there ever was a question with two answers, that would be it.

I think you can love your child so much that that love prevents you from setting clear limits and boundaries, from establishing effective structures and a sense of routine and order, which I believe children thrive on. The word *discipline* has harsh connotations for some parents, but in reality the word means 'to teach'. And to teach is to love.

My daughter Esme is two years old. The first years of her life have whizzed by and I've learned a lot as a first-time parent, especially about sleeping. Dr Weissbluth helped me get Esme sleeping through the night by five months or so. Lately, though, our pleasant, orderly, structured bedtime routine seems to be deteriorating. Her bedtime is creeping later and later, and sometimes she's not asleep until nine or ten at night, and then, because she always gets her twelve hours, she'll sleep the next morning until 10:00. My husband jokes that it's like having a two-year-old teenager. I'm lucky to have a sympathetic husband. In fact, maybe he's a little like me – too sympathetic. Lately we find ourselves echoing each other, saying, 'We don't want to break her spirit,' even though we intended to set limits and provide healthy discipline.

Self-esteem

How does one's sense of self develop? True self-esteem stems from the experience of competence and appropriate functioning. Self-esteem is a genuine sense of one's self as worthy of nurturing and protection. This allows us the capability of growth and development. As one's self-esteem is reinforced, a sense of competence leads to further increases in self-esteem. This positive spiral starts slowly and reinforces itself. This is a universal process occurring in both parents and baby.

'When do I feed him?' 'Is she getting enough milk?' 'Do I pick her up?' 'How do I stop this crying?' All of these questions are the beginning of creating a dance between parent and child. With the help of experience, innate abilities and intuition, these questions become easier to answer and parents become more confident. Experience and knowledge often make parenting the second and third child easier. Therefore, as our children grow, our competence as parents increases.

Infants are born with the capacity to organise experience, progressing to higher levels as they mature. Babies' brains are programmed to work towards competency and efficiency. This ability expands as the child experiences more situations and develops the capacity to tolerate a wide range of stimuli. All exploration must be done in the context of a loving caregiver. Through the regulation of physiological functioning, emotional understanding and interest in the world, infants grow. A baby who sleeps well and is well fed is more available to explore the world around her.

Babies respond to cause and effect. As the mother or father coos and talks with their baby, he smiles and makes noises back. The parents' continued responses to vocalisation encourage more vocal production. Direct eye contact with your infant also encourages this dialogue.

A child psychiatrist described how each infant needs a caregiver who can 'attune' to the infant. Emotional attunement is a three-step process done by the baby's caregiver. First, the caregiver *matches*, labels, or identifies the infant's internal feeling state: the baby is hungry, tired or sad. Then there is a *recognition* that the internal feeling state is different from the overt behaviour, crying. Last, the caregiver *responds* to convey emotional resonance: 'You are upset because you are hungry.' Attunement is not like looking in a mirror, imitating the behaviour ('You're crying'); rather, it is reading the cues of the internal feeling state: yes, the infant is crying and this is what it means. A mother of a six-week-old hears her son's cry knowing it is a hunger cry. When her baby smells her and feels that his mother is about to start breast-feeding, he quickly settles down, knowing that his dinner is coming. This rhythm was created by a repetition of a sequence that mum and baby learned. A wet-nappy cry can be differentiated from a hunger cry. As the caregiver responds to the baby's signal, babies become more organised, learn cause and effect, and feel more competent.

Babies will respond differently to their fathers, mothers, siblings and baby-sitters. Infants grow in the context of parents who try the best they can to be empathetic and to help develop their child's strengths and ideals. Early in life a child soaks up praise. 'My child is the prettiest, smartest, cleverest, or strongest' can be choruses sung to our children. Tending to their needs with warm smiles is all part of this loving attitude.

Your baby brings much to this equation, for she is born with her own innate level of tolerance and range for stimulation and arousal. Babies vary in endowment and maturation rates. This variability creates differences in how they experience initial and subsequent events. A mother or father each comes with his or her own endowments. How the baby-caregiver unit is formed varies greatly and creates the social environment of the child. This powerful unit brings changes to all parties.

Let's return to Esme's request for one more story at night.

'One More Story' (Continued)

I needed to examine who was really having trouble sticking to our bedtime routine – daughter or mother. Could it be that I was having more trouble putting her down than she was having going down?

Could it be that I was holding on, clinging to her at the very time when I most needed to encourage an easy transition from day to night, from play to rest, from being together to being alone, for both of us, for the purposes of healthy rest and healthy separation? It hit me with a jolt that *I* was the one who didn't want to put that warm cuddly bundle down into her cot, to let go, say good night, shut her door and leave her; that *I* was the one suffering from separation anxiety. My mind raced. When had I made this leap from viewing bedtime as a useful, necessary, peaceful break in the time I spent with my daughter to a rockier separation?

Once I realised that much, everything tumbled out. There were a million reasons – some very simple, some more complex. Since she's been older, she's been so much fun to be with. Every day she understands a new concept; every second there's something new to learn, look at, point to, pronounce. She adores her books – she'll throw aside any toy if she can read instead, and I'm as excited and stimulated by all of this growth as she is. Because I'm proud of how much she's absorbing, 'One more story, Mummy' secretly pleases me.

Good-Enough Parenting

Parental confidence can make the parenting job much easier, even despite the inevitable problems and pitfalls of child rearing. We all make mistakes. This is why a prominent paediatrician called parenting 'good enough', meaning that there is no one style of parenting that is perfect. The first time the parent misses a messy nappy does not 'damage' a child. However, repeated failures of misreading the child's signal will have an impact. The emotional microenvironment is growth-promoting or growth-inhibiting, depending on the caregiver's ability to read her child's affective state. It is the pattern of daily response, not the moment-to-moment response, that a baby internalises and forms memories of. Missing one signal in an infant's life will not cause permanent damage as long as the parent learns and does not repeat the same mistakes. Good-enough parenting includes maintaining a child's arousal within a moderate range that is high enough to maintain interactions but not so intense as to cause avoidance or distress. Optimal stimulation produces a balance between positive feelings and awareness and internal tension. Too much stimulation, like tickling, can quickly become unpleasantly intense if not properly dosed. Lack of proper regulation by parents prevents the emergence of a system to cope with heightened levels of arousal and discomfort. Sleep is just one example where a child needs to develop internal regulation.

A child must have the conviction that her surroundings are secure, providing pleasure and satisfaction while preventing or balancing anxiety. This includes both bodily needs and emotional needs. With mother as a secure base, the baby is free to explore the world. Babies who are securely attached to their caregivers respond more positively to peers and teachers later in life. A baby's security manifests itself by a balance of interest, curiosity, pleasure and exploration of the environment.

The protective response, innate to most caregivers, is sometimes interpreted as 'Never frustrate your child'. This is virtually impossible. Babies need to learn to tolerate frustration and learn self-soothing techniques to calm themselves and prepare them for life's inevitable obstacles. Gentle limits are the way to do this. A dilemma occurs when a parent needs to step away to promote growth. When babies learn to walk, first they creep along the furniture and then they hold on to a hand. Eventually both baby and caregiver must let go so that independent walking will occur. Both parent and child feel anxiety at this separation. Struggles appear as each development task, such as rolling over, sitting, standing and talking, is mastered. This is normal and may consist of an increase in fussiness or frustration experienced by both baby and caregiver. As each new step occurs, challenges and tensions are introduced, resolved and mastered.

When do caregivers step away? Sometimes adults have the tendency to infer adult meanings from the child's actions. It is important to remember that a baby may not be feeling or experiencing what the adult feels. We cannot 'read' an infant's mind. Too often adults have a tendency to *project their own feelings on to the baby* and not really listen to or attune to their baby. The grandmother who is cold tells her granddaughter to put on a sweater. This assumption that we know what is going on in an infant's internal world can lead to conflicts in parenting if we project instead of attune. Try to understand your baby's needs and not confuse them with your own.

The wise mother of twenty-month-old Esme learned that *she* did not want to put her daughter down to say good night. She realised that loving her child 'too much' had got in the way of setting healthy limits.

Development of Internal Controls

Infants learn internal regulation, a balance between inhibitory and excitatory control, from the routines and regularity of their environment. Development and regulation of physiological needs such as hunger, thirst, sleep, elimination and tactile stimulation happen almost intuitively. Each developmental milestone is subject to regulation from the environment, especially the family. Having a 'night owl' baby does not lead to a normalised routine. This baby must be slowly synchronised to the world's sleep/wake cycle. Healthy emotional development occurs with appropriate regulation of developmental tasks by the family. As parents regulate infants, infants internalise this as self-regulation.

When adults provide the necessary skills to help an infant complete a task successfully there is an increase from the child's current knowledge to a higher level. Initially it may be as simple as picking up a crying infant. Later, we tie our child's shoes until she learns that skill herself. But we do not tie her shoes forever. Nor do we forever pick up a crying child. Gradually we must withdraw our support so the child can function independently. The capacity to use small amounts of anxiety, excitement and curiosity as a signal allows babies to more fully explore the world.

Babies cry in order to communicate all of their needs.

Calming babies leads to positive attachments and feelings of safety for the infant. Crying does not necessarily mean distress; rather, it can be a simple communication about a wet nappy or a signal to play. A mother of an eight-month-old relates that her baby cries to get her to come into her bedroom at night. The minute the baby sees her mum she smiles with delight. This mother had the wisdom to recognise her daughter's cries not as signalling distress but as asking her mother to come and play.

There are many ways, short of holding or feeding a baby, to stop their crying. Helping them learn self-soothing can come in many forms. The key is creating a balance between frustration and comfort. The frustration element provides an opportunity for the child to grow and develop skills. Too much frustration is disorganising, but having no frustration prevents a child from learning. To soothe crying babies who are preverbal (under fourteen or fifteen months), waiting several seconds before picking them up can be helpful. Alternatively, handing a child an object or a favourite blanket can be a soothing technique. If your baby is still distressed, patting her on the back gently or stroking her may work. As your child becomes older, soothing words can be quite useful. All these methods are the beginning of a journey in teaching your child self-regulation. These rudimentary steps to self-regulation bring about less fussiness and less crying. The result maximises the baby's growing competence and self-control.

Saying No Helps Your Child

Many of us grew up believing that discipline means humiliation, shame, guilt and an occasional swat on the bottom. Today we interpret discipline in a way that is true to its Latin root, which means 'to teach'. Setting limits should be done with reason and firmness, in a positive, loving environment. Teaching self-soothing is as important as teaching language or social skills.

When do we start setting these limits for a child? We start this process very early. Waiting a few moments to pick up your crying child or talking slowly to her while preparing food are the beginnings of teaching an infant to wait and to learn expectations of routines. Even babies learn routines quickly. Most can settle themselves when hearing their caregiver's steps or the tone of a voice. The baby stops crying or fussing. Most limits should be simple rules spoken in advance so that children know what to expect. If your tendency is to always jump to do things for your child, to protect your child from feeling frustrated or from experiencing failure, you will not be teaching him techniques he will need for the future. The progress is gradual and is part of the challenge of parenting.

Families are not democracies. Parents are in charge and have ultimate authority. Unlike past generations, when child rearing was done in a more autocratic society in which the father had supreme rights, today limits are presented by both parents to create order. When limits were presented in an autocratic manner, fear and intimidation, not learning and understanding, ruled the family. Yes, family members should have mutual respect and principles of equality, but this does not imply that children have an equal say. A baby changes the family balance, creating a new equilibrium. Parents must take charge and make decisions in the best interest of the child even though it might cause distress. No one lets an infant or a child ride in a car without a safety seat. Even if the child protests, families usually stay firm on this rule. Other limits sometimes have to be invoked in the same way as the seat belt law – firmly and confidently.

Behaviour can be modified. Our culture, family and society influence the norms and values of behaviour standards. One of the first steps in changing behaviour is to first understand the behaviour. Once a limit is set, you cannot expect children to simply accept it or consider it normal. We do not say to infants 'Don't cry.' We show them soothing techniques: a dummy, a thumb, a blanket.

When a child enters the toddler stage, the learning of *no* signals the beginning of the child's ability to do symbolic thinking. The toddler, becoming more adept at communicating his needs, begins to collide with his caregiver's wishes. This conflict leads to frustration and rage. This rage must be negotiated carefully, because it has the potential to disrupt the child's sense of well-being and safety. This does not mean that limits should not be dispensed. Parents have to be very clear and present limits in a calm, soothing voice and stand their ground despite pleas for them to waver. If you have already encouraged a positive and protective environment, the child looks at these limits as an extension of that protection.

It is never too late to say no to your child. A thirteen-year-old girl with long-standing night-time difficulties came to my office for evaluation. Her history revealed that she had never been taught to sleep through the night. She had wandered from room to room, disrupting her parents' sleep, since the age of fifteen months. Her parents felt she must be up for a 'reason' and that she needed them at night. They thought that setting limits on this would be too frustrating for her, and so they waited for her to grow out of it. This child did not have anything psychologically wrong with her; she had just never been taught the skills of learning to sleep. Treatment consisted of education regarding sleep habits and then 'forcing' her to stay in her room while her parents stayed by the door so she could not exit. After experiencing the anxiety and learning self-soothing techniques, she (and her parents) slept through the night for the first time in over ten years. Sleeping in their own beds for several nights created renewed energy and positive relationships. Taking pride in their accomplishment increased their feelings of competence.

My Child Has Sleep Problems. What Do We Do Now?

So your child does not sleep. The beauty and the joy of seeing your child loses its lustre when seen through weary eyes. Sleep deprivation creates difficulties for both the parent and the child. How does letting a child cry at night or keeping him in his room when he is obviously distressed help him develop self-esteem?

A child awakens for many reasons – illness, trauma, a disturbance in the nap schedule. A friend came to me when her child became afraid to sleep at night after they were robbed. My friend herself, however, was still frightened, traumatised and afraid to sleep. I told her that when her fears relaxed, her son would sleep again. She called me up several weeks later to explain that all were sleeping better in their own beds because the thief had been captured. Babies who are ill or scared will awaken, but only temporarily. If more than several nights go by and your child is still waking, this behaviour has become a habit and is no longer a cry for help. Listen to your intuition and experience; recognise that limits must be gently introduced.

It is common to want to avoid the unpleasant situation of teaching your child to sleep. None of us wants to hear our child cry. However, the longer you delay correcting the sleep problem, the more difficult it will be to remedy. Recall that all developmental steps proceed with some frustration and difficulty. The brain needs order and predictability to develop and form neuronal connections. As Dr Weissbluth explains, a child's sleep disruption creates disorder at the highest level.

Parents need to support each other in training their children. In my own situation, our first child failed to learn on his own to sleep through the night. Being a child psychiatrist had taught me about nurturing and reducing frustration, but not about parenting. Thus, believing the standard theories learned during my training, I feared that I would 'damage' my child. I was unable to let him cry initially, despite my glazed eyes and grumpy disposition. When our son was thirteen months old, my husband recognised that he was up for the secondary gain of being with us. Together we decided that sleep needed to be encouraged for the health and welfare of the entire family. My husband and I held and comforted each other through that difficult night while we let him cry. He held me back when I wanted to go in to comfort the baby. We both stayed up and listened to the crying, reminding each other that this, too, was part of the 'joy' of parenting. After a few nights, we slept peacefully, continuing our growth as a family.

It is a common misbelief that awakening is a signal that a child has unmet psychological needs. This leads to parental guilt and blame. Stop this line of thought immediately!

You may be uncertain whether letting your child cry will damage her permanently. Letting your child cry is neither punitive nor withholding if you think about it as training a physiological need. It is important to understand the context of your actions. You are not a 'bad' parent if you let your child cry. Teaching a child to sleep is not ignoring his needs. Infants and young children do not appear to remember crying spells; however, they do begin to remember repeated behaviours from carers that form a pattern. If you have been protecting and doling out frustration in small doses during the day, the child internalises this protection. In teaching a child to sleep, the parent's goal is to reward good behaviour, in this case sleeping, without inadvertently rewarding poor behaviour, that is, waking.

When Other Issues Get in the Way

Child's Issues

Some children are born with difficult temperaments. Raising a child who is challenging stresses the system. A difficult-to-care-for infant erodes the reserve of parents by excessive crying and demanding. These children tend to have more problems sleeping and then to react more extremely to stimuli, leading parents to be more extreme in their own reactions. You may find yourself short-tempered, exhausted and frustrated. A simple *no* becomes a tantrum. Giving your child a blue balloon instead of a yellow one could trigger a major meltdown, leading to a feeling of defeat. Remember, the trick to parenting these children is to become more flexible and leave more time to prepare or to plan transitions. It is always important to look for the positive aspects of each child. The stubborn infant may transform into a persistent or ambitious adult.

Setting limits and sticking to them is extremely important, especially with challenging children. These children may not respond immediately, so you *must* be flexible. If you say 'no playing with your food', the difficult infant may take an extra swipe before stopping. Avoid the power struggles and appreciate that she is obeying. Unfortunately, because many of these children learn slowly, directions and corrections must be repeated over and over until learning takes place.

Some children are not endowed with all their learning processes intact. For example, children with auditory processing deficits may not use the spoken word for comfort, requiring more physical contact. Children who have difficulty reading nonverbal cues will respond better to verbal commands. Parents usually find ways to compensate for their child's deficits. Frustration tolerance may be harder to measure in these children. Always, a gentle push towards competence must occur. Children endowed differently still need to be taught frustration tolerance despite the challenges it poses to parents.

Parents' Issues

Having a child stirs up many personal issues that, if not understood, can interfere with parenting. If a parent cannot act in the infant's best interest, there will be specific disruptions that inhibit growth. Some parents lack the ability to read their baby's signals. When children do not have their signals read, they are at risk to develop 'primitive strategies', meaning that they tend to cry and become more unable to self-soothe. Once these strategies are in place, they are continuously repeated because the baby or young child *learns to cry to get what he wants*. These maladaptive strategies will need to be unlearned in a more supportive setting later in life. Fortunately, there are several books and tapes to help parents learn about normal development. Once parents learn, they can teach their baby.

Some parents bend over backwards to appease their child: 'I want to avoid the strict parenting that I received.' This may lead to the absence of limits. Parents who are too sensitive to their child's needs risk enabling their child to become too dependent on their carer. These children do not learn to read their own signals and require an adult to do it for them.

Children crave order, and setting limits is one way to that end. Harsh commands, physical punishment or power assertion produces children who have higher levels of guilt and exhibit parent-pleasing behaviour. It is even worse when, after becoming too harsh or letting your child cry too long, you quickly rush to hug your child. This sends a very mixed message to your child. Your child starts to think that crying is what you need to do to be hugged.

Some parents like their children to remain in one developmental stage because they themselves have certain needs that were never adequately met. For example, keeping a child up at night may fulfil a parent's need for closeness. Here the child is forced to ignore her own need to sleep in order to accommodate her parent's misreading: 'I know you are up because you missed me. I am here now.' Like the grandmother who is cold and asks her granddaughter to put on a sweater, the mother who is lonely imagines that her daughter is lonely, too, and so she keeps her baby up with her late at night and hinders the child's sleep. The baby gets conflicting information and may not know what to read – her own signal or her caregiver's. The child may then have difficulties integrating new information because skills to manage this situation have not been taught.

Let's continue with Esme's mother's story. Note where she writes, 'I now miss having my mother as a grandmother to my daughter . . . I also miss having her be a mother to me.'

'One More Story' (Continued)

Bedtime is a special time – sitting in the rocking chair, holding her in her jammies, the night tape playing softly, the whole house quiet, no phone, no distractions, no interruptions, no pressures or time constraints. It's a time of intense, focused interaction with my daughter. Not that I don't have plenty of time with her during the day – I'm a writer and I work at home two or three half-days a week. But only at bedtime does she really let me cuddle with her, hold her – during the day she's too busy running around playing and never wants to sit still. At night she strokes my hair, wiggles my nose, asks me to sing silly songs, reads her favourite stories one more time. We have so much fun together! I love our quiet time as much as she does, and I'm very guilty of letting it go on and on, into five, six, seven songs or books, another minute, another cuddle, until we're both exhausted.

My husband and I discussed the complex reasons for my attachment to my daughter. I was very close to my own mother, although not so much physically, which is probably why I value that cuddle time in the rocking chair. My mother died seven years ago, when she was only fifty. I was on the cusp of my marriage and I went through a very difficult mourning period. I still miss her a lot, and having a child has made that loss even sharper. I now miss having my mother as a grandmother to my daughter. I miss sharing my baby with her. I also miss having her be a mother to me. I don't want to lay the burden of having to be everything for me on my child. My own mother, who had a difficult relationship with *her* mother, did that to me, which is perhaps why I have separation anxiety to begin with. And, again, I don't want to love my child so much that I'm unable to establish consistent, clear boundaries and rules effectively.

Marriage Issues

Babies establish a new equilibrium in families. The couple is no longer alone, and the role of parent must be established. The importance of social and emotional support to the developing child must be emphasised. A positive emotional climate influences a baby's development. If the parents cannot create this support, development of the child may be hindered. Without support for both parents, caregivers are more likely to engage in dysfunctional parenting with their children.

If adult intimacy needs are not being met by a marriage or the relationship is not supportive or is stressful, parenting tasks become difficult. Either partner may turn to their child to meet those needs. Toddlers exposed to parental conflict develop a negative response to this tension and are at risk to become aggressive towards peers. Infants as young as one year can sense this distress and develop an emotional response to it. Mothers and fathers may demonstrate two different regulatory patterns. Often in conflict-filled marriages, mothers become over-involved with their infants and fathers tend to withdraw and not be as affectively responsive to their children. Both responses may be damaging to a child's sense of security and competence in the future.

When both parents work together, as did Esme's parents, sleep problems are more easily solved. Note where Esme's mother writes, 'And of course, when Esme goes to bed earlier, I have more time to enjoy a nice dinner with my husband.'

'One More Story' (Conclusion)

As we cleaned the kitchen, my husband and I had a real heart to heart. He was proud that I saw my own part in our bedtime battles and acknowledged that it was not much easier for him when he put her down. We made an agreement that from now on the new bedtime would be 8:00 sharp, with a goal of moving it to 7:30 and even to 7:00 in two weeks. That would be the final curtain call, no ifs, ands or buts. But how to help mum stick to the rules?

Dr Weissbluth suggested setting a kitchen timer for an allotted time at the beginning of the bedtime routine, say thirty minutes or one hour. My husband and I agreed to try one hour – which would include bath, brushing teeth, nappy, jammies, story and cuddling. The timer, Dr Weissbluth said, would act as a signal for the child (and mother!) to understand that the bedtime routine together was over.

The first night the *ding* of the timer seemed to come incredibly fast. Both my husband and I were enjoying singing an alphabet song to Esme, and we all three turned to look at the timer in a kind of dumb-faced shock. It seemed such an intrusive little fellow! Esme was curious and asked what the bell was for. 'Time for bed,' we said, a little reluctantly. 'Lights out'. But neither my husband nor I moved a muscle to put her in bed. We did hurry along our song, however, and limit our reading to two books instead of four or five. But the time had seemed to go so fast! We were both amazed at how poorly we'd organised that hour from bath to bed.

We resolved to do better the next night. Again that meddlesome little bell seemed to ring too soon, but this time not as much. Setting the timer had helped us make better use of the early time – in the bath, brushing teeth and putting on jammies – so we'd have more time for stories. Again Esme was interested in the bell. 'Time for bed. Lights out,' we said. Esme smiled. She actually smiled. My daughter thought this little strategy was a delightful game!

'Okay, Mummy. Cot,' she said. Dumbfounded, I stopped rocking. We still spent a minute having the animals call her, one by one, into her bed, but one minute was a whole lot less than before.

On subsequent nights, the timer became our friend. Without a doubt, it added a sense of structure to our bedtime routine and helped us organise our time.

There have been a few nights when that bell still seems intrusive, when I want to read 'one more story' as much as my daughter does. I realise that another part of my separation anxiety is that I felt I was an intelligent child who didn't receive as much stimulation as I might have. Fortunately, my parents made books very available – I didn't have a lot of toys, though I always had books – but I had to learn from them on my own. I have trouble limiting Esme's 'reading' simply because I don't want to give up an opportunity for a potential learning experience that I perceive myself not having had when I was a child.

So, with a little probing and the help of a plastic kitchen timer, we've turned our lives around. It's just amazing to see Esme respond to new limits with a kind of pride and resourcefulness.

And, of course, when Esme goes to bed earlier, I have more time to enjoy a nice dinner with my husband, talk about our work or our child, rent a video, whatever. And in the daytime, her naps are more regular, her moods are sunnier and her appetite improved. Another trick I've learned is to build in more focused playtime during the day. Instead of jumping up to answer the phone when Esme and I are playing with Mr Potato Head, I let it ring. I also allow for more reading time during the day, so that one of our favourite activities is not saved up just for bedtime.

Now, when I hear those words 'one more story', I know that to respond with a 'No. Tomorrow is another day' does not mean I don't love my child. Quite the contrary.

> P. S. As the weeks have gone by, there have been a few nights when I have forgotten to turn the timer on. Esme runs to get it off the bookshelf and says, 'Mummy! Timer!' She has a special place on the second shelf where she likes to put it while it ticks away (I think it gives her a sense of control to place it within her reach). And when it rings, if we're in the middle of the story, she asks me to 'please finish'. I find that to be a reasonable request, partly because I know I'm in control now, so I don't get all freaked-out about it being too late. And so we finish our story and then I remind her that the timer went off a minute ago. She studies me very seriously and says, 'Okay, Mummy. Time for nite-nite.'

Summary

Parenting is a process that reinforces itself: As confidence grows, so does a parent's feeling of competence. One of the most important concepts to remember is that there will be times when you will want to give less attention – even if this causes crying, *even at night* – in order for your child to develop skills of independence and self-soothing. Crying, in this context, does not damage self-esteem. Rather, the end result is heightened competence in your child and in *you*.

CHAPTER 13

The Pros and Cons of Other Approaches to Sleep Problems

Notions, theories, and opinions on how to prevent or solve sleep problems abound. Let's look at some published ideas and see how they stand up to the facts about children's sleep habits that we've just explored together in this book.

Proper Association with Falling Asleep

Richard Ferber's Theory

A child associates certain conditions with falling asleep, such as being held in a parent's arms, lying on a living room sofa or rocking in a swing. When put to sleep in a cot or bed, those certain conditions are missing upon awakening, so the child has difficulty returning to sleep. The progressive approach is to not respond to the baby's cry at night for a brief period of time, say five minutes. After the child has cried for five minutes, the parents return and stay in the room two to three minutes but do not pick up or rock the child. This is thought to reassure the parents and the child that all is well. Parents then leave, whether the child is asleep or not, whether crying or not, and return in ten minutes for the same brief interaction, if needed. After leaving, parents would return again after fifteen minutes of crying for a brief curtain call. They would return every fifteen minutes for a brief encounter until the child fell asleep during one of their fifteen-minute absences. If there is no crying or mild whimpering, then there is no return. If the child awoke later that night with hard crying, parents would repeat the original progressive routine of five, ten and then fifteen minutes of delay in response time. The second night would be a repeat performance, except the progression would be ten, fifteen and twenty minutes. The third night would be fifteen, twenty and twenty-five minutes, and so on. The child learns to associate her bed or cot with falling asleep and returning to sleep.

My Comment

Whether we call this method 'developing proper association' or 'learning self-soothing skills', I'm sure it can work. The general problem is that it's very difficult to maintain any time schedule in the middle of the night for several nights in a consistent fashion – frustration and exhaustion often override planning and patience.

Unrestricted Breast-feeding and the Family Bed

William Sears's Theory

Unrestricted breast-feeding and the family bed are how to get your baby or child to sleep.

My Comment

Beware of writers who have never had the opportunity to study sleeping and who have a strong personal opinion regarding parenting. You are a good parent if you practise 'attachment parenting', which by definition includes 'natural mothering', which is unrestricted breast-feeding and sharing sleep in a family bed. This is in contrast to 'detachment parenting', which involves 'escape mothering', which is the term used for mothers who wish to pursue a career outside the home. The use of these terms is not surprising when you realise that La

Leche League International, a breast-feeding support group, published the original book. As a father whose four sons were breast-fed and as a paediatrician in practice with a full-time certified lactation consultant, I certainly support breast-feeding. But there is more to being a parent than just the method of feeding.

Over-reliance on vague psychological terms and unsupported psychological mechanisms serves the sole purpose of advancing the author's cause. For example: 'An unfulfilled need is never completely erased; it is only temporarily suppressed and will flare up again in a different way.' Advocating unrestricted breast-feeding and the family bed is the main message. To be fair, the author does have one sentence in the entire book where he states, 'The sleeping arrangement whereby all three of you (mother, father and baby) sleep best is the right one for your individual family.' But he basically ignores the enormous individuality of temperament differences, experience of the parents, and age-specific sleep patterns of children.

What does the author suggest you do if 'natural methods of night-time parenting' fail? Try another, presumably 'unnatural' method? No! The author says to use the strong hypnotic prescription drug chloral hydrate to knock out your child. Yet there is not one good study that supports this practice.

Summary

The major problems with these other methods are that insufficient or no attention is given to the importance of prevention or treatment of sleep problems by focusing on naps and schedules. There is more to healthy sleep habits than not waking at night. Children who don't sleep well usually have developed this pattern as a result of parental mismanagement. Too much attention, irregularity, or inconsistency in bedtime 'policy' and routines can interfere with the development of healthy sleep habits, and accepting this responsibility is the first step in developing a treatment plan.

You may be uncertain as to whether you want to try a

gradual, 'fading' approach or an abrupt, 'cold turkey' extinguishing approach. If I were exclusively a specialist doing research on sleep problems and providing consultative services, I could devote a great deal of time to coaching parents and helping them maintain their resolve to carry through with a gradual approach. As a general-practice paediatrician, though, I find that the time demands of a busy office make it more difficult for me to be as available for this as I would like to be. So when you try to decide between the gradual approach versus an abrupt approach in putting to rights your child's sleep habits, consider not only your own resolve but also the external supports that you know you can count on.

Many parents start with a gradual approach, see partial success, but then get worn down and recognise their evolving inconsistency. Feeling a bit more confident and competent, many parents then shift directions to a more abrupt approach. But some parents cannot even start to correct their child's sleeping problems at all, because the same personal stresses that created the unhealthy sleep habits in the first place – revolving around the child's emerging independence, marital discord and other problems with the parents – are still present. To maintain or develop healthy sleep habits for your child, have the courage to do what is best for the child. In less time than you think, you will wind up with a loving home, a happy, well-rested child and well-rested parents.

References

Chapter 1. Why Healthy Sleep Is So Important

Bernstein, D., Emde, R., and Campos, J. (1973). REM sleep in four-month infants under home and laboratory conditions. *Psychosomatic Medicine, 35,* 322–329.

Coons, S., and Guilleminault, C. (1982). Development of sleep-wake patterns and non–rapid eye movement sleep stages during the first six months of life in normal infants. *Pediatrics, 69,* 793–798.

Emde, R. N., and Metcalf, D. R. (1970). An electroencephalographic study of behavioural rapid eye movement states in the human newborn. *Journal of Nervous and Mental Disorders, 150,* 376–386.

Fish, B. (1963). The maturation of arousal and attention in the first months of life: A study of variations in age development. *Journal of the American Academy of Child Psychiatry, 2,* 253–270.

Harper, R. N., Leake, B., Miyahana, L., Mason, J., Hoppenbrouwers, T., Sterman, M. B., and Hodgman, J. (1981). Temporal sequencing in sleep and waking states during the first six months of life. *Experimental Neurology, 72,* 294–307.

Jacklin, C. N., Snow, M. E., Cozahapt, M., and Maccoby, E. E. (1980). Sleep pattern development from 6 through 33 months. *Journal of Pediatric Psychology, 5,* 295–302.

Klein, K. E., Hermann, R., Kuklinski, P., and Hans, M. W. (1977). Circadian performance rhythms: Experimental studies in air operations. In R. R. Mackie (ed.), *Vigilance: Theory, Operational Performance and Physiological Correlants* (NATO Conference Series III, Human Factors, Vol. 3). New York: Plenum Press.

Salzarulo, P., and Chevalier, A. (1983). Sleep problems in children and their relationship with early disturbances of the waking-sleep rhythms. *Sleep, 6,* 47–51.

Schulz, H., Salzarulo, P., Fagioli, I., and Massetani, R. (1983). REM latency: Development in the first year of life. *Electroencephalography and Clinical Neurophysiology, 56,* 316–322.

Still, G. F. (1931). *The History of Pediatrics.* London: Oxford University Press.

Sundell, C. E. (1922). Sleeplessness in infants. *Practitioner, 109,* 89–92.

Chapter 2. Healthy Sleep and Sleep Strategies

Sleep Duration: Night and Day

Anders, T. F., Carksadon, M. A., and Dement, W. C. (1980). Sleep and sleepiness in children and adolescents. *Pediatric Clinics of North America, 27,* 29–43.

Anders, T. F., and Keener, M. A. (1985). Developmental course of night-time sleep-wake patterns in full-term and premature infants during the first year of life: Part I. *Sleep, 8,* 173–192.

Anders, T. F., Keener, M. A., and Kramer, H. (1985). Sleep-wake state organisation, neonatal assessment and development in premature infants during the first year of life: Part II. *Sleep, 8,* 193–206.

Cobb, K. (2002). Missed ZZZ's, more disease: Skimping on sleep may be bad for your health. *Science News, 7,* 152–154.

Parmelee, A. H., Schulz, H. R., and Disbrow, M. A. (1961). Sleep patterns of the newborn. *Journal of Pediatrics, 58,* 241–250.

Parmelee, A. H., Wenner, W. H., and Schulz, H. R. (1964). Infant sleep patterns: From birth to 16 weeks of age. *Journal of Pediatrics, 65,* 576–582.

Randazzo, A. C., Muehlbach, M. L., Schweitzer, P. K., and Walsh, J. K. (1998). Cognitive function following acute sleep restriction in children ages 10–14. *Sleep, 21,* 861–868.

Shimada, M., Takahashi, K., Segawa, M., Higurashi, M., Samejim, M., and Horiuchi, K. (1999). Emerging and entraining patterns of the sleep-wake rhythm in preterm and term infants. *Brain & Development, 21,* 468–473.

Weissbluth, M. (1981). Sleep duration and infant temperament. *Journal of Pediatrics, 99,* 817–819.

Weissbluth, M. (1984). Sleep duration, temperament, and Conners' ratings on three-year-old children. *Journal of Developmental and Behavioral Pediatrics, 5,* 120–123.

Weissbluth, M., Poncher, J., Given, G., Schwab, J., Mervis, R., and Rosenburg, M. (1981). Sleep durations and television viewing. *Journal of Pediatrics, 99,* 486–488.

Naps

Coons, S., and Guilleminault, C. (1984). Development of consolidated sleep and wakeful period in relation to the day/night cycle in infancy. *Developmental Medicine and Child Neurology, 26,* 169–176.

Daiss, S. R., Bertelson, A. D., and Benjamin, L. T. (1986). Napping versus resting: Effects on performance and mood. *Psychophysiology, 23,* 82–88.

Emde, R. N., and Walken, S. (1961). Longitudinal study of infant sleep: Results of 14 subjects studied at monthly intervals. *Psychophysiology, 13,* 456–461.

Folkard, S., Hume, K. I., Minors, D. S., Waterhouse, J. M., and Watson, F. L. Independence of the circadian rhythm in alertness from the sleep-wake cycle. *Nature, 313,* 678–679.

Larson, M., Gunnar, M. R., and Hertsgaard, L. (1991). The effects of morning naps, car trips, and maternal separation on adrenocortical activity in human infants. *Child Development, 62,* 362–372.

Mahowald, M. W., and Schenck, C. H. (1992). Dissociated states of wakefulness and sleep. *Neurology, 42* (Suppl. 6), 44–52.

Marks, G. A., Shaffery, J. P., Oksenberg, A., Speciale, S. G., and Roffwarg, H. P. (1995). A functional role for REM sleep in brain maturation. *Behavioral Brain Research, 69,* 1–11.

Minors, D. S., and Waterhouse, J. M. (1984). The sleep-wakefulness rhythm, exogenous and endogenous factors (in man). *Experientia, 40,* 410–416.

Sandyk, R. (1992). Melatonin and maturation of REM sleep. *International Journal of Neuroscience, 63,* 105–114.

Watamura, S., Sebanc, A., and Gunnar, M. (2002). Rising cortisol at child care: Relations with nap. *Developmental Psychobiology, 40,* 33–42.

Weissbluth, M. (1995). Naps in children: 6 months–7 years. *Sleep, 18,* 82–87.

Wladimorva, G. (1993). Study of cyclic structure of daytime sleep in normal infants aged 2 to 12 months. *Acta physiologica et pharmacoligica Bulgarica, 9,* 62–69.

Sleep Consolidation

Bonnet, M. M. (1985). Effect of sleep disruption on sleep, performance, and mood. *Sleep, 8,* 11–19.

Coons, S., and Guilleminault, C. (1985). Motility and arousal in near-miss sudden infant death syndrome. *Journal of Pediatrics, 107,* 728–732.

Martin, S. E., Engleman, H. M., Deary, I. J., and Douglas, N. J. (1996). The effect of sleep fragmentation on daytime function. *American Journal of Respiratory and Critical Care Medicine, 153,* 1328–1332.

Stepanski, E., Lamphere, J., Badia, P., Zorick, F., and Roth, T. (1984). Sleep fragmentation and daytime sleepiness. *Sleep, 7,* 18–26.

Weissbluth, M., Davis, A. T., and Poncher, J. (1984). Night waking in 4- to 8-month-old infants. *Journal of Pediatrics, 104,* 477–480.

Sleep Schedule, Timing of Sleep

Abe, K., Sasaki, H., Takebayashi, K., Seki, F., and Roth, T. (1978). The development of circadian rhythms of human body temperature. *Journal of Interdisciplinary Cycle Research, 9,* 210–216.

Czeisler, C. A., Weitzman, E. D., and Moore-Ede, M. C. (1980). Human sleep: Its duration and organisation depend on its circadian phase. *Science, 210,* 1264–1267.

Dinges, D. F., Pack, F., Williams, K., Gillen, K. A., Powell, J. W., Ott, G. E., Aptowicz, D., and Pack, A. I. (1997). Cumulative sleepiness, mood disturbance, and psychomotor vigilance performance decrements during a week of sleep restricted to 4–5 hours per night. *Sleep, 20,* 267–277.

Dreyfus-Brisac, C., and Monod, N. (1965). Sleep of premature and full term neonates – A polygraphic study. *Proceedings of the Royal Society of Medicine, 58,* 6–7.

Emde, R. N, Swedberg, J., and Suzuki, B. (1975). Human wakefulness and biological rhythms after birth. *Archives of General Psychiatry, 32,* 780–783.

Lodemore, M., Petersen, S. A., and Wailoo, M. P. (1991). Development of night temperature rhythms over the first six months of life. *Archives of Disease in Childhood, 66,* 521–524.

Louis, J., Cannard, C., Bastuji, H., and Challamel, M.-J. (1997). Sleep ontogenesis revisited: A longitudinal 24-hour home polygraphic study on 15 normal infants during the first two years of life. *Sleep, 20,* 323–333.

Onishi, S., Miyazawa, G., Nishimura, Y., Sugiyama, S., Yamakawa, T., Inagaki, H., Katoh, T., Itoh, S., and Isobe, K. (1983). Postnatal development of circadian rhythm in serum cortisol levels in children. *Pediatrics, 72,* 399–404.

Reppert, S. M. (1985). Maternal entrainment of the developing circadian system. *Annals of the New York Academy of Science, 453,* 162–169.

Sadeh, A. (1997). Sleep and melatonin in infants. *Sleep, 20,* 185–191.

Weissbluth, M. (1982). Modification of sleep schedule with reduction of night waking: A case report. *Sleep, 5,* 262–266.

Sleep Regularity

Acebo, C., and Carskadon, M. A. (2002). Influence of irregular sleep patterns on waking behaviour. In M. A. Carskadon (ed.), *Adolescent Sleep Patterns: Biological, Social, and Psychological Influences*, 220–235. Cambridge: Cambridge University Press.

Bates, J. E., Viken, R. J., Alexander, D. B., Beyers, J., and Stockton, S. (2002). Sleep and adjustment in preschool children: Sleep diary reports by mothers relate to behaviour reports by teachers. *Child Development, 73,* 62–74.

Sleep Position, SIDS

Ponsouby, A. L., Dwyer, M. B., Gibbons, L. E., Cochran, J. A., and Wang, Y. G. (1993). Factors potentiating the risk of sudden infant death syndrome associated with the prone position. *New England Journal of Medicine, 329,* 377–382.

Breast-feeding versus Bottle-feeding and Family Bed versus Cot

Elias, M. F., Nicolson, N. A., Bora, C., and Johnston, J. (1986). Sleep/wake patterns of breast-fed infants in the first 2 years of life. *Pediatrics, 77,* 322–329.

Hayes, M. J., Parker, K. G., Sallinen, B., and Davare, A. A. (2001). Bedsharing, temperament, and sleep disturbance in early childhood. *Sleep, 24,* 657–662.

Hunsley M., and Thoman, E. B. (2002) The sleep of co-sleeping infants when they are not co-sleeping: Evidence that co-sleeping is stressful. *Developmental Psychobiology, 40,* 14–22.

Klackenberg, G. (1982). Sleep behaviour studied longitudinally. *Acta Paediatrica Scandinavia, 71,* 501–506.

Latz, S., Wolf, A. W., and Lozoff, B. (1999). Cosleeping in context. Sleep practices and problems in young children in Japan and the United States. *Archives of Pediatrics & Adolescent Medicine, 153,* 339–346.

Lozoff, B., Wolf, A. W., and Davis, N. S. (1984). Co-sleeping in urban families with young children in the United States. *Pediatrics, 74,* 171–182.

Lozoff, B. L., Wolf. A. W., and Davis, N. S. (1985). Sleep problems seen in pediatric practice. *Pediatrics, 75,* 477–483.

Okami, P., Weisner, T., and Olmstead, R. (2002). Outcome correlates of parent-child bedsharing: An eighteen-year longitudinal study. *Journal of Developmental & Behavioral Pediatrics, 23,* 244–253.

Rosenfeld, A. A., Wenegrant, A. O., Haavik, D. K., Wenegrant, B. C., and Smith, C. R. (1982). Sleeping patterns in upper-middle-class families when the child awakens ill or frightened. *Archive of General Psychiatry, 39,* 943–947.

Solid Foods and Feeding Habits

Beal, V. A. (1964). Termination of night feeding in infancy. *Journal of Pediatrics, 75,* 690–692.

Deisher, R. W., and Goers, S. S. (1954). A study of early and later introduction of solids into the infant diet. *Journal of Pediatrics, 45,* 191–199.

Grunwaldt, E., Bates, T., and Guthrie, D. (1960). The onset of sleeping through the night in infancy: Relation to introduction of solid food in the diet, birth weight and position in the family. *Pediatrics, 26,* 667–668.

Jones, N. B., Brown, M. F., and MacDonald, L. (1978). The association between perinatal factors and later night waking. *Developmental Medicine and Child Neurology, 20,* 427–434.

Lavie, P., Kripke, D. F., Hiatt, J. F., and Harrison, J. (1978). Gastric rhythms during sleep. *Behavioral Biology, 23,* 526–630.

Parmelee, A. H., Wenner, W. H., and Schulz, W. R. (1964). Infant sleep patterns from birth to 16 weeks of age. *Journal of Pediatrics, 65,* 576–582.

Robertson, P. M. (1974). Solids and 'sleeping through'. *British Medical Journal, 1,* 200.

Salzarulo, P., Fagioli, I., Salomon, F., and Riccour, C. (1979). Alimentation continué et rhythmic veille-sommeil chez l'enfant. (Continuous feeding and the waking-sleeping rhythm in children.) *Archives Françaises de Pédiatrie* (Suppl.), *36,* 26–32.

Schultz, H., Salzarulo, P., Fagioli, I., and Massetani, R. (1983). REM latency: Development in the first year of life. *Electroencephalography and Clinical Neurophysiology, 56,* 316–322.

Schulz, H., Massetani, R., Fagioli, I., and Salzarulo, P. (1985). Spontaneous awakenings from sleep in infants. *Electroencephalography and Clinical Neurophysiology, 61,* 267–271.

Wright, P., MacLeod, M. A., and Cooper, M. J. (1983). Waking at night: The effect of early feeding experience. *Child Care Health Development, 9,* 309–319.

The Effects of Healthy Sleep: Sleep Patterns, Intelligence, Learning and School Performance

Anders, T. F., Keener, M. A., and Kraemer, H. (1985). Sleep-wake state organisation, neonatal assessment and development in premature infants during the first year of life: Part II. *Sleep, 8,* 193–206.

Bonnet, M. H. (1985). Effect of sleep disruption on sleep, performance, and mood. *Sleep, 8,* 11–19.

Busby, K., and Pikik, R. T. (1983). Sleep patterns in children of superior intelligence. *Journal of Child Psychology and Psychiatry, 24,* 587–600.

Dahl, R. E., Pelhan, W. E., and Wierson, M. (1991). The role of sleep disturbances in attention deficit disorder symptoms: A case study. *Journal of Pediatric Psychology, 16,* 229–239.

Deneberg, V. H., and Thoman, E. B. (1981). Evidence for a functional role for active (REM) sleep in infancy. *Sleep, 4,* 185–191.

Dunst, C. J., and Lingerfelt, B. (1985). Maternal ratings of temperament and operant learning in two- to three-month-old infants. *Child Development, 56,* 555–563.

Fibiger, W., Singer, G., Miller, A. J., Armstrong, S., and Datar, M. (1984). Cortisol and catecholamine changes as functions of time-of-day and self-reported mood. *Neuroscience Biobehavioural Reviews, 8,* 523–530.

Hayasaki, Y. (1927). On the sleeping hours at school, children of 6 to 20 years. *Psychological Abstracts, 1,* 439.

Johs, M. W., Gay, T. J. A., Masterton, J. P., and Bruce, D. W. (1971). Relationship between sleep habits, adrenocortical activity and personality. *Psychosomatic Medicine, 33,* 499–508.

Matheny, A. D., and Dolan, A. B. (1974). Childhood sleep characteristics and reading achievement. *JSAS Catalog of Selected Documents in Psychology, 4,* 76.

Minde, K., Faucon, A., and Falkner, S. (1994). Sleep problems in toddlers: Effects of treatment on their daytime behaviour. *Journal of the American Academy of Child & Adolescent Psychiatry, 33,* 1114–1121.

Terman, L. M. (1925). *Genetic studies of genius:* Vol. 1. *Mental and physical traits of a thousand gifted children.* Palo Alto: Stanford University Press.

Weissbluth, M. (1981). Sleep duration and infant temperament. *Journal of Pediatrics, 99,* 817–819.

Weissbluth, M. (1984). Sleep duration, temperament, and Conners' ratings of 3-year-old children. *Journal of Developmental and Behavioral Pediatrics, 5,* 120–123.

Weissbluth, M. (1985). How sleep affects school performance. *Gifted Children Monthly, 6,* 14–15.

Chapter 3. Sleep Problems and Solutions

Mood and Performance

Beltramini, A. U., and Hertzog, M. E. (1983). Sleep and bedtime behaviour in preschool-aged children. *Pediatrics, 71,* 153–158.

Dement, W. C., and Carskadon, M. A. (1982). Current perspectives on daytime sleepiness: The issues. *Sleep, 5* (Suppl. 2), S56–S66.

Dixon, K. N., Monroe, L. J., and Jakim, S. (1981). Insomniac children. *Sleep, 4,* 313–318.

Fibiger, W., Singer, G., Miller, A. J., Armstrong, S., and Datar, M. (1984). Cortisol and catecholamine changes as functions of time-of-day and self-reported mood. *Neuroscience Biobehavioural Reviews, 8,* 523–530.

Gaillard, J. M. (1985). Neurochemical regulation of the states of alertness. *Annals of Clinical Research, 17,* 175–184.

Gunner, M. R., Malone, S., Vance, G., and Fisch, R. O. (1985). Coping with aversive stimulation in the neonatal period: Quiet sleep and plasma cortisol levels during recovery from circumcision. *Child Development, 56,* 824–834.

Harrison, G. A. (1985). Stress, catecholamines, and sleep. *Aviation, Space and Environmental Medicine, 56,* 651–653.

Hauri, P., and Olmstead, E. (1980). Childhood-onset insomnia. *Sleep, 3,* 59–65.

Hicks, R. A., and Pellegrini, R. J. (1977). Anxiety levels of short and long sleepers. *Psychological Reports, 41,* 569–570.

Johs, M. W., Gay, T. J. A., Masterton, J. P., and Bruce, D. W. (1971). Relationship between sleep habits, adrenocortical activity and personality. *Psychosomatic Medicine, 33,* 499–508.

Kales, A., Bixler, E. O., Vela-Bueno, A., Cadieux, R. J., Soldatos, C. R., and Kales, J. D. (1984). Biopsychobehavioural correlates of insomnia: Part III. Polygraphic findings of sleep difficulty and their relationship to psychopathology. *International Journal of Neuroscience, 23,* 43–56.

Lucey, D. R., Hauri, P., and Snyder, M. L. (1981). The wakeful 'Type A' student. *International Journal of Psychosomatic Research, 101,* 333–337.

Price, V. A., Coates, T. J., Thoresen, C. E., and Grinstead, O. A.

(1978). Prevalence and correlates of poor sleep among adolescents. *American Journal of Diseases of Children, 132,* 583–586.

Simonds, J. F., and Parraga, H. (1982). Prevalence of sleep disorders and sleep behaviours in children and adolescents. *Journal of the American Academy of Child Psychiatry, 4,* 383–388.

Sundell, C. E. (1922). Sleeplessness in infants. *Practitioner, 109,* 89–92.

Tan, T. L., Kales, J. D., Kales, A., Soldatos, C. R., and Bixler, E. O. (1984). Biopsychobehavioural correlates of insomnia: Part IV. Diagnosis based on DSM III. *American Journal of Psychiatry, 141,* 357–362.

Excessive Daytime Sleepiness

Hoddes, E., Zarcone, V., Smythe, H., Phillips, R., and Dement, W. C. (1973). Quantification of sleepiness: A new approach. *Psychophysiology, 10,* 431–436.

Stepanski, E., Lamphere, J., Badia, P., Zorick, F., and Roth, T. (1984). Sleep fragmentation and daytime sleepiness. *Sleep, 7,* 18–26.

Night Waking, Difficulty Staying Asleep

Coulter, D. L., and Allen, R. J. (1982). Benign neonatal sleep myoclonus. *Archives of Neurology, 39,* 191–192.

Earls, F. (1980). Prevalence of behaviour problems in 3-year-old children. *Archives of General Psychiatry, 37,* 1153–1157.

Fukumoto, M., Muchozuki, N., Tekeishi, M., Nomura, Y., and Segawa, M. (1981). Studies of body movements during night sleep in infancy. *Brain and Development, 3,* 37–43.

Karacan, I., Wolff, S. M., Williams, R. L., Hurscl, C. J., and Webb, W. B. (1968). The effects of fever on sleep and dream patterns. *Psychosomatics, 9,* 331–339.

Oster, J., and Nelson, A. (1974). Growing pains: A clinical investigation of a school problem. *Acta Paediatrica Scandinavia, 61,* 329–334.

Radbill, S. X. (1965). Teething in fact and fancy. *Bulletin of the History of Medicine, 39,* 339–345.

Richman, N. (1981). A community survey of characteristics of

1- to 2-year-olds with sleep disruption. *American Academy of Child Psychiatry, 20,* 281–291.

Tasanen, A. (1969). General and local effects of the eruption of deciduous teeth. *Annales de Paediatrac Fenniae, 14* (Suppl. 29).

Weissbluth, M. (1982). Modification of sleep schedule with reduction of night waking: A case report. *Sleep, 5,* 262–266.

Weissbluth, M., Christoffel, K. K., and Davis, A. T. (1984). Treatment of infantile colic with dicyclomine hydrochloride. *Journal of Pediatrics, 104,* 951–955.

Weissbluth, M., Davis, A. T., and Poncher, J. (1984). Night waking in 4- to 8-month-old infants. *Journal of Pediatrics, 104,* 477–480.

Chapter 4. Sleep, Extreme Fussiness/Colic and Temperament

Aldrich, C. A., Sung, C., and Knop, C. (1945). The crying of newly born babies: Part II. The individual phase. *Journal of Pediatrics, 27,* 89–96.

Barr, R. G. (1989). Feeding and temperament as determinants of early infant crying/fussing behaviour. *Pediatrics, 84,* 14–521.

Bates, J. E., Viken, R. J., Alexander, D. B., Beyers, J., and Stockton, S. (2002). Sleep and adjustment in preschool children: Sleep diary reports by mothers relate to behaviour reports by teachers. *Child Development, 73,* 62–74.

Blum, N. J., Taubman, B., Tretina, L., and Heyward, R. Y. (2002). Maternal ratings of infant intensity and distractibility. Relationship with crying during the second month of life. *Archives Pediatrics and Adolescent Medicine, 156,* 286–290.

Boon, W. H. (1982). The crying baby. *Journal of the Singapore Paediatric Society, 24,* 145–147.

Brazelton, T. B. (1962). Crying in infancy. *Pediatrics, 29,* 579–588.

Breslow, L. (1957). A clinical approach to infantile colic: A review of 90 cases. *Journal of Pediatrics, 50,* 196–206.

Canivet, C., Jakobsson, I., and Hagander, B. (2000). Infantile colic. Follow-up at four years of age: Still more 'emotional'. *Acta Paediat, 89,* 13–17.

Carey, W. B. (1972). Clinical application of infant temperament measurements. *Journal of Pediatrics, 81,* 823–828.

Carey, W. B. (1985). Temperament and increased weight gain in infants. *Journal of Developmental and Behavioral Pediatrics, 3,* 128–131.

Carey, W. B., and McDevitt, S. C. (1978). Revision of the infant temperament questionnaire. *Pediatrics, 61,* 735–739.

Clifford, T. J., Campbell, M., Speechley, K. N., and Gorodzinsky, F. (2002). Sequelae of infant colic. Evidence of transient infant distress and absence of lasting effects on maternal mental health. *Archives of Pediatric and Adolescent Medicine, 15,* 1183–1188.

Clifford, T. J., Campbell, M. K., Speechley, K. N., and Gorodozinsky, F. (2002). Infant colic. Empirical evidence of the absence of an association with source of early infant nutrition. *Archives of Pediatric and Adolescent Medicine, 156,* 1123–1128.

Collins, D. D., Scoggin, C. H., Zwillich, C. W., and Welf, J. U. (1978). Hereditary aspects of decreased hypoxic response. *Journal of Clinical Investigations, 62,* 104–110.

Crockenberg, S. B., and Smith, P. (1982). Antecedents of mother-infant interaction and infant-irritability in the first three months of life. *Infant Behavior and Development, 5,* 105–119.

DeVries, M. (1984). Temperament and infant mortality among the Masai of East Africa. *American Journal of Psychiatry, 141,* 1189–1194.

Dunst, C. J., and Lingerfelt, B. (1985). Maternal ratings of temperament and operant learning in 2- to 3-month-old infants. *Child Development, 56,* 555–563.

Emde, R. N., Gaensbauer, T. J., and Harman, P. J. (1976). Emotional expression in infancy: A biobehavioural study. *Psychological Issues, 10,* 1–200.

Etzel, B. C., and Gewirtz, J. L. (1967). Experimental modification of caretaker-maintained high-rate operant crying in a 6- and 20-week old infant (Infans tyrannotearus): Extinction of crying with reinforcement of eye contact and smiling. *Journal of Experimental Child Psychology, 5,* 503–517.

Freedman, D. G. (1979). Ethnic differences in babies. *Human Nature, 2,* 36–43.

Garrison, M. M., and Christakis, D. A. (2000). A systematic review of treatments for infant colic. *Pediatrics, 106,* 184–190.

Giganti, F., Fagioli, I., Ficca, G., and Salzarulo, P. (2001). Polygraphic investigation of 24-hr waking distribution in infants. *Physiology and Behavior, 73,* 621–624.

Heine, R. G., Cameron, D. J. S., Chung, W. C., Hill, D. J., and Catto-Smith, A. G. (2002). Cause & effect of unhappy coexistence. GERD does not cause crying. *Journal of Pediatrics, 140,* 14–19.

Hill, D. J., and Hosking, C. S. (2000). Infantile colic and food hypersensitivity. *Journal of Pediatric Gastroenterology and Nutrition, 30,* (Suppl.), S67–S76.

Hunziker, U. A., and Barr, R. G. (1986). Increased carrying reduces infant crying: A randomized controlled trial. *Pediatrics, 77,* 641–648.

Illingworth, R. S. (1954). 'Three months' colic. *Archives of Diseases of Children, 29,* 167–174.

Illingworth, R. S. (1955). Crying in infants and children. *British Medical Journal, 1,* 75–78.

Karelitz, S., Fisichelli, V. R., Costa, J., Karelitz, R., and Rosen- feld, L. (1964). Relation of crying activity in early infancy to speech and intellectual development at age three years. *Child Development, 35,* 769–777.

Keefe, M. R., Kotser, A. M., Froese-Fretz, A., and Curtin, M. (1996). A longitudinal comparison of irritable and nonirritable infants. *Nursing Research, 45,* 4–9.

Keener, M. A., Zeanah, C. H., and Anders, T. F. (1988). Infant temperament, sleep organisation, and night-time parental interventions. *Pediatrics, 81,* 762–771.

Kirjavainen, J., Kirjavainen, T., Huhtala, V., Lehtonen, L., Korvenranta. H., and Kero, P. (2001). Infants with colic have a normal sleep structure at 2 and 7 months of age. *Journal of Pediatrics, 138,* 218–223.

Kurtoglu, S., Uzum, K., Hallac, I. K., and Coskun, A. (1997). 5-Hydroxy-3-indole acetic acid levels in infantile colic: Is serotoninergic tonus responsible for this problem? *Acta Paediatric, 86,* 764–765.

Lehtonen, L., Korhonen, T., and Korvenranta, H. (1994). Temperament and sleeping patterns in colicky infants during the first year of life. *Journal of Developmental and Behavioral Pediatrics, 15,* 416-420.

Lester, B. M., and Bookydis, C. F. Z. (eds.) (1985). *Infant Crying*. New York: Plenum Press.

Lounsbuery, M. L., and Bates, J. E. (1982). The cries of infants of differing levels of perceived temperamental difficultness: Acoustic properties and effects on listeners. *Child Development, 53,* 677–686.

Matheny, A. P., Wilson, R. S., Dolan, A. B., and Krantz, J. Z. (1985). Behavioral contrasts in twinships: Stability and patterns of differences in childhood. *Child Development, 52,* 579–588.

Meyer, J. E., and Thaler, M. M. (1971). Colic in low birthweight infants. *American Journal of Diseases of Children, 122,* 25–27.

Monnier, M., and Gaillard, J. M. (1980). Biochemical regulation of sleep. *Experientia, 36,* 21–24.

Novosad, C., Freudigman, K., and Thoman, E. B. (1999). Sleep patterns in newborns and temperament at eight months: A preliminary study. *Journal of Developmental and Behavioral Pediatrics, 20,* 99–105.

O'Connor, L. H., and Feder, H. H. (1984). Estradiol and progesterone influence a serotonin mediated behavioural syndrome (myoclonus) in female guinea pigs. *Brain Research, 293,* 119–125.

Ogden, T. H. (1985). The mother, the infant and the matrix: Interpretations of aspects of the work of Donald Winnocott. *Contemporary Psychoanalysis, 21,* 346–371.

Olafsdottir, E., Forshei, G., and Markestad, T. (2001). Randomised controlled trial of infantile colic treated with chiropractic spinal manipulation. *Archives of Disease in Childhood, 84,* 138–141.

Papousek, M., and von Hofacker, N. (1998). Persistent crying in early infancy: A non-trivial condition of risk for the developing mother-infant relationship. *Child: Care, Health and Development, 24,* 395–424.

Parmelee, A. H., Jr. (1997). Remarks on receiving the C. Anderson Aldrich Award. *Pediatrics, 59,* 389–395.

Paulozzi, L., and Sells, M. (2002). Variation in homicide risk during infancy – United States, 1989–1998. *Morbidity and Mortality Report, 51,* 187–189.

Pierce, P. (1948). Delayed onset of 'three months' colic in premature infants. *American Journal of Diseases of Children, 75,* 190–192.

Raiha, H., Lehtonen, L., Korhonen, T., and Korvenranta, H. (1996). Family life 1 year after infantile colic. *Archives of Pediatric and Adolescent Medicine, 150,* 1032–1036.

Rautava, P., Lehtonen, L., Helenius, H., and Sillanpaa, M. (1995). Infantile colic: Child and family three years later. *Pediatrics, 96,* 43–47.

Rebelsky, F., and Black, R. (1972). Crying in infancy. *Journal of Genetic Psychology, 121,* 49–57.

Reijneveld, S. A., Brugman, E., and Hirasing, R. A. (2001). Excessive infant crying: The impact of varying definitions. *Pediatrics, 108,* 893–897.

Richman, N., Douglas, J., Hunt, H., Lansdown, R., and Levere, R. (1985). Behavioral methods in the treatment of sleep disorders – A pilot study. *Journal of Child Psychology and Psychiatry, 26,* 581–590.

Scher, A., Epstein, R., Sadeh, A., Tirosh, E., and Lavie, P. (1992). Toddlers' sleep and temperament: Reporting bias or a valid link: A research note. *Journal of Child Psychology and Psychiatry and Allied Disciplines, 33,* 1249–1254.

Scher, A., Tirosh, E., and Lavie, P. (1998). The relationship between sleep and temperament revisited: Evidence for 12-month-olds: A research note. *Journal of Child Psychology and Psychiatry and Allied Disciplines, 39,* 785–788.

Schulz, H., Salzarulo, P., Fagioli, I., and Massetani, R. (1983). REM latency: Development in the first year of life. *Electroencephalography and Clinical Neurophysiology, 56,* 316–322.

Shaver, B. A. (1974). Maternal personality and early adaptation as related to infantile colic. In P. M. Schereshefsky and L. J. Yarrow (eds.), *Psychological Aspects of a First Pregnancy and Early Postnatal Adaptation* (209–215). New York: Raven Press.

Snow, M. E., Jacklin, C. N., and Maccoby, E. E. (1980). Crying episodes and sleep-wakefulness transitions in the first 26 months of life. *Infant Behavior and Development, 3,* 387–394.

St. James-Roberts, I., Conroy, S., and Hurry, J. (1997). Links between infant crying and sleep-waking at six weeks of age. *Early Child Development, 48,* 143–152.

St. James-Roberts, I., and Plewis, I. (1996). Individual differences, daily fluctuations, and developmental changes in amounts of infant waking, fussing, crying, feeding, and sleeping. *Child Development, 67,* 2527–2540.

Stahlberg, M.-R. (1984). Infantile colic: Occurrence and risk factors. *European Journal of Pediatrics, 143,* 108–111.

Stenger, K. (1956). Therapy of spastic bronchitis. *Med Klin, 51,* 1451–1455.

Stifter, C. A., and Braungart, J. (1992). Infant colic: A transient condition with no apparent effects. *Journal of Applied Developmental Psychology, 13,* 447–462.

Sullivan, C. E., Murphy, E., Kozar, L. F., and Phillipson, E. A. (1979). Ventilatory responses to CO_2 and lung inflation in tonic versus phasic REM sleep. *Journal of Applied Physiology: Respiration, Environment and Exercise Physiology, 47,* 1304–1310.

Tandon, P., Gupta, M. L., and Barthwal, J. P. (1983). Role of monoamine oxidase-B in medroxyprogesterone acetate (17-acetoxy-6 gamma-methyl-4-pregnene-4-3, 20-dione) induced changes in brain dopamine levels in rats. *Steroids, 42,* 231–239.

Thomas, A., Chess, S., and Birch, H. G. (1968). *Temperament and Behavior Disorders in Childhood.* New York: New York University Press.

Watanabe, K., Inokuma, K., and Nogoro, T. (1983). REM sleep prevents sudden infant death syndrome. *European Journal of Pediatrics, 140,* 289–292.

Webb, W. B., and Campbell, S. S. (1983). Relationship in sleep characteristics in identical and fraternal twins. *Archives of General Psychiatry, 40,* 1093–1095.

Weissbluth, L., and Weissbluth, M. (1992). Infant colic: The effect of serotonin and melatonin on circadian rhythms in the intestinal smooth muscle. *Medical Hypotheses, 39,* 164–167.

Weissbluth, M. (1981). Infantile colic and near-miss sudden infant death syndrome. *Medical Hypotheses,* 7, 1193–1199.

Weissbluth, M. (1981). Sleep duration and infant temperament. *Journal of Pediatrics, 99,* 817–819.

Weissbluth, M. (1982). Chinese-American infant temperament and sleep duration: An ethnic comparison. *Developmental and Behavioral Pediatrics, 3,* 99–102.

Weissbluth, M. (1982). Modification of sleep schedule with reduction of night waking: A case report. *Sleep, 5,* 262–266.

Weissbluth, M. (1984). Sleep duration, temperament, and Conners' ratings of three-year-old children. *Journal of Developmental and Behavioral Pediatrics, 5,* 120–123.

Weissbluth, M. (1984). *Crybabies.* New York: Arbor House.

Weissbluth, M. (1986). Infant colic. In S. S. Gellis and B. M. Kagan (eds.), *Current Pediatric Therapy,* 12th ed. (765–767). Philadelphia: W. B. Saunders.

Weissbluth, M. (1987). Sleep and the colicky infant. In *Sleep and Its Disorders in Children,* edited by C. Guilleminault. (129–140). New York: Raven Press.

Weissbluth, M. (1995). Colic. In *Principles and Practice of Sleep Medicine in the Child,* edited by R. Ferber and M. H. Kryger. (75–78). Philadelphia: W. B. Saunders.

Weissbluth, M., Brouillette, R. T., Liu, K., and Hunt, C. E. (1982). Sleep apnea, sleep duration, and infant temperament. *Journal of Pediatrics, 101,* 307–310.

Weissbluth, M., Christoffel, K. K., and Davis, A. T. (1984). Treatment of infantile colic with dicyclomine hydrochloride. *Journal of Pediatrics, 104,* 951–955.

Weissbluth, M., Davis, A. T., and Poncher, J. (1984). Night waking in 4- to 8-month-old infants. *Journal of Pediatrics, 104,* 477–480.

Weissbluth, M., and Green, O. C. (1984). Plasma progesterone concentration and infant temperament. *Journal of Developmental and Behavioral Pediatrics, 5,* 251–253.

Weissbluth, M., Hunt, C., Brouillette, R. T., Hanson, D., David, R. J., and Stein, I. M. (1985). Respiratory patterns during sleep and temperament ratings in normal infants. *Journal of Pediatrics, 106,* 688–690.

Weissbluth, M., and Liu, K. (1983). Sleep patterns, attention span, and infant temperament. *Journal of Developmental and Behavioral Pediatrics, 4,* 34–36.

Weissbluth, M., and Weissbluth, L. (1992). Colic, sleep inertia, melatonin and circannual rhythms. *Medical Hypotheses, 38,* 224–228.

Wessel, M. A., Cobb, J. C., Jackson, E. B., Harris, G. S., and Detwiler, A. C. (1954). Paroxysmal fussing in infants, sometimes called 'colic'. *Pediatrics, 14,* 421–434.

White, B. P., Gunnar, M. R., Larson, M. C., Donzella, B., and Barr,

R. C. (2000). Behavioral and physiological responsivity, sleep, and patterns of daily cortisol production in infants with and without colic. *Child Development, 71,* 862–877.

Williams, C. D. (1959). The elimination of tantrum behaviour by extinction procedures. *Journal of Abnormal and Social Psychology, 59,* 269.

Wolke, D., Gray, P., and Meyer, R. (1994). Excessive infant crying: A controlled study of mothers helping mothers. *Pediatrics, 94,* 322–332.

Wolke, D., and Meyer, R. (1995). Co-morbidity of crying and feeding problems with sleeping problems in infancy: Concurrent and predictive associations. *Early Development and Parenting, 4,* 191–207.

Wolke, D, Rizzo, P., and Woods, S. (2002). Persistent infant crying and hyperactive problems in middle childhood. *Pediatrics, 109,* 1054–1060.

Zeskind, P. S., and Huntington, L. (1984). The effects of within-group and between-group methodologies in the study of perceptions of infant crying. *Child Development, 55,* 1658–1665.

Chapter 5. Months One to Four

Christophersen, E. (2002). Diagnosis and management of sleep problems. In *Treatments That Work with Children.* Washington, D.C.: American Psychological Association.

Etzel, B. C., and Gewirtz, J. L. (1967). Experimental modification of caretaker-maintained high-rate operant crying in a 6- and 20-week-old infant (Infans tyrannotearus): Extinction of crying with reinforcement of eye contact and smiling. *Journal of Experimental Child Psychology, 5,* 303–317.

Fagan, J. W., Ohr, P. J., Fleckenstein, L. K., and Ribner, D. R. (1985). The effects of crying on long-term memory in infancy. *Child Development, 56,* 1584–1592.

Leach, Penelope (1978). *Your Baby and Child from Birth to Five.* New York: Alfred A. Knopf.

Maziade, M., Boudreault, M., Cote, R., and Thivierage, J. (1986). Influence of gentle birth delivery procedures and other perinatal circumstances on infant temperament: Developmental and social implications. *Journal of Pediatrics, 108,* 134–136.

McGraw, K., Hoffman, R., Harker, C., and Herman, J. H. (1999). The development of circadian rhythms in a human infant. *Sleep, 22,* 303–310.

Spock, Benjamin. (1983). *Baby and Child Care.* New York: Pocket Books.

Chapter 6. Months Five to Twelve

Caren, S., and Searleman, A. (1985). Birth stress and self-reported sleep difficulty. *Sleep, 8,* 222–226.

Dinges, D. F., and Broughton, R. J. (1989). *Sleep and Alertness: Chronobiological, Behavioral, and Medical Aspects of Napping.* New York: Raven Press.

Douglas, J., and Richman, N. (1984). *My Child Won't Sleep.* Hammondsworth, Middlesex, England: Penguin Books.

France, K. G., Blampied, N. M., and Wilkinson, P. (1991). Treatment of infant sleep disturbance by trimeprazine in combination with extinction. *Journal of Developmental and Behavioral Pediatrics, 12,* 308–314.

France, K. G. (1992). Behavior characteristics and security in sleep-disturbed infants treated with extinction. *Journal of Pediatric Psychology, 17,* 467–475.

Hirschberg, J. C. (1957). Parental anxieties accompanying sleep disturbance in young children. *Bulletin of the Menninger Clinic, 21,* 129–139.

Hiscock, H., and Wake, M. (2002). Randomised controlled trial of behavioural infant sleep intervention to improve infant sleep and maternal mood. *British Medical Journal, 324,* 1062–1072.

Hiscock, H., and Wake, M. (2001). Infant sleep problems and postnatal depression: A community based study. *Pediatrics, 107,* 1317–1322.

Klastskin, E. H., Jackson, E. B., and Wilkin, L. C. (1956). The influence of degree of flexibility in maternal care practices on early child behaviour. *American Journal of Orthopsychiatry, 26,* 79–93.

Lewis, M. (1997) *Altering Fate: Why the Past Does Not Predict the Future.* New York: The Guilford Press.

Mahler, M. S. (1972). On the first three subphases of the separation-individuation process. *International Journal of Psycho-Analysis, 53,* 333–338.

Peiyoong, L., Hiscock, H., Wake, M., and Epi, G. D. (2003). Outcomes of infant sleep problems: A longitudinal study of sleep, behaviour, and maternal well-being. *Pediatrics.* In press.

Richman, N., Douglas, J., and Hunt, H. (1985). Behavioral methods in the treatment of sleep disorders: A pilot study. *Journal of Child Psychology and Psychiatry, 26,* 581–590.

Thomas, A., and Chess, S. (1984). Genesis and evolution of behavioural disorders: From infancy to early adult life. *American Journal of Psychiatry, 141,* 1–9.

Webb, W. B., and Agnew, H. W. (1974). Regularity in the control of the free-running sleep-wakefulness rhythm. *Aerospace Medicine, 45,* 701–704.

Weissbluth, M. (1982). Modification of sleep schedule with reduction of night waking: A case report. *Sleep, 5,* 262–266.

Winnicott, D. W. (1965). The capacity to be alone. In D. W. Winnicott, *The Maturational Processes and Facilitating Environment* (29–36). New York: International Universities Press.

Chapter 7. Months Thirteen to Thirty-six

Gutelius, M. E., and Kirsch, A. D. (1977). Controlled study of child health supervision: Behavioral results. *Pediatrics, 60,* 294–304.

Howarth, E., and Hoffman, M. S. (1984). A multidimensional approach to the relationship between mood and weather. *British Journal of Psychology, 75,* 5–23.

Kahyama, J., Shiike, T., and Hasegawa, T. (2000). Young children who are late sleepers sleep less than early sleepers. *Sleep, 23* (Abstract Suppl. 2), A198–A199.

Largo, R. H., and Honziker, U. A. (1984). A developmental approach to the management of children with sleep disturbances in the first three years of life. *European Journal of Pediatrics, 142,* 170–173.

Lozoff, B., Wolf, A. W., and Davis, N. S. (1985). Sleep problems seen in pediatric practice. *Pediatrics, 75,* 477–483.

Lyons, J. T., and Oates, R. K. (1993). Falling out of bed: A relatively benign occurrence. *Pediatrics, 92,* 125–127.

Richman, N. (1981). A community survey of one- to two-year-olds with sleep disruptions. *Journal of the American Academy of Child Psychiatry, 20,* 281–291.

Scher, A., Tirosh, E., and Lavie, P. (1998). The relationship between sleep and temperament revisited: Evidence for 12-month-olds: A research note. *Journal of Child Psychiatry and Allied Disciplines, 39,* 785–788.

Van Tassel, E. B. (1985). The relative influence of child and environmental characteristics on sleep disturbances in the first and second years of life. *Journal of Developmental and Behavioral Pediatrics, 6,* 81–86.

Williams, C. D. (1959). Case report: The elimination of tantrum behaviour by extinction procedures. *Journal of Abnormal and Social Psychology, 59,* 269.

Chapter 8. Preschool Children

Atkinson, E., Vetere, A., and Grayson, K. (1995). Sleep disruption in young children. The influence of temperament on the sleep patterns of pre-school children. *Child: Care, Health and Development, 21,* 233–246.

Bates, J. E., Viken, R. J., Alexander, D. B., Beyers, J., and Stockton, S. (2002). Sleep and adjustment in preschool children: Sleep diary reports by mothers relate to behaviour reports by teachers. *Child Development, 73,* 62–74.

Christophersen, Edward R. (1998). *Beyond Discipline: Parenting That Lasts a Lifetime*, 2nd ed. (127–128). Shawnee Mission, Kansas: Overland Press.

Clarkson, S., Williams, S., and Silva, P. A. (1986). Sleep in middle childhood – a longitudinal study of sleep problems in a large sample of Dunedin children aged 5–9 years. *Australian Paediatric Journal, 22,* 31–35.

Cullen, K. J. (1976). A 6-year controlled trial of prevention of children's behaviour disorders. *Journal of Pediatrics, 88,* 662–666.

Fukuda, K., and Sakashita, Y. (2002). Sleeping pattern of kindergartners and nursery school children: Function of daytime nap. *Perceptual and Motor Skills, 94,* 219–228.

Gregory, A. M., and O'Connor, T. G. (2002). Sleep problems in childhood: A longitudinal study of developmental change and association with behavioural problems. *Journal of the American Academy of Child & Adolescent Psychiatry, 41,* 954–971.

Jones, D. P. H., and Verduyn, C. M. (1983). Behavioral management of sleep problems. *Archives of Diseases of Children, 58,* 442–444.

Kohyama, J., Shiike, T., Ohinata-Sugimoto, J., and Hasegawa, T. (2002). Potentially harmful sleep habits of 3-year-old children in Japan. *Journal of Developmental and Behavioral Pediatrics, 23,* 67–70.

Lavigne, J. V., Arend, R., Rosenbaum, D., Smith, A., Weissbluth, M., Binns, H. J., and Christoffel, K. K. (1999). Sleep and behaviour problems among preschoolers. *Journal of Developmental and Behavioral Pediatrics, 20,* 164–169.

Manber, R., Bootzin, R. R., Acebo, C., and Carskadon, M. A. (1996). The effects of regularising sleep-wake schedules on daytime sleepiness. *Sleep, 19,* 432–441.

Mantz, J., Muzet, A., Neiss, R. (1995). Sleep in 6-year-old children: Survey in school environment. *Archives of Pediatrics, 21,* 215–220.

Minde, K., Popiel, K., Leos, N., Falkner, S., Parker, K., and Handley-Derry, M. (1993). The evaluation and treatment of sleep disturbances in young children. *Journal of Child Psychology and Psychiatry, 34,* 521–533.

Owens-Stively, J., Frank, N., Smith, A., Hagino, O., Spirito, A., Arigan, M., and Alario, A. J. (1997). Child temperament, parenting discipline style, and daytime behaviour in childhood sleep disorders. *Journal of Developmental and Behavioral Pediatrics, 18,* 314–321.

Richman, N., Douglas, J., Hunt, H., Lansdown, R., and Levere, R. (1985). Behavioral methods in the treatment of sleep disorders – A pilot study. *Journal of Child Psychology and Psychiatry, 26,* 581–590.

Sekine, Y., Yamagami, T., Handa, K., Saito, T., Nanre, S., Kawaminami, K., Tokui, N., Yoshida, K., and Kagamimori, S. (2002). A dose-response relationship between short sleeping hours and childhood obesity: Results of the Toyama Birth Cohort Study. *Child: Care, Health and Development, 28,* 163–170.

von Kries, R., Toschke, A. M., Wurnser, H., Sauerwald, T., and Koletsko, B. (2002). Reduced risk for overweight and obesity in 5- and 6-year-old children by duration of sleep – a cross sectional study. *International Journal of Obesity and Related Metabolic Disorders, 26,* 710–716.

Witting, W., Mirmiran, M., Bos, N. P., and Swaab, D. F. (1993). Effect of light intensity on diurnal sleep-wake distribution in young and old rats. *Brain Research Bulletin, 30,* 157–162.

Wright, L., Woodcock, J., and Scott, R. (1970). Treatment of sleep disturbance in a young child by conditioning. *Southern Medical Journal, 63,* 174–176.

Chapter 9. School Children and Adolescence

Acebo, C., and Carskadon, M. A. (2002). Influence of irregular sleep patterns on waking behaviour. In M. A. Carskadon (ed.), *Adolescent Sleep Patterns. Biological, Social, and Psychological Influences,* (220–235). Cambridge: Cambridge University Press.

Anders, T. E., Carskadon, M. A., Dement, W. C., and Harvey, K. (1978). Sleep habits of children and the identification of pathologically sleepy children. *Child Psychiatry and Human Development, 9,* 56–63.

Anderson, D. R. (1979). Treatment of insomnia in a 13-year-old boy by relaxation training and reduction of parental attention. *Journal of Behavioral Therapy and Experimental Psychiatry, 10,* 263–265.

Asnes, R. S., Sautulli, R., and Beuporad, J. R. (1981). Psychogenic chest pain in children. *Clinical Pediatrics, 20,* 788–792.

Backeland, F., and Lasky, R. (1966). Exercise and sleep patterns in college athletes. *Perceptual and Motor Skills, 23,* 1203–1207.

Blader, J. C., Kopewicz, H. S., Abikoff, H., and Foley, C. (1997). Sleep problems of elementary school children: A community survey. *Archives of Pediatrics and Adolescent Medicine, 151,* 473–480.

Bootzin, R. R., and Perlis, M. L. (1992). Nonpharmacologic treatments of insomnia. *Journal of Clinical Psychiatry, 53,* 27–41.

Bootzin, R. (1972). A stimulus control treatment for insomnia. *Proceedings of the American Psychological Association, 7,* 395–396.

Carskadon, M. A. (2002). *Adolescent Sleep Patterns. Biological, Social, and Psychological Influences.* Cambridge: Cambridge University Press.

Carskadon, M. A., Vieiera, C., and Acebo, C. (1993). Association between puberty and delayed phase preference. *Sleep, 16,* 258–262.

Czeisler, C. A., Weitzman, E. D., Moore-Ede, M. C., Zimmerman,

J. C., and Knaver, R. S. (1980). Human sleep: Its duration and organisation depend on its circadian phases. *Science, 210,* 1264–1267.

Dollinger, S. J. (1985). Effects of a paradoxical intervention on a child's anxiety about sleep- and sports-related performance. *Perceptual and Motor Skills, 61,* 83–86.

Epstein, R., Chillag, N., and Lavie, P. (1998). Stating times of school: Effects on daytime functioning of fifth-grade children in Israel. *Sleep, 21,* 250–256.

Espie, C. A., and Lindsay, W. R. (1985). Paradoxical intention in the treatment of chronic insomnia. *Behavioral Research and Therapy, 23,* 703–709.

Fallone, G. P., Seiffer, R., Acebo, C., and Carskadon, M. A. (2000). Prolonged sleep restriction in 11- and 12-year-old children: Effects on behaviour, sleepiness, and mood. *Sleep, 23,* (Suppl.), A28.

Fukuda, K., and Ishihara, K. (2002). Routine evening naps and night-time sleep patterns in junior high and high school students. *Psychiatry and Clinical Neurosciences, 56,* 229–230.

Gau, S. F., and Soong, W. T. (1995). Sleep problems of junior high school students in Taipei. *Sleep, 18,* 667–673.

Hauri, P., and Fisher, J. (1986). Persistent psychophysiologic (learned) insomnia. *Sleep, 9,* 38–53.

Hicks, R. A., and Pellegrini, R. J. (1991). The changing sleep habits of college students. *Perceptive Motor Skills, 72,* 1106.

Kahn, A., Van de Merckt, C., Rebuffat, E., Mozin, M. J., Sottiaux, M., Blum, D., and Hennart, P. (1989). Sleep problems in healthy preadolescents. *Pediatrics, 84,* 542–546.

Kirmil-Gray, K., Eagleston, J. R., Gibson, E., and Theresen, C. E. (1985). Sleep disturbances in adolescents: Sleep quality, sleep habits, beliefs about sleep, and daytime functioning. *Journal of Youth and Adolescence, 13,* 375–384.

Liu, X., Sun, Z., Uchiyama, M., Shibui, K., and Kim, K. (2000). Prevalence and correlates of sleep problems in Chinese schoolchildren. *Sleep, 23,* 1053–1062.

Liu, X., Uchiyama, M., Okawa, M., and Kurita, H. (2000). Prevalence and correlates of self-reported sleep problems among Chinese adolescents. *Sleep, 23,* 27–34.

Manni, R., Ratti, R. T., Marchioni, E., Castelovo, G., Murelli, R., Sartori, I., Galimberti, C. A., and Tartara, A. (1997). Poor sleep in adolescents: A study of 869 17-year-old Italian secondary school students. *Journal of Sleep Research, 6,* 44–49.

Morrison, D. N., McGee, R., and Stanton, W. R. (1992). Sleep problems in adolescence. *Journal of American Academy of Child and Adolescent Psychiatry, 31,* 94–99.

Nicassio, P. M., and Buchanan, D. C. (1981). Clinical application of behaviour therapy for insomnia. *Comprehensive Psychiatry, 22,* 512–521.

Price, V. A., Coates, T. J., Thoresen, C. E., and Grinstead, O. A. (1978). Prevalence and correlates of poor sleep among adolescents. *American Journal of Diseases of Children, 132,* 582–586.

Randazzo, A. C., Muehlbach, M. J., Schweitzer, P. K., and Walsh, J. K. (1998). Cognitive function following acute sleep restriction in children ages 10–14. *Sleep, 21,* 861–868.

Randazzo, A. C., Schweitzer, P. K., and Walsh, J. K. (1998). Cognitive function following 3 nights of sleep restriction in children 10–14. *Sleep, 21* (Suppl.), A249.

Reid, A., Maldonado, C. C., and Baker, F. C. (2002). Sleep behaviour of South African adolescents. *Sleep, 25,* 423–427.

Roberts, R. E., Roberts, C. R., and Chen, I. G. (2002). Impact of insomnia on future functioning of adolescents. *Journal of Psychosomatic Research, 53,* 561–569.

Sadeh, A., Gruber, R., and Raviv, A. (2002). Sleep, neurobehavioural functioning, and behaviour problems in school-aged children. *Child Development, 73,* 405–417.

Delayed Sleep Phase Syndrome

Czeisler, C. A., Richardson, G. S., Coleman, R. M., Zimmerman, J. C., Moore-Ede, M. C., Dement, W. C., and Weitzman, E. D. (1981). Chronotherapy: Resetting the circadian clocks of patients with delayed sleep phase insomnia. *Sleep, 4,* 1–21.

Weitzman, E. D., Czeisler, C. A., Coleman, R. M., Spielman, A. J., Zimmerman, J. C., and Dement, W. C. (1981). Delayed sleep phase syndrome: A chronobiological disorder with sleep-onset insomnia. *Archives of General Psychiatry, 38,* 737–746.

Kleine-Levin Syndrome

Ferguson, B. G. (1986). Kleine-Levin syndrome: A case report. *Journal of Child Psychological Psychiatry, 27,* 275–278.

Waller, D. A., Jarriel, S., Erman, M., and Emslie, G. (1984). Recognizing and managing the adolescent with Kleine-Levin syndrome. *Journal of Adolescent Health Care, 5,* 139–141.

Fibromyalgia Syndrome

Anthony, K. K., and Schanberg, L. E. (2001). Juvenile primary fibromyalgia syndrome. *Current Rheumatology Reports, 3,* 165–171.

Buskila, D., Neumann, L., Hershman, E., Gedalia, A., Press, J., and Sukenik, S. (1995). Fibromyalgia syndrome in children – An outcome study. *Journal of Rheumatology, 22,* 525–528.

Mikkelsson, M., Sourander, A., Piha, J., and Salminen, J. J. (1997). Psychiatric symptoms in preadolescents with musculoskeletal pain and fibromyalgia. *Pediatrics, 100,* 220–227.

Reid, G. J., Lang, B. A., and McGrath, P. J. (1997). Primary juvenile fibromyalgia: Psychological adjustment, family functioning, coping, and functional disability. *Arthritis and Rheumatism, 40,* 752–760.

Roizenblatt, S., Tufik, S., Goldenberg, J., Pinto, L. R., Hilaria, M. O., and Feldman, D. (1997). Juvenile fibromyalgia: Clinical and polysomnographic aspects. *Journal of Rheumatology, 24,* 579–585.

Siegel, D. M., Janeway, D., and Baum, J. (1998). Fibromyalgia syndrome in children and adolescents: Clinical features at presentation and status at follow-up. *Pediatrics, 101,* 377–382.

Drugs and Diet to Help Us Sleep

Camfield, C. S., Chaplin, S., Doyle, A. B., Chapiro, S. H., Cummings, C., and Camfield, P. R. (1979). Side effects of phenobarbital in toddlers: Behavioral and cognitive aspects. *Journal of Pediatrics, 95,* 361–365.

Kahn, A., Mozin, M. J., Casimir, G., Montauk, L., and Blum, D. (1985). Insomnia and cow's milk allergy in infants. *Pediatrics, 76,* 880–884.

Kolata, G. (1982). Food affects human behaviour. *Science, 218,* 1209–1210.

Norvenius, G., Widerlov, E., and Lonnerholm, G. (1979). Phenylpropanolamine and mental disturbances. *Lancet, 1,* 1367–1368.

Roehrs, T. A., Tietz, E. I., Zorick, F. J., and Roth, T. (1984). Daytime sleepiness and antihistamines. *Sleep, 7,* 137–141.

Russo, R. M., Gururaj, V. J., and Allen, E. J. (1976). The effectiveness of diphenhydramine HCl in pediatric sleep disorders. *Journal of Clinical Pharmocology, 16,* 284–285.

Ryo, J. E. (1985). Effects of maternal caffeine consumption on heart rate and sleep time in breast-fed infants. *Developmental Pharmacology and Therapeutics, 8,* 355–363.

Schneider-Helmert, D., and Spinweber, C. L. (1986). Evaluation of L-tryptophan for treatment of insomnia. *Psychopharmacology, 89,* 1–7.

Spring, B., Maller, O., Wurtman, J., et al. (1982–1983). Effects of protein and carbohydrate meals on mood and performance: Interactions with sex and age. *Journal of Psychiatric Research, 17,* 155–167.

Yogman, M. W., and Zeizel, S. H. (1985). Nutrients, neurotransmitters and infant behaviour. *American Journal of Clinical Nutrition, 45,* 352–360.

Chapter 10. Special Sleep Problems

Sleepwalking

Archbold, K. H., Pituch, K. J., Panabi, P., and Chervin, R. D. (2002). Symptoms of sleep disturbances among children at two general pediatric clinics. *Journal of Pediatrics, 140,* 97–102.

Hublin, C., Kaprio, J., Partinen, M., Hejjila, K., and Koskenvu, M. (1997). Prevalence and genetics of sleepwalking: A population-based twin study. *Neurology, 48,* 177–181.

Kales, A., Soldatos, C. R., Caldwell, A. B., Kales, J. D., Humphrey, F. J., Charney, D. S., and Schweitzer, P. K. (1980). Somnambulism: Clinical characteristics and personality patterns. *Archives of General Psychiatry, 37,* 1406–1410.

Neveus, T., Cnattingius, S., Olsson, U., and Hetta, J. (2001). Sleep habits and sleep problems among a community sample of schoolchildren. *Acta Paediatrica, 90,* 1365–1367.

Klackenberg, G. (1982). Somnambulism in childhood – Prevalence, course, and behavioural correlations. *Acta Paediatrica Scandinavia, 71,* 495–499.

Sleep Talking

Reimao, R., and Lefevre, A. B. (1980). Prevalence of sleep-talking in childhood. *Brain Development, 2,* 353–357.

Night Terrors

DiMario, F. J., Jr., and Emery, E. S. 3d. (1987). The natural history of night terrors. *Clinical Pediatrics, 26,* 505–511.

Kales, J. D., Kales, A., Soldatos, C. R., Chamberlain, K., and Martin, E. D. (1979). Sleep walking and night terrors related to febrile illness. *American Journal of Psychiatry, 136,* 1214–1215.

Weissbluth, M. (1984). Is drug treatment of night terrors warranted? *American Journal of Diseases of Children, 138,* 1086.

Nightmares

Cason, H. (1935). The nightmare dream. *Psychological Monographs, 46* (5, Whole No. 209).

Cellucci, A. J., and Lawrence, P. S. (1978). Individual differences in self-reported sleep – Variable correlations among nightmare sufferers. *Journal of Clinical Psychology, 34,* 721–725.

Mindell, J. A., and Barrett, K. M. (2002). Nightmares and anxiety in elementary-aged children: Is there a relationship? *Child: Care, Health and Development, 28,* 317–322.

Smedje, H., Broman, J. E., and Hetta, J. (2001). Short-term prospective study of sleep disturbances in 5- to 8-year-old children. *Acta Paediatrica, 90,* 1456–1463.

Head Banging and Body Rocking

Abe, K., Oda, N., and Amatomi, M. (1984). Natural history and predictive significance of head-banging, head-rolling and breath-holding spells. *Developmental Medicine and Child Neurology, 26,* 644–648.

Leung, A. K., and Robson, W. L. (1990). Head banging. *Journal of the Singapore Paediatric Society, 32,* 12–17.

Bruxism

Reding, G. R., Rubright, W. C., and Zimmerman, S. O. (1966). Incidence of bruxism. *Journal of Dental Research, 45,* 1198–1204.

Reding, G. R., Zepelin, H., and Monroe, L. J. (1968). Personality study of nocturnal teeth grinders. *Perceptual and Motor Skills, 26,* 523–531.

Reding, G. R., Zepelin, H., Robinson, J. E., Smith, V. H., and Zimmerman, S. O. (1968). Sleep pattern of bruxism: A revision. *Psychophysiology, 4,* 396.

Weideman, C. L., Busch, D. L., Yan-Go, F. L., Clark, G. T., and Gornbein, J. A. (1996). The incidence of parasomnias in child bruxers versus nonbruxers. *American Academy of Pediatric Dentistry, 18,* 456–460.

Narcolepsy

Challamel, M. J., Mazzola, M. E., Nevsimalova, S., Cannard, C., Louis, J., and Revol, M. (1994). Narcolepsy in children. *Sleep, 17* (Suppl. 8), S17–S20.

Wise, M. S., and Lynch, J. (2001). Narcolepsy in children. *Seminars in Pediatric Neurology, 8,* 198–206.

Yoss, R. E., and Daly, D. D. (1960). Narcolepsy in children. *Pediatrics, 77,* 1025–1033.

Poor-Quality Breathing (Allergies and Snoring)

Ali, N. J., Pitson, D. J., and Stradling, J. R. (1993). Snoring, sleep disturbances, and behaviour in 4- to 5-year olds. (1993). *Archives of Disease in Childhood, 68,* 360–366.

Ali, N. J., Pitson, D. J., and Stradling, J. R. (1994). Natural history of snoring and related behaviour problems between the ages of 4 and 7 years. *Archives of Disease in Childhood, 71,* 74–76.

Anderson, O. W. (1950). The management of 'infantile insomnia'. *Journal of Pediatrics, 38,* 394–401.

Ballenger, W. L. (1914). *Diseases of the Nose, Throat and Ear.* Philadelphia: Lea and Febiger.

Brouillette, R., Hansen, D., David, R., Klemka, L., Szatkowski, A., Ferbach, S., and Hung, C. (1984). A diagnostic approach to suspected obstructive sleep apnea in children. *Journal of Pediatrics, 105,* 10–14.

Brown, S. L., and Stool, S. E. (1982). Behavioral manifestations of sleep apnea in children. *Sleep, 5,* 200–201.

Butte, W., Robertson, C., and Phelan, P. (1985). Snoring in children: Is it pathological? *Medical Journal of Australia, 143,* 335–336.

Chervin, R. D., Archbold, K. H., Dillon, J. E., Panahi, P., Pituch, K. J., Dahl, R. E., and Guilleminault, C. (2002). Inattention, hyperctivity, and symptoms of sleep-disordered breathing. *Pediatrics, 109,* 449–456.

Chervin, R. D., Dillon, J. E., Bassetti, C., Ganoczy, D. A., and Pituch, K. J. (1997). Symptoms of sleep disorders, inattention, and hyperactivity in children. *Sleep, 20,* 1185–1192.

Flemming, B. M. (1925). A study of sleep of young children. *Journal of the American Association of University Women, 19,* 25–28.

Goldstein, N. A., Fatima, M., Campbell, T. F., and Rosenfeld, R. M. (2002). Child behaviour and quality of life before and after tonsillectomy and adenoidectomy. *Archives of Otolaryngology – Head and Neck Surgery, 128,* 770–775.

Gozal, D. (1998). Sleep-disordered breathing and school performance. *Pediatrics, 102,* 616–620.

Guilleminault, C., Winkle, R., Korobkin, R., and Simmons, B. (1982). Children and nocturnal snoring: Evaluation of the effects of sleep related respiratory resistive load and daytime functioning. *European Journal of Pediatrics, 139,* 154–171.

Guilleminault, C., Pelaya, R., Leger, D., Cler, A., and Bocian, R. C. V. (1996). Recognition of sleep-disordered breathing in children. *Pediatrics, 98,* 871–882.

Guilleminault, C., and Dement, W. C. (1977). 235 cases of excessive daytime sleepiness. *Journal of Neurological Sciences, 31,* 13–27.

Guilleminault, C., Eldridge, F. L., Simmons, F. B., and Dement, W. C. (1976). Sleep apnea in eight children. *Pediatrics, 58,* 23–31.

Kahn, A., Mozin, J., and Casimir, G. (1985). Insomnia and cow's milk allergy in infants. *Pediatrics, 76,* 880–884.

Klein, G. L., Ziering, R. W., Girsh, L. S., and Miller, M. F. (1985). The allergic irritability syndrome: Four case reports and a position statement from the Neuroallergy Committee of the American College of Allergy. *Annals of Allergy, 55,* 22–24.

Kravath, R. E., Pollack, C. D., and Borowiecki, B. (1977). Hypoventilation during sleep in children who have lymphoid airway obstruction treated by nasopharyngeal tube and T and A. *Pediatrics, 59,* 865–871.

Lind, M. G., and Lundell, B. (1982). Tonsillar hyperplasia in children: A cause of obstructive sleep apneas, CO_2 retention, and retarded growth. *Archives of Otolaryngology, 108,* 650–654.

Mangat, D., Orr, W. C., and Smith, R. O. (1977). Sleep apnea, hypersomnolence, and upper airway obstruction secondary to adenotonsillar enlargement. *Archives of Otolaryngology, 103,* 383–386.

Mauer, K. W., Staats, B. A., and Olsen, K. D. (1983). Upper airway obstruction and disordered nocturnal breathing in children. *Mayo Clinic Proceedings, 58,* 349–353.

Owens, J., Opipari, L., Nobile, C., and Spirito, A. (1998). Sleep and daytime behaviour in children with obstructive sleep apnea and behavioural sleep disorders. *Pediatrics, 102,* 1178-1184.

Weissbluth, M., Davis, A. T., and Poncher, J. (1984). Night waking in 4- to 8-month-old infants. *Journal of Pediatrics, 104,* 477–480.

Weissbluth, M., Davis, A. T., Poncher, J., and Reiff, J. (1983). Signs of airway obstruction during sleep and behavioural, developmental, and academic problems. *Journal of Developmental and Behavioral Pediatrics, 4,* 119–121.

Locating the Problem

Brouillette, R., and Thach, B. T. (1979). A neuromuscular mechanism maintaining extrathoracic airway patency. *Journal of Applied Physiology: Respiration, Environment, Exercise and Physiology, 46,* 772–779.

Brouillette, R., Fernbach, S. K., and Hunt, C. E. (1982). Obstructive sleep apnea in infants and children. *Journal of Pediatrics, 100,* 31–40.

Chokroverty, S. (1980). Phasic tongue movements in human rapid-eye-movement sleep. *Neurology, 30,* 665–668.

Felman, A. H., Loughlin, G. M., Leftridge, C. A., and Cassisi, N. J. (1979). Upper airway obstruction during sleep in children. *American Journal of Respiration, 133,* 213–216.

Haponik, E. F., Smith, P. L., Bohlman, M. E., Allen, R. P., Goldman,

S. M., and Bleecker, E. R. (1983). Computerized tomography in obstructive sleep apnea: Correlation of airway size with physiology during sleep and wakefulness. *American Review of Respiratory Diseases, 127,* 221–226.

Remmers, J. E., deGroot, W. J., Sauerland, E. K., and Anch, A. M. (1978). Pathogenesis of upper airway occlusive during sleep. *Journal of Applied Physiology: Respiration, Environment, Exercise and Physiology, 44,* 931–938.

Wilkinson, A. R., McCormick, M. S., Freeland, A. P., and Pickering, D. (1981). Electrocardiographic signs of pulmonary hypertension in children who snore. *British Medical Journal, 282,* 1579–1581.

Finding the Answers

McGeary, G. D. (1981). Help a snorer. *Journal of the American Medical Association, 245,* 1729.

Simmons, F. B., Guilleminault, C., Dement, W. C., and Tilkian, A. G. (1977). Surgical management of airway obstruction during sleep. *Laryngoscope, 87,* 326–338.

Enjoying the Cure

Guilleminault, C., Winkle, R., Korobkin, R., and Simmons, B. (1982). Children and nocturnal snoring: Evaluation of the effects of sleep-related respiratory resistive load and daytime functioning. *European Journal of Pediatrics, 139,* 165–171.

Hyperactive Behaviour

Busby, K., Firestone, P., and Pivik, R. T. (1981). Sleep patterns in hyperkinetic and normal children. *Sleep, 4,* 366–384.

Conners, C. K. (1974). Rating scale for use in drug studies with children. *Psychopharmacology Bulletin, 10,* (Special Issue), 24.

Greenhill, L., Puig-Antich, J., Goetz, R., Hanlon, C., and Davies, M. (1983). Sleep architecture and REM sleep measures in pre-pubertal children with attention deficit disorder with hyper-activity. *Sleep, 6,* 91–101.

Porrino, L. J., Rapoport, J. L., Behar, D., Sceery, W., Ismond, D. R., and Bunney, W. E. (1983). A naturalistic assessment of the motor activity of hyperactive boys. *Archives of General Psychiatry, 40,* 681–687.

Simonds, J. F., and Parraga, H. (1984). Sleep behaviours and disorders in children and adolescents evaluated at psychiatric clinics. *Journal of Developmental and Behavioral Pediatrics, 5,* 6–10.

Weissbluth, M. (1984). Sleep duration, temperament, and Conners' ratings of 3-year-old children. *Journal of Developmental and Behavioral Pediatrics, 5,* 120–123.

Weissbluth, M., and Liu, K. (1983). Sleep patterns, attention span, and infant temperament. *Journal of Developmental and Behavioral Pediatrics, 4,* 34–36.

Seasonal Affective Disorder

Carskadon, M. A., and Acebo, C. (1993). Parental reports of seasonal mood and behaviour changes in children. *Journal of the American Academy of Child and Adolescent Psychiatry, 32,* 264–269.

Glod, C. A., Teicher, M. H., Polcari, A., McGreenery, C. E., and Ito, Y. (1997). Circadian rest-activity disturbances in children with seasonal affective disorder. *Journal of the American Academy of Child and Adolescent Psychiatry, 36,* 188–195.

Swedo, S. E., Allen, A. J., Glod, C. A., Clark, C. H., Teicher, M. H., Richter, D., Hoffman, C., Hamburger, S. D., Dow, S., Brown, C., and Rosenthal, N. E. (1997). A controlled trial of light therapy for the treatment of pediatric seasonal affective disorder. *Journal of the American Academy of Child and Adolescent Psychiatry, 36,* 816–821.

Bed-wetting

Bader, G., Neveus, T., Kruse, S., and Sillen, U. (2002). Sleep of primary eneuretic children and controls. *Sleep, 25,* 579–583.

Chapter 11. Special Events and Concerns

Twins, Triplets and More

Linkowki, P. (1994). Genetic influences on EEG sleep and the human circadian clock: A twin study. *Pharmacopsychiatry, 27,* 7–10.

Injuries

Belechri, M., Petridou, E., and Trichopoulos, D. (2002). Bunk versus conventional beds: A comparative assessment of fall injury risk. *Journal of Epidemiology and Community Health, 56,* 413–417.

Carey, W. B. (1972). Clinical application of infant temperament measurement. *Journal of Pediatrics, 81,* 823–828.

Richman, N. A. (1981). A community survey of 1- to 2-year-olds with sleep disruptions. *Journal of the American Academy of Child Psychiatry, 20,* 281–291.

Weissbluth, M. (1981). Sleep duration and infant temperament. *Journal of Pediatrics, 5,* 817–819.

Weissbluth, M. (1984). Sleep duration, temperament, and Conners' ratings of 3-year-old children. *Journal of Developmental and Behavioral Pediatrics, 5,* 120–123.

Overweight, Exercise and Diet

Butte, N. F., Jensen, C. L., Moon, J. K., Glaze, D. G., and Frost, J. D. (1992). Sleep organisation and energy expenditure of breast-fed and formula-fed infants. *Pediatric Research, 32,* 514–519.

Carey, W. B. (1985). Temperament and increased weight gain in infants. *Journal of Developmental and Behavioral Pediatrics, 6,* 128–131.

deVries, M. W. (1984). Temperament and infant mortality among the Masai of East Africa. *American Journal of Psychiatry, 141,* 1189–1194.

Neumann, M., and Jacobs, K. W. (1992). The relationship between dietary components and aspects of sleep. *Perceptive Motor Skills, 75,* 873–874.

Sekine, Y., Yamagami, T., Handa, K., Saito, T., Nanre, S., Kawaminami, K., Tokui, N., Yoshida, K., and Kagamimori, S. (2002). A dose-response relationship between short sleeping hours and childhood obesity: Results of the Toyama Birth Cohort Study. *Child: Care, Health and Development, 28,* 163–170.

von Kries, R., Toschke, A. M., Wurnser, H., Sauerwald, T., and Koletsko, B. (2002). Reduced risk for overweight and obesity in 5- and 6-year-old children by duration of sleep – a cross sectional study. *International Journal of Obesity and Related Metabolic Disorders, 26,* 710–716.

Youngstedt, S. D., O'Connor, P. J., and Dishman, R. K. (1997). The effects of acute exercise on sleep: A quantitative synthesis. *Sleep, 20,* 203–214.

Child Abuse

Arvola, T., Tahvanainedn, A., and Isolauri, E. (2000). Concerns and expectations of parents with atopic infants. *Pediatric Allergy and Immunology, 11,* 183–188.

Kemp, A. S. (1999). Atopic eczema: its social and financial costs. *Journal of Pediatrics, 35,* 229–231.

Reuveni, H., Chapnick, G., Tal, A., and Tarasiuk, A. (1999). Sleep fragmentation in children with atopic dermatitis. *Archives of Pediatrics and Adolescent Medicine, 153,* 249–253.

Chapter 12. Competent Parents, Competent Child, by Karen Pierce, M.D.

Basch, M. F. (1988). *Understanding Psychotherapy: The Science Behind the Art.* New York: Basic Books.

Brazelton, T. B., and Cramer, B. G. (1990). *The Earliest Relationship.* Reading, Massachusetts: Addison-Wesley Company.

Caplan, L. (1978). *Oneness and Separateness.* Oak Park, Illinois: La Leche.

Siegel, D. J. (1999). *The Developing Mind: Toward a Neurobiology of Interpersonal Experience.* New York: The Guilford Press.

Stern, D. N. (1990). *Diary of a Baby.* New York: Basic Books.

Chapter 13. The Pros and Cons of Other Approaches to Sleep Problems

Sears, W. (1995). *Nighttime Parenting: How to Get Your Baby and Child to Sleep.* New York: New American Library.

Index

– *A* –
abuse, 434–35
accident-prone children, 431–32
Action Plans for Exhausted Parents, xiii, xxii
  back sleeping, 107
  bedtimes, 241, 307, 337
  colicky babies, 184–86
  crying, 109–10, 135–36, 191, 242
  daytime correction of night-time behaviours, 357
  disturbed sleep, 134–36
  door locks, 357
  family beds *vs.* cots, 108, 187
  fears, 337
  feeding, 108, 188
  healthy sleep, 106–7
  infants, older (thirteen to thirty-six months), 337
  light, 306
  naps, 135, 190, 241–42, 306–7, 337
  newborns, 240–43
  one- to two-hour window, 240–41
  overtiredness, 241
  post-colic stage, 188–91, 306
  preschoolers, 357
  routines, 108
  schedules, 135
  sleep consolidation, 190, 241
  sleep logs, 135
  sleep rules, 337
  sleep training, 188
  soothing, 107–8, 135, 240–41
  temperament, 186–88
  wake-up time, 135
activity levels, 162, 178–79
  See also attention deficit hyperactivity disorder (ADHD)
adaptability, 61, 162–64
  naps, 32
  preschoolers, 151–52, 340–41
adenoids, 383–86, 389
adolescents, 360–68
  bedtimes, 49, 363–64
  chronic mononucleosis, 368
  chronotherapy, 371
  daytime sleepiness, 361–62
  delayed sleep phase syndrome, 365–66, 370–71
  depression and anxiety, 356, 370, 373, 397
  diet, 372–73
  duration of sleep, 20–23, 26, 362–63
  exercise, 367, 370
  falling asleep, 362, 368–69
  fibromyalgia syndrome, 366–67
  hormone changes, 362
  illness and injuries, 364, 366–67
  Kleine-Levin syndrome, 366
  mental function, 363–64
  naps, 361
  narcolepsy, 382
  nightmares, 380
  night waking, 362
  prescription medications, 371–73
  school performance, 363–64
  seasonal affective disorder (SAD), 397
  sleep schedules, 370–71
  sleepwalking, 377–78
  stimulus control treatment, 369–70
  temporal control treatment, 369–70
  wakefulness, 26
  wake-up time, 360–65
adoption, 428–30
adrenaline, xviii, 112–13
ages. *See* newborns; infants, young (five to twelve months); infants, older (thirteen to thirty-six months); preschoolers; schoolchildren; adolescents
airway obstruction, xiii, 380, 386, 389–93, 396*f*
alcohol use, 40
alertness. *See* wakefulness
allergies, 290–91, 355, 377, 382–84, 392

American Academy of Pediatrics, 79
anxiety, 373
  adolescents, 356, 370, 373, 397
  schoolchildren, 359–60
  separation, 264–65, 267, 335
apnoea. *See* airway obstruction
arousals. *See* fragmented sleep; night waking
atopic dermatitis, 435
attention deficit hyperactivity disorder (ADHD), xix, 62, 393–96
  breathing problems, 389, 394–95
  cumulative sleepiness, 54
  disturbed sleep, 396*f*
  links with colic/fussiness, 394–95
  restlessness, 393
  sleep-disordered breathing (SDB), 389
  temperament, 152
attention span, 20, 24, 60, 163–64
  naps, 32
  post-colic stage, 182
  REM-sleep, 59–60
  sleep schedules, 45

– B –

Bates, John, 151, 342–43, 351
baths, 370
beanbag chairs and pillows, 159
bedrooms, 133–34
beds
  falling from, 432
  family beds, 78–80, 86–87, 131, 134, 330, 455–56
  staying in/getting up from, 132–33, 319–23
  transition to, from cots, 134, 170–72, 177, 316–17, 399–400
bedtimes, 6, 44*f*
  adolescents, 49, 363–64
  biological rhythms, 336
  clocks, 331–32
  consistency, 260–61
  crying, 33–36, 261
  daytime sleepiness, 125
  four-month stage, 170–72
  infants, older (thirteen to thirty-six months), 308–10, 315–16, 332–36
  infants, young (five to twelve months), 259–62, 267, 271
  late, 130
  naps, 32–33, 127–30
  newborns, 203–4, 218, 234
  obesity, 343
  older children, 260
  parenting, 61–62, 300
  preschoolers, 49–50, 349–51
  routines, 75, 344–45, 444–46
  schedules, 47–48, 260–61, 279–83
  schoolchildren, 260, 358–60, 425–27
  wake-up time, 119–20
  work and careers, 425–27
bed-wetting, 384, 386, 398
behaviours, xix, 8
  bedtime variability, 49
  colicky babies, 140
  depression and anxiety, 356, 370, 373, 397
  difficult temperament, 165
  discipline, 443–45
  disturbed sleep, 396*f*
  nine month stage, 266–67
  oppositional, 115
  preschoolers, 342–43, 351
  reinforcement, 320–21, 326–27, 334–35
  self-agency, 266–67, 318
  setting limits, 436–45
  sleep rules, 325–27, 353–54
  See also attention deficit hyperactivity disorder (ADHD); temperament
biofeedback, 368
biological rhythms, xvi, 15–16, 50–53, 195
  bedtimes, 336
  colicky babies, 168
  difficult temperament, 165
  digestion, 140
  disorganised sleep, 51–52
  early maturation, 245–46
  infants, younger (five to twelve months), 245–46
  naps, 26–27, 29, 31
  newborns, 50–51, 197
  post-colic stage, 178, 250–53
  shift-work, 51–52
  sleep schedules, 45, 145–46, 245–46
  temporal control, 336
  twenty-five-hour cycles, 55–57
  See also consolidation of sleep
body rocking, 381
body temperature rhythms, 50–51
Bootzin, Richard R., 369–70
brain growth. *See* mental function
Brazelton, Barry, 141
breast-feeding
  colicky babies, 87–98
  consolidation of sleep, 46, 77, 170–72
  duration of sleep, 17, 42
  frequency, 94–95
  fussiness, 76–77, 83–87
  home offices, 421
  post-colic stage, 177
  soothing, 67–68
  sudden infant death syndrome (SIDS), 76–77
  at ten to twelve months, 270

breast-feeding (*cont'd*)
unrestricted, 455–56
using bottled breast milk, 85–86, 92, 96
breathing problems, xiii, 40, 377
airway obstruction, 380, 386, 389–93
allergies, 382–93
disturbed sleep, 396*f*
duration of sleep, 386–89
enlarged tonsils and/or adenoids, 383–86, 389–93
links with attention deficit hyperactivity disorder (ADHD), 394–95
night waking, 386–89
obesity, 391–92
pulmonary hypertension, 391
sleep-disordered breathing (SDB), 389
surgery, 391–92
bruxism, 381–82

– *C* –
caffeine, 40
cars. *See* motion sleep
Carskadon, Mary, 363–64
Cartwright, Rosalind, 370
case studies
adolescents, 364–65
adopted infants, 428–30
bedtimes, 33–36, 333–34
child care staffs, 10–11
colicky babies, 94–98, 154–56
extinction crying system, 212–14
home offices, 422
morning naps, 252–53
naps, 36–39, 228–29, 238–39
night feeding, 100–103
post-colic baby, 166, 180–81
re-establishing naps, 127–30
six-week stage, 205–9
sleep schedules, 216–18
travel and sleep regularity, 56–57, 416–17
twins, 401–6, 410
changes in routine, 133, 289–90
adoption, 428–30
daylight saving time, 399
extinction system, 212
illness and injuries, 417–19, 430–34
moving, 412–14
naps, 239–40, 268–69
night terrors, 379
travel, 55–57, 178, 414–17
travel problems, 55–57
work schedules, 419–28
changing sleep habits. *See* learning to sleep; retraining of sleep habits
chemicals. *See* hormones that affect sleep
Chess, Stella, 164–65, 277–78
child abuse, 434–35
chronic mononucleosis, 368
chronotherapy, 371
circadian timing system. *See* biological rhythms
circumcision, 114
clocks, 331–32, 353–54
cognitive function. *See* mental function
cold-turkey approach. *See* extinction system
colic/extreme fussiness, 18, 84–98
activity levels, 178–79
behaviour, 140
biological rhythms, 168
causes of, 140–41
descriptions of, 139–40
duration of sleep, 143–46
environmental stimulation, 178–79
extinction systems, 211–15
four-month stage, 172–75
links with attention deficit hyperactivity disorder (ADHD), 394–95
motion sleep, 155–56, 158–59
newborns, 138–60, 222–24
night waking, 145, 149–52, 161
post-colic sleep, 149–52, 160–61
prescription medications for, 147
soothing, 153, 158–59, 223–24
temperament, 146–49, 166–75
wakefulness, 145–46
See also fussiness
common fussiness. *See* fussiness
consolidation of sleep, 14, 39–44, 190, 336
biological rhythms, 51–52
at four months, 171–74
naps, 46–48, 50–51, 77, 121–30, 224–29
night sleep, 46, 50–51, 77, 141, 231
temperament, 148
Consumer Product Safety Commission, 79
controlled crying systems, 11–12, 104–6, 168–69, 176, 214–15
cortisol secretion, 50–52, 59, 112–14, 140–41
cosleeping. *See* family beds
cots, 78–80, 86–87
post-colic stage, 177
staying in/getting out of, 132–33, 319–23
transition to beds, 134, 170–72, 177, 316–17, 399–400
twins, 411
crib tents, 132–33, 323–24, 400
crying, xxi, 141–42, 152–53, 273–79
attachment theories, 274–75
bedtimes, 33–36, 261

crying (*cont'd*)
  check and console system, 215
  controlled crying systems, 11–12, 104–6, 168–69, 176, 214–15
  difficult temperament, 165
  duration of sleep, 20
  extinction system, 104–6, 211–14, 261–62, 297–305, 457
  naps, 249–50
  newborns, 196, 211–14, 220–22
  night sleep, 261, 312
  'no cry' systems, 168–69, 176
  post-colic stage, 176, 253–54
  psychological aspects, 447–49
  sleep deficits, 144
  vomiting, 301, 307
  See also fussiness; retraining of sleep habits
cumulative sleepiness, 53–55, 116

– *D* –
daycare, 124
day/night confusion, 18, 230–31
daytime correction of bedtime problems, 349–51
daytime sleep. *See* naps
daytime sleepiness, xxi
  adolescents, 361–62
  bedtimes, 125
  breathing problems, 384, 386
  cumulative, 53–55, 55, 116
  daytime, 111, 116, 118–20, 125
  fragmented sleep, 41–42
  nap problems, 121–30
  wake-up time, 119–21
delayed sleep phase syndrome, 365–66, 370–71
Dement, William C., xix, 6, 384–85
depression and anxiety, 116
  adolescents, 356, 370, 373, 397
  mothers of colicky babies, 141
  postpartum depression, 66, 84, 85, 105
  role of sleep problems, 272–75
dermatitis, 435
development. *See* newborns; infants, young (five to twelve months); infants, older (thirteen to thirty-six months); preschoolers; schoolchildren; adolescents
dicyclomine hydrochloride, 147
diet. *See* feeding
disease. *See* illness and injuries
disrupted sleep. *See* fragmented sleep; night waking
dissociated states of wakefulness and sleep. *See* sleep inertia
disturbed sleep, xvi, 111–18, 291–93, 396*f*
  fears, 314–15
  hormone levels, 112–14
  newborns, 18
door locks, 133, 324, 352–53
Douglas, Jo, 300–301
dreams, 379–81
drowsiness, 49, 63, 70–71, 210
duration of sleep, 14, 16–26
  adolescents, 20–23, 26, 362–63
  breast-feeding, 17, 42
  breathing problems, 386–89
  colicky babies, 143–46
  crying, 20
  fussiness, 20, 24
  genetic factors, 407, 410–11
  infants, older (thirteen to thirty-six months), 19–26, 42, 259–60
  infants, younger (five to twelve months), 259–60, 287–88
  naps, 22*t*, 29–30, 42, 60, 248
  newborns, 16–19, 196, 201, 230
  night sleep, 23*t*
  post-colic stage, 181–84
  preschoolers, 342–43
  schoolchildren, 358
  temperament, 148–49
  total sleep, 21*t*

– *E* –
ear infections, 294, 383–84
eczema, 435
environmental stimulation, 71, 75, 174–75, 178–79
  colicky babies, 178
  good stimulation, 250
  motion, 37, 41–42, 234
  naps, 287
  newborns, 18–19
  night waking, 148–49
  noise, 287
  overstimulation, 226–27
  REM sleep, 59
  soothing, 64
  wake-up time, 119
  See also light
exercise programmes, 367–70, 373, 432–34
extinction system, 104–6, 211–15, 261–62, 297–305, 457
extreme fussiness/colic. *See* colic/extreme fussiness

– *F* –
fading system, 295–97
falling asleep, 368–69
  adolescents, 362
  drowsiness, 49, 63, 70–71, 210
  schoolchildren, 359–60
  See also soothing
family beds, 78–80, 86–87, 131, 134
  unrestricted, 455–56

wake-up time, 330
fathers, 65–67
colicky babies, 158
soothing, 77, 105, 237
work and careers, 425–28
See also parenting
fatigue. *See* overtiredness
fears, 131–32
infants, older (thirteen to thirty-six months), 314–15
preschoolers, 354
schoolchildren, 359
feeding, 68, 293
breast *vs.* bottle, 76–78, 83–87
children and adolescents, 372–73
colicky babies, 87–92
failure to thrive, 77
food allergies, 383, 386–87, 392
at four months, 170–72
frequency, 99–103
gastro-oesophageal reflux, 141
hypersensitivity to food, 141
infants, younger (five to twelve months), 262–64, 266–67
milk allergies, 372–73, 387, 392
newborns, 17–18, 87–92, 170–72, 198
night sleep, 99–103, 203
night waking, 171
post-colic stage, 173–74
solids, 99–103
stomach cramps, 140
temperament, 140
tooth decay, 293, 331
weight problems, 77, 385–86, 391–92, 432–34
See also breast-feeding
Ferber, Richard, 454–55
fibromyalgia syndrome, 366–67
fight-or-flight response, xviii, 113
food allergies, 383, 386, 387, 392
four month stage, 160–66, 170–75
See also newborns
fragmented sleep, 41–42, 49
See also night waking
Frischer, Laya, 165–66
fussiness, xiii, 5–6, 59–60
breast-feeding, 76–77, 87–98
crying, 141–42
duration of sleep, 20, 24
extreme *vs.* common, 80–87
family beds, 79
at four months, 170–72
hunger, 142
links with attention deficit hyperactivity disorder (ADHD), 394–95
newborns, 59–60, 98, 142–43, 170–72, 184, 204–18, 230
night waking, 171–72
at six-weeks, 98, 142–43, 184, 204–18
sleep inertia, 27–28
soothing, 70, 73–74, 105
See also colic/extreme fussiness; crying; daytime sleepiness

– *G* –
gender differences
bed-wetting, 398
fibromyalgia syndrome, 366–67
night waking, 290–91
genetic factors, 195
duration of sleep, 407, 410–11
sleepwalking, 378
Genetic Studies of Genius (Terman), 61–62
graduated extinction. *See* controlled crying systems
growing pains, 294
Guilleminault, Christian, 6, 384–85

– *H* –
head banging, 381
health, 52
homeostatic control mechanism, 15
hormones that affect sleep, 112–18, 232–33
adolescents, 362
adrenaline, xviii, 112–13
cortisol, 50–52, 59, 112–13, 140–41
melatonin, 18, 29, 51, 140, 159, 372
progesterone, 59
serotonin, 140, 168
hunger, 41
See also feeding
hyperactivity. *See* attention deficit hyperactivity disorder (ADHD); restlessness
hyper-alert states, 113–15

– *I* –
Illingworth, Dr, 139
illness and injuries, 52
adolescents, 364
allergies, 382–84
atopic dermatitis, 435
changes in routine, 417–19
disturbed sleep, 316
ear infections, 294, 383–84
eczema, 435
enlarged tonsils and/or adenoids, 383–86, 389–93
headaches, 360, 384, 386
night waking, 318, 417–19
schoolchildren, 360
snoring, 388
infant homicides, 141
infants, older (thirteen to thirty-six months)
bedtimes, 308–10, 332–36

infants, older (*cont'd*)
  behaviours, 318
  communication skills, 444–45
  crib tents, 323–24
  daytime sleepiness, 318
  disturbed sleep, 314–15
  door locks, 324
  duration of sleep, 19–26, 42, 259–60
  fears, 314–15
  Jack-in-the-Box Syndrome, 319–23, 344
  naps, 29–30, 308–14, 327–30
  night waking, 312, 317–23, 332–36
  separation anxiety, 335
  sleep consolidation, 312
  sleep rules, 325–27
  sleep schedules, 45–48, 315–16
  thirteen- to fifteen-month stage, 308–11
  transitions from cot to bed, 314, 316–17
  twenty-two- to thirty-six-month stage, 313–17
  wake-up time, 330–32
infants, younger (five to twelve months), 244–307
  adoption, 428–30
  afternoon naps, 257–58
  bedtimes, 259–62, 279–83
  biological rhythms, 245–46
  changes in routine, 265, 289–90
  chronic fatigue, 291–92
  crying, 273–75, 276–79
  deprivation of naps, 283–87
  disturbed sleep, 291–93
  duration of sleep, 259–60, 287–88
  extinction system, 261–62, 297–305
  fading system, 295–97
  feeding, 262–64, 266–67
  forced awakening, 248, 259
  four month stage, 160–66, 170–75
  head banging, 381
  intervals of wakefulness, 247–48
  learning to sleep, 12, 246–63, 286–87, 305
  lights, 287
  morning naps, 248–57
  naps, 248–60, 283–87
  night waking, 262–63, 266–67, 279, 290–95
  nine-month stage, 266–67
  scheduled awakenings, 298
  self-soothing, 299
  separation anxiety, 264–65
  sleep maturation process, 269–70
  sleep schedules, 254–56
  snoring and/or mouth breathing, 387
  soothing, 265–66
  ten- to twelve-month stage, 267–71
  wakefulness, 247–48, 256–57
  wake-up time, 247, 288–89, 298
  See also newborns
infections. *See* illness and injuries
insecurity of attachment, xx, 441
  See also separation anxiety
insomnia, 116–17
intelligence. *See* mental function
intensity, 163–64
internal clocks. *See* biological rhythms
Internal Timing System, 16
irritability. *See* fussiness

– J –
Jack-in-the-Box Syndrome, 319–23, 344
jet-lag syndrome, 49, 51
  See also biological rhythms

– K –
Kirjavainen, J., 143–44
Kleine-Levin syndrome, 366

– L –
lactation consultants, 93
La Leche League International, 455–56
learning disabilities. *See* school performance
learning to sleep, xxi, 6, 131
  crying, xviii
  daytime correction of bedtime problems, 349–51
  at four months, 171–74
  infants, younger (five to twelve months), 12, 246–63, 286–87, 305
  naps, 31–32
  newborns, 71, 171–74, 200, 210–11
  night waking, 130–31
  post-colic sleep, 150–52, 250–53
  progressive approach, 454–55
  re-establishing naps, 126–30
  self-soothing skills, 153, 160, 182, 228, 277, 343, 442–43
  setting limits, 436–45, 448–50
  See also consolidation of sleep; night waking; retraining of sleep habits
Lewis, Michael, 275–76
light, 15, 18–19, 287
  crossing time zones, 414
  day/night confusion, 18, 230–31
  fears of the dark, 131–32
  naps, 287
  wakefulness, 253
  wake-up time, 330
limit setting, 436–45, 448–50
locks, 133, 324, 352–53

– M –
Mahler, Margaret S., 277
massage, 69
medications. *See* prescription medications

meditative relaxation, 368
melatonin, 18, 29, 51, 140, 159, 372
mental function, xix, 6, 24–26, 59–62
  adolescents, 363–64
  attention span, 20, 24, 32, 45, 59–60, 163–64, 182
  communication development, 444–45
  cumulative sleepiness, 54
  depression, 116, 272–75
  distractibility, 164
  overstimulation, 441
  overtiredness, 341–42
  post-colic stage, 179
  routines, 446
  sleep maturation process, 14–17, 269–70
  sleep schedules, 45
  See also learning to sleep; school performance
Minde, Klaus, 66–67
mood, xix, 8, 163, 164
  disturbed sleep, 112–18
  overtiredness, 341
  sleep schedules, 45
  snoring, 384–85
  See also temperament
mother-infant distress syndrome, 174
mothers
  anxiety and colicky babies, 141
  attachment theories, 274–75
  depression related to infant sleep problems, 272–75
  lactation, 88
  natural mothering theory, 455–56
  post-colic stage, 182–83
  postpartum depression, 66, 84, 85, 105
  separation problems, 182–83, 264–65
  support systems for, 85–86
  temperament, 147–48
  work and careers, 419–28
motion sleep, 37, 41–42, 234
  colicky babies, 155–56, 158–59
  prevention, 256
  See also restlessness
mouth breathing. *See* breathing problems
moving, 412–14
multiple births, 400–412
My Child Won't Sleep (Douglas and Richman), 300–301
myths about sleeping, xvi, 6–7, 9–10, 455–56

– *N* –
naps, 14, 19–39, 22*t*, 190
  adaptability, 32
  adolescents, 361
  afternoon, 123–24, 244–59, 257–58
  attention span, 32
  bedtime schedules, 32–33, 127–30
  biological rhythms, 26–27, 29, 31
  changes in routine, 125–26
  circadian timing system, 26–27
  crying, 249–50
  daytime sleepiness, 121–30
  deprivation of, 268–69, 283–87
  duration of sleep, 22*t*, 29–30, 42, 60, 248
  frequency, 29–30
  infants, older (thirteen to thirty-six months), 267, 311–14, 327–30
  infants, younger (five to twelve months), 248–59, 267–71
  learning to sleep, 31–32
  light, 287
  morning, 121–23, 224–29, 248–57, 311–12
  optimal wakefulness, 28
  organisation of, 46–48, 50–51, 77, 121–30, 224–30, 236–37, 244–66
  post-colic sleep, 250–53
  preschoolers, 338–43, 355–56
  re-establishment of, 313–14, 330, 355–56
  refusal to nap, 126–30
  REM sleep, 28–29
  schedules, 226–29, 339, 355–56
  sleep inertia, 27–28
  sleep maturation process, 269–70
  third naps, 124–25, 172, 244, 246, 258–59, 267
  time of day, 31
narcolepsy, 28, 382
National Committee to Prevent Child Abuse, 435
'natural' sleep habits, 6–7, 9–10, 455–56
neurological development. *See* mental function
newborns, xiii, 69, 185–243
  bedtimes, 203–4, 218, 234
  biological rhythms, 50–51, 197
  colicky babies, 138–60, 222–24
  crying, 196, 211–14, 220–22
  disturbed sleep, 18
  drowsiness, 63, 70–71, 210
  duration of sleep, 16–19, 196, 201, 230
  environment, 18–19, 219, 231
  feeding, 17–18, 87–92, 198, 203
  first week, 197–200
  four month stage, 160–66, 170–75, 224–29
  fussiness, 59–60, 98, 142–43, 170–72, 204–18, 230
  home offices, 421–24

newborns (*cont'd*)
learning to sleep, 71, 200, 210–11
melatonin, 51
multiple births, 400–412
nap organisation, 46–48, 121–30, 224–32, 236–37
night sleep organisation, 204–5, 231
night waking, 203–4
one- to two-hour window, 63, 70–71, 104–5, 121–22, 196, 219–20, 232–34
overtiredness, 198–99, 232–33
position, 57–59
second to fourth week, 201–4
seventh to eighth week, 218–24
sixth week, 98, 142–43, 184, 199, 204–18
sleep inertia, 27–28
sleep schedules, 45–48, 215–18, 232–34
snoring and/or mouth breathing, 387
social learning, 18, 46, 60–61, 204
soothing, 196, 199, 228, 235–40
sucking, 200
wakefulness, 17, 50, 59, 63, 70–71, 104–5
See also colic/extreme fussiness
nightmares, 379–81
night sleep, 20, 24, 46
crying, 261, 312
daytime correction of bedtime problems, 349–51
development of, 17, 46, 50–51, 77, 141, 148
duration of sleep, 23*t*
feeding, 99–103, 203
fragmented sleep, 42
getting out of bed, 132–33, 319–23
morning wake-up time, 43*f*
preschoolers, 345–55
schedules, 49–57
See also bedtimes; learning to sleep
night terrors, xx, 28, 378–79
night waking, 99–103, 130–31
adolescents, 362
breathing problems, 385–89
colicky babies, 145, 149–52, 161
extinction system, 297–304
fading system, 295–97
feeding, 171
fussiness, 171–72
illness, 417–19
infants, older (thirteen to thirty-six months), 317–23, 332–36
infants, younger (five to twelve months), 262–63, 266–67, 279, 290–95
newborns, 203–4
post-colic sleep, 149–52, 161, 181–84
preschoolers, 345–55
schoolchildren, 359–60
sleep schedules, 279
temperament, 148–49
'no cry' systems, 168–69
non-REM sleep, 59–60
night terrors, 379
physical restoration, 29
young infants, 245
nursing. *See* breast-feeding

– *O* –
obesity, 343, 391
See also weight problems
Ogden, T. H., 183
oppositional behaviour, 115
optimal wakefulness. *See* wakefulness
organisation of sleep. *See* consolidation of sleep
overstimulation, 226–27
overtiredness, xviii, 5–6, 9, 53, 113–15, 316
brain development, 341–42
chronic fatigue, 291–92
cumulative sleepiness, 53–55
day/night confusion, 5
newborns, 198–99
preschoolers, 339
restlessness, 291–93
vs. drowsiness, 63

– *P* –
paradoxical intention, 368
parenting, xvi, xxi–xxii, 345–55
anger, 185
attachment parenting theory, 455–56
bedtimes, 61–62, 300, 425–27
child abuse, 434–35
confidence, 440–42
conflicts, 450–53
consistency, 235–40, 249, 260–61, 345–55
control, 275–76
discipline, 443–45
disturbed sleep, 396*f*
fathers' roles, 65–67, 77, 105, 158, 237, 425–28
multiple births, 400–412
night waking, 148–49, 152–53, 320–21
post-colic stage, 174, 181–84
reading baby's signals, 438–42, 448–50
reinforcement of sleep problems, 271–75, 290–91, 334–35, 346–49
self-esteem, 438–40
setting limits, 436–45, 448–50
sleep rules, 325–27, 353–54

sleep schedules, 30, 32, 37, 181–84, 327–28
social interactions, 320–21
soothing, 74, 159–60
training programs, 11–12
work and careers, 419–28
See also Action Plans for Exhausted Parents
Parents Without Partners, 435
Parmelee, A. H., Jr., 150
partial airway obstruction, 290–91
See also breathing problems
persistence. *See* attention span
personality. *See* temperament
Pickwickian syndrome, 391
post-colic stage, 149–53, 160–61, 177–84
biological rhythms, 178
crying, 176, 253–54
duration of sleep, 181–84
feeding, 173–74
naps, 250–53
night waking, 181–84, 290–95
sleep schedules, 181–84
soothing, 174–75
premature infants, 16, 46, 139
preschoolers, 338–57
activities and schedules, 339, 355–56
adaptability, 340–41
bedtimes, 49–50, 349–51
behaviour, 342–43
daytime correction of bedtime problems, 349–51
depression and anxiety, 356
duration of sleep, 342–43
fears, 354
Jack-in-the-Box Syndrome, 344
naps, 338–43, 355–56
night sleep, 345–55
night waking, 345–55
self-soothing skills, 343, 349–50
sleep rules, 353–54
sleep schedules, 344–45
social learning, 341
soothing, 343–45
temperament, 339–42
prescription medications
for adolescents, 371–73
allergy medications, 372
antidepressants, 367
antihistamines, 371, 392
for colic, 147
decongestants, 372, 392
night terrors, 379
phenobarbital, 371
professional help, 13, 93
progressive approach to learning to sleep, 454–55
progressive relaxation, 368
protective arousals, 40
pulmonary hypertension, 391

– Q –

quiet alertness. *See* wakefulness

– R –

regulatory mechanisms of sleep, 15
relaxation programmes, 369–70, 373
REM sleep
brain development, 29
environment, 59
naps, 28–29, 31, 252
newborns, 59, 245
See also non-REM sleep
research, xvi–xvii, 9
bedtimes, 358
duration of sleep, 19–25, 358
maternal depression, 272–75
mental function, 60–62
naps, 30–31
night waking, 317–18, 346–49
schoolchildren, 358–59
restlessness, 291–93, 366–67
attention deficit hyperactivity disorder (ADHD), 393
breathing problems, 385–86, 388
retraining of sleep habits, xviii, 12, 286–87
check and console system, 215
controlled crying systems, 11–12, 104–6, 168–69, 176, 214–15
daytime correction of bedtime problems, 349–51
extinction system, 104–6, 211–14, 261–62, 297–305, 457
fading system, 295–97
'no cry' systems, 168–69, 176
progressive approach (Ferber), 454–55
re-establishment of naps, 126–30, 313–14, 330, 355–56
silent return to sleep, 133
stimulus control treatment, 315, 336, 369–70
temporal control treatment, 336, 369–70
rhythmicity, 162
Richman, Naomi, 300–301

– S –

schedules for sleeping, 14, 45–57
adolescents, 370–71
bedtimes, 47–48, 260–61, 279–83
biological rhythms, 45, 50–53, 145–46
consistency, 249
infants, older (thirteen to thirty-six months), 315–16

schedules for sleeping (*cont'd*)
infants, younger (five to twelve months), 246*f*, 254–56, 271
naps, 123–24, 226–29
newborns, 215–18, 232–34
night waking, 279
post-colic sleep, 150–52, 181–84
preschoolers, 344–45
routines, 75, 344–45, 444–46
sleep signals, 52–53
temporal control, 336
twins, 407–8
See also changes in routine; overtiredness
schoolchildren, 358–60
aches and pains, 360
anxiety, 359–60, 372–73
bedtimes, 260, 358–60, 425–27
bed-wetting, 398
diet, 372–73
duration of sleep, 358
falling asleep, 359–60, 368–69
fears, 359
night terrors, 378–79
night waking, 359–60
prescription medications, 371–73
seasonal affective disorder (SAD), 397
sleepwalking, 377–78
school performance, xix, 24, 59–62
adolescents, 363–64
auditory processing deficits, 448
breathing problems, 384, 391–92
cumulative sleepiness, 54
fatigue, 54, 356
nonverbal learning disabilities, 448
preschoolers, 343, 351
sleep-disordered breathing (SDB), 389
temperament, 152, 448
See also attention deficit hyperactivity disorder (ADHD)
Science News, 52
seasonal affective disorder (SAD), 397
security of attachment, xxii, 441
See also separation anxiety
self-suggestion, 368
sensitivity, 164, 166
separation anxiety
infants, older (thirteen to thirty-six months), 335
infants, younger (five to twelve months), 264–65, 267
insecurity of attachment, xx, 441
serotonin, 140, 168
setting limits, 436–45, 448–50
shift work, 51–52
siblings, 131, 316–17, 399–412
SIDS. *See* sudden infant death syndrome (SIDS)
silent return to sleep, 133
sixteen- to twenty-one-month stage, 311–12
six-week stage, 98, 142–43, 184, 199, 204–18
skin problems, xiii, 435
sleep-disordered breathing (SDB), 389
See also breathing problems
sleep inertia, 27–28
sleepiness. *See* daytime sleepiness
sleeplessness. *See* overtiredness
sleep logs, 12, 118, 222, 420
sleep mode, xix–xx
sleep position, 57–59
sleep rhythms. *See* biological rhythms
sleep rules, 133, 325–27, 353–54
sleep signals, 52–53
sleep talking, 378
sleep training. *See* learning to sleep
sleepwalking, 28, 377–78
snoring, xiii, 377, 384–93
airway obstruction, 380, 389–93
allergies, 382–84
enlarged tonsils and/or adenoids, 383–86, 389–93
obesity, 391
sudden infant death syndrome (SIDS), 387
surgery, 391–92
social learning, 60–61, 224
infants, younger (five to twelve months), 160, 244–45
newborns, 18, 46, 204
preschoolers, 341
society's expectations. *See* myths about sleeping
soothing, 63–73
breast-feeding, 87–92
colicky babies, 153, 158–59, 223–24
consistency, 235–40
drowsiness, 49, 63, 70–71, 210
fears, 315
fussiness, 70, 73–74, 105
infants, younger (five to twelve months), 265–66, 270
massage, 69
medical remedies, 72–73
newborns, 196, 199
'no cry' systems, 168–69
parenting, 74, 159–60
post-colic stage, 174–75
preschoolers, 343–45
resources, 73–74
rhythmic/rocking motions, 68, 381
self-soothing skills, 153, 160, 182, 198, 228, 277, 343, 441–43
smiling, 224
sucking, 67–68, 142, 159
swaddling, 68–69, 159

St. James-Roberts, Dr, 143–44
Stanford Sleepiness Scale, 119
stimulus control treatment, 315, 336, 369–70
stomach sleeping, 57–58
sucking, 67–68, 142, 159, 200
sudden infant death syndrome (SIDS), 40
  breast feeding, 76–77
  family beds, 79
  sleep position, 57–58
  snoring, 387
Sundell, Charles E., 8–9
sunlight. *See* light
swaddling, 68–69, 159

– T –

teeth grinding, 381–82
teething, 293
temperament, xviii, 80–83, 153, 161–64
  approach/withdrawal, 162, 164
  colicky babies, 146–49, 166–75
  difficult, 164–65
  disturbed sleep, 396*f*
  duration of sleep, 148–49
  feeding, 140
  four-month point, 160–66
  preschoolers, 151–52, 339–42
  setting limits, 447–48
  See also fussiness
temporal control treatment, 336, 369–70
ten- to twelve-month stage, 267–71
  See also infants, younger (five to twelve months)
Terman, Lewis M., 61–62
therapy, 13, 93
thirteen- to fifteen-month stage, 308–11
Thomas, Alexander, M.D., 161, 164–65, 277–78
time of day
  changing time zones, 414–17
  daylight saving time, 399
  naps, 31
timing. *See* schedules for sleeping
toddlers. *See* infants, older (thirteen to thirty-six months)
tonsils, 383–86, 389
training. *See* learning to sleep
trampoline devices, 159
travel, 55–57, 178
  changing time zones, 414–17
  sleep disruptions, 133
tryptophan, 159, 372
twenty-five-hour cycles, 55–57
twenty-two- to thirty-six-month stage, 313–17
twins, triplets, and more, 400–412

– U –

U.S. Consumer Product Safety Commission, 79

– V –

variable bedtimes, 49–50
vomiting, 301, 307

– W –

wakefulness, 30
  activity levels, 162
  adolescents, 26
  alertness, xix–xx, 8, 11, 28, 115, 351, 441
  colicky babies, 145–46
  gradations of, 118–19
  hyper-alert states, 113–15
  infants, younger (five to twelve months), 247–48, 256–57
  light, 253
  morning naps, 250–52
  naps, 28, 250–52
  newborns, 17, 50, 59, 63, 70–71, 104–5
  one- to two-hour window, 63, 70–71, 104–5, 121–22, 196, 219–20, 232–34
  optimal, 28
  sleep inertia, 27–28
  young adults, 351
wake-up time, 43*f*, 48, 75
  adolescents, 360–65
  forced awakenings, 248, 259
  infants, older (thirteen to thirty-six months), 330–32
  infants, younger (five to twelve months), 247
  scheduled, 298
  sleep problems, 119–22, 125, 288–89
  too early, 119–21, 125
  too late, 122
  using clocks, 331–32
water beds, 159
weight problems, 77, 385–86, 391–92, 432–34
Weissbluth, Linda, 140
Wessel, M. A., 139–40, 142, 146–47
Williams, Carl D., 333–34
Winnicott, D. W., 277
Wolke, D., 150, 152

– Y –

young infants. *See* infants, younger (five to twelve months); newborns

About the Author

A paediatrician for thirty years, DR MARC WEISSBLUTH is also a leading researcher on sleep and children. He founded the original Sleep Disorders Center at Chicago's Children's Memorial Hospital in 1985 and is a Professor of Clinical Paediatrics at Northwestern University School of Medicine. Dr Weissbluth discovered that sleep is linked to temperament and that sleeping problems are related to infant colic. His landmark seven-year study on the development and disappearance of naps highlighted the importance of daytime sleep. In addition to his own research, he has written chapters on sleep problems in textbooks for paediatricians, has lectured extensively to parent groups, and has appeared on *Oprah*. Dr Weissbluth is the father of four sons, two grandsons and, thankfully, one granddaughter – and they are all good sleepers. Dr Weissbluth has been married for thirty-eight years to Linda, and she has provided both inspiration and original ideas for this book.